From Statistics to Neural Networks

Theory and Pattern Recognition Applications

NATO ASI Series

Advanced Science Institutes Series

A series presenting the results of activities sponsored by the NATO Science Committee, which aims at the dissemination of advanced scientific and technological knowledge, with a view to strengthening links between scientific communities.

The Series is published by an international board of publishers in conjunction with the NATO Scientific Affairs Division

A Life Sciences **B Physics**	Plenum Publishing Corporation London and New York
C Mathematical and Physical Sciences **D Behavioural and Social Sciences** **E Applied Sciences**	Kluwer Academic Publishers Dordrecht, Boston and London
F Computer and Systems Sciences **G Ecological Sciences** **H Cell Biology** **I Global Environmental Change**	Springer-Verlag Berlin Heidelberg New York London Paris Tokyo Hong Kong Barcelona Budapest

NATO-PCO DATABASE

The electronic index to the NATO ASI Series provides full bibliographical references (with keywords and/or abstracts) to more than 30000 contributions from international scientists published in all sections of the NATO ASI Series. Access to the NATO-PCO DATABASE compiled by the NATO Publication Coordination Office is possible in two ways:

- via online FILE 128 (NATO-PCO DATABASE) hosted by ESRIN, Via Galileo Galilei, I-00044 Frascati, Italy.
- via CD-ROM "NATO Science & Technology Disk" with user-friendly retrieval software in English, French and German (© WTV GmbH and DATAWARE Technologies Inc. 1992).

The CD-ROM can be ordered through any member of the Board of Publishers or through NATO-PCO, Overijse, Belgium.

Series F: Computer and Systems Sciences, Vol. 136

From Statistics to Neural Networks

Theory and Pattern Recognition Applications

Edited by

Vladimir Cherkassky

Department of Electrical Engineering, University of Minnesota
Minneapolis, MN 55455, USA

Jerome H. Friedman

Department of Statistics, Stanford University
Stanford, CA 94309, USA

Harry Wechsler

Computer Science Department, George Mason University
Fairfax, VA 22030, USA

Springer-Verlag
Berlin Heidelberg New York London Paris Tokyo
Hong Kong Barcelona Budapest
Published in cooperation with NATO Scientific Affairs Division

Proceedings of the NATO Advanced Study Institute From Statistics to Neural Networks, Theory and Pattern Recognition Applications, held in Les Arcs, Bourg Saint Maurice, France, June 21–July 2, 1993

CR Subject Classification (1991): G.3, I.5, I.2.6, I.2.10

ISBN-13: 978-3-642-79121-5 e-ISBN-13: 978-3-642-79119-2
DOI: 10.1007/978-3-642-79119-2

Library of Congress Cataloging-in-Publication Data. NATO Advanced Study Institute From Statistics to Neural Networks, Theory, and Pattern Recognition Applications (1993: Bourg-Saint-Maurice, France). From statistics to neural networks: theory and pattern recognition applications/edited by Vladimir Cherkassky, Jerome H. Friedman, Harry Wechsler. p. cm. – (NATO ASI series. Series F, Computer and systems sciences; v. 136) 1. Neural networks (Computer science) 2. Pattern recognition systems. I. Cherkassky, Vladimir S. II. Friedman, J. H. (Jerome H.) III. Wechsler, Harry. IV. Title. V. Series. QA76.87.N382 1993 006.3'1–dc20 94-34254

Softcover reprint of the hardcover 1st edition 1994

Typesetting: Camera ready by editors
SPIN 10130792 45/3140 - 5 4 3 2 1 0 - Printed on acid-free paper

Preface

The NATO Advanced Study Institute From Statistics to Neural Networks, Theory and Pattern Recognition Applications took place in Les Arcs, Bourg Saint Maurice, France, from June 21 through July 2, 1993. The meeting brought together over 100 participants (including 19 invited lecturers) from 20 countries.

The invited lecturers whose contributions appear in this volume are: L. Almeida (INESC, Portugal), G. Carpenter (Boston, USA), V. Cherkassky (Minnesota, USA), F. Fogelman Soulie (LRI, France), W. Freeman (Berkeley, USA), J. Friedman (Stanford, USA), F. Girosi (MIT, USA and IRST, Italy), S. Grossberg (Boston, USA), T. Hastie (AT&T, USA), J. Kittler (Surrey, UK), R. Lippmann (MIT Lincoln Lab, USA), J. Moody (OGI, USA), G. Palm (Ulm, Germany), B. Ripley (Oxford, UK), R. Tibshirani (Toronto, Canada), H. Wechsler (GMU, USA), C. Wellekens (Eurecom, France) and H. White (San Diego, USA).

The ASI consisted of lectures overviewing major aspects of statistical and neural network learning, their links to biological learning and non-linear dynamics (chaos), and real-life examples of pattern recognition applications. As a result of lively interactions between the participants, the following topics emerged as major themes of the meeting:
(1) Unified framework for the study of Predictive Learning in Statistics and Artificial Neural Networks (ANNs);
(2) Differences and similarities between statistical and ANN methods for non-parametric estimation from examples (learning);
(3) Fundamental connections between artificial learning systems and biological learning systems.

These major themes are summarized below:

Predictive Learning and Statistics

A learning system is a computer program that constructs rules for predicting values for some property of a real system (response/output), given the values of other properties (predictors/inputs) of that system. In contrast to expert systems which attempt to organize the knowledge of human experts in the particular field, predictive learning systems attempt to construct useful prediction rules purely by processing data taken from past successfully solved cases; that is, cases for which the values of both the response and predictors have been determined. Learning systems are generic programs that do not contain any domain specific knowledge. All information is presumed to be contained in the supplied data. It is the job of the learning algorithm to (automatically) extract and organize that information to obtain an accurate prediction rule.

Methodology and theory for computer learning have been traditionally developed in the fields of applied mathematics (multivariate function approximation), statistics (multiple regression and classification), and engineering (pattern recognition). Recently renewed interest and excitement has been generated by research in artificial intelligence (machine learning) and biologically motivated methods for data modeling (artificial neural networks), both in terms of widened applications and methodological development.

For the most part the leading developments in each of these fields has progressed independently of the corresponding developments in the other fields. There has been relatively little cross-referencing of the respective literatures. Many important "discoveries" in one field were in fact well known in others that study the predictive learning problem. A goal of this ASI was to bring together leading researchers and practitioners from these respective fields so that participants could learn their respective views of the problem and its solutions.

Since statistics is one of the oldest disciplines to study data based learning, it has perhaps seen the greatest duplication of its approaches in other fields. To quote B. Efron "Statistics has been the most successful information science, and those who ignore it are condemned to reinvent it." However it is also true that statistics has been slow to embrace modern (computer oriented) approaches to the problem. This reluctance is based largely on its history that has shaped the attitudes of those who are educated in the discipline.

Statistics was invented to study the limits of inference from data. That is, to what extent a collection of measurements actually characterizes the system under study, or is simply an artifact of a particular (random) sample taken from that system. To quote R. A. Fisher "It is the scientist (user), not the statistician, who constructs the structural model. It is the role of the statistician to study the inferential limitations of that model under various uncertainty (error) mechanisms." This involves the construction of probability models for the error mechanism and probability calculus to perform the inference. In this sense the statistician is often cast in the role of the messenger with bad news, since his main role is to inform the user of the limitations associated with what he wants to do, rather than the most optimistic opportunities. Statistical answers tend to be vague and highly qualified.

In the past the clients of statisticians were from the "softer" sciences (medicine, psychology, political science, economics, etc.) where sample sizes are small, noise levels very high and the issue is often whether there is any signal at all. In these settings inference from such data must be done with great care. This was the basis of the "scientific method". Statisticians are trained to be very careful and to always understate the strengths of methods they propose and stress the weaknesses. Only methods that have been extensively validated mathematically, and over a long period of use, are proposed for application.

This very cautious approach has caused statistics to evolve into a very scholarly mathematically oriented discipline that is initially suspicious of new ideas, often with good reason. As with all good things, caution and resistance to new ideas can be overdone. There is a large market for successful predictive learning methods and computers are here to stay. Monte Carlo methods can be used to validate new procedures for which the mathematics becomes too difficult for direct solution. Large data bases generated by systems for which the signal to noise is high are now being routinely produced, especially in engineering and the physical sciences. For such data traditional statistical tools are not flexible enough to extract all the available information. The challenges associated with these types of data underlie the motivations of neural network and machine learning approaches.

In the field of statistics a small cadre of researchers has also taken up these challenges, sometimes producing surprisingly similar methods. For example, projection pursuit is quite similar to (feedforward) neural networks and recursive partitioning (CART) is nearly identical to many decision tree induction methods in machine learning. The statisticians attending this ASI are among those at the forefront of this effort. They bring with them a shared excitement for the new challenges associated with modern approaches to predictive learning, along with the care and scholarship that has traditionally characterized the field of statistics.

Statistical Versus ANN Methods for Learning from Examples

There is a range of conflicting opinions on the utility of ANNs for statistical inference. On one extreme, high expectations of neural network enthusiasts are usually caused by their statistical ignorance. On the other hand, negative attitude towards empirical neural network research on the part of some statisticians can be traced to the view that algorithmic approaches are inferior to analytical proofs. Some of the tension between the two fields is caused by the difference in research methodology. ANN researchers focus first on developing an algorithm for solving a particular application problem, while statisticians concentrate first on theoretical assumptions/analysis, implementation being a secondary issue. The following differences between the two approaches have been noted during this ASI:

Problem/model complexity. Usually (but not always) ANNs deal with large amount of training data (i.e. thousands of samples), whereas statistical methods use much smaller training samples. Hence, ANN models usually have higher complexity (number of parameters or weights) than statistical methods.

Goals of modeling. In statistics, the usual goal is *interpretability*, which favors structured models (i.e. classification trees and linear regression). In ANN research, the main objective is *generalization/prediction*. Hence, the ANN models usually have little, if any, interpretability. However, for many high-dimensional problems even structured methods are difficult to interpret, due to large model size (i.e. large classification tree). Interpretation of complex models produced by adaptive methods can be enhanced by computer visualization techniques.

Comparisons and search for the best method. Most statistical and ANN methods are asymptotically "good", i.e. can guarantee faithful estimates when the number of training samples grows very large. Unfortunately, the real world provides finite and usually sparse data sets. For such ill-posed problems, asymptotic performance is irrelevant, and the best method should conform to the properties of data at hand. Hence, no single method dominates all others for all possible data

sets. The real research goal is not to find the best method, but to characterize the class of functions/mappings (along with assumptions about the noise, smoothness etc.) for which a given method works best. Another important relevant problem is characterization of real data sets from important application domains.
Batch vs. flow-through processing. Most statistical methods utilize the whole training set (batch mode), whereas ANNs favor iterative processing (one sample at a time) known as flow-through methods in statistics. Iterative ANN processing requires many presentations of training data and uses slow computational paradigm (gradient descent). Statistical methods are usually much faster.
Computational complexity and usability. Since statistical methods extract information from the entire training set, they tend to be more computationally complex and difficult to use by non-statisticians. ANN methods tend to be simple computationally, albeit at the expense of recycling (multiple presentation) of the training data. Hence, ANN methods can be easily understood and applied by novice users. Also, hardware implementations favor simpler ANN methods.
Robustness and quality of prediction estimates. ANN methods appear more robust than statistical ones with respect to parameter tuning. Even suboptimal choice of parameters (network size, learning rate etc.) usually gives reasonable results. Another important aspect of robustness is the quality of prediction estimates produced by a modeling method, i.e. providing confidence intervals for prediction estimates. Confidence intervals are routinely provided in statistical methods, but usually are lacking in ANN application studies. Usually, the quality of solutions generated by ANNs cannot be guaranteed. This is partly due to the "black box" structure of ANNs. More work needs to be done to make them more transparent.

Towards Intelligent Information Processing: Biological Connections

Whereas the connection between artificial networks and statistical inference is generally well understood, the relationship/relevance of predictive learning framework to biological pattern recognition is not so clear. However, several common principles underlying the operation of ANNs and biological perceptual systems can be identified as discussed next.
Problem/system complexity. A key characteristic of intelligent behavior is the visual ability to sense, perceive and interpret the environment. Most perceptual (e.g. visual) tasks are complex mostly because they are under-constrained (or ill-posed). At the same time, human visual system exhibits robust performance, despite limited and slow computational resources. Perceptual systems are inherently more complex than (artificial) data-driven methods. It is widely believed that the human perceptual system handles complexity through the use of Active and Selective Perceptual strategies. The term Active Selective Perception means that the observer learns where to search for the data and what type of data to use for processing. ANNs and statistical methods do not have yet such attentive capabilities.
Representation bias. The basic tasks performed by biological neural networks involve learning adaptive mappings for approximating/mapping sensory input sig-

nals. The task of finding optimal signal representations is fundamental to any biological task (such as cognition and classification), and is arguably even more important than higher-level learning. Biological studies suggest representation of the sensory input through decomposition using local (kernel) bases ("receptive fields"). The problem of representation corresponds to selection of basis function in function approximation and predictive learning. Since various data modeling methods differ primarily in the choice of the basis functions, this problem also corresponds to the problem of model selection in predictive learning. Even though statistical studies suggest that there is no single best method/representation that dominates others for every possible data set, biological systems clearly favor local representations. This may be a biological cue to statisticians: pay more attention to local adaptive methods. Examples of local methods that do not have adequate statistical interpretation include wavelets and fuzzy inference systems (where each fuzzy rule can be interpreted as a local basis function). A particular challenging problem is to re-examine the curse of dimensionality, as it relates to local methods and real-world recognition problems. Even though theoretical limitations of local methods in high-dimensional spaces are well-known in statistics, empirical evidence provided by biological systems suggests that for many practical applications the curse of dimensionality is not relevant. It is most likely that assumptions underlying theoretical treatment of the curse do not hold for many real applications, possibly because of locality.

Hybrid systems. The complexity of biological neural systems and the wide range of tasks involved in perception require a large repertoire of intelligent modules. Hence, an advanced perceptual system should be able to develop hybrid adaptation systems driven by multistrategy learning schemes. It appears that employing hybrid learning systems accounts for success of several successful connectionist applications. The analogy between perception and ANNs is evident in the system approach used in the development of full fledged perceptual systems. The bottom-up ("data-driven") part corresponds to preprocessing and feature extraction. Once the features are derived, image classification ("understanding and classification") takes place. The top-down ("model-driven") part corresponds to post-processing ("disambiguation") and active selective perception ("priming") using global regularization constraints. This perceptual architecture is characteristic of hybrid systems where modularity is functionally defined. One important conclusion reached during this ASI was that future intelligent systems based on ANN technology should be task-driven and that their functionality could be enhanced by modular design using hybrid systems approaches and multistrategy learning.

Even though most lectures address one of the above themes, it became clear during the meeting that there was a strong connection between several of the topics. This lead to numerous discussions both in the formal setting (during lectures and panel discussions) and informal personal interactions between the participants.

The feedback from the participants regarding the contents of presented lectures and the social contacts during this meeting was very positive. This ASI was made possible by the efforts of the organizing committee: Vladimir Cherkassky (University of Minnesota, USA), Francoise Fogelman Soulie (LRI, France), Harry Wechsler (George Mason University, USA) and Christian Wellekens (Eurecom, France). We are grateful for financial support provided by the North

Atlantic Treaty Organization, Scientific Affairs Division, and for the matching funds provided by the US Office of Naval Research (ONR) and the US Advanced Research Projects Agency (ARPA).

Finally, special thanks are due to Filip Mulier from the University of Minnesota who spent endless hours on organization of the ASI and provided invaluable assistance in editing this volume.

July 1994

Vladimir Cherkassky, Minneapolis (Director)
Jerome H. Friedman, Stanford (Co-director)
Harry Wechsler, Fairfax (Co-director)

Contents

In the case of several authors, * indicates who presented the paper

An Overview of Predictive Learning and Function Approximation

Jerome H. Friedman

Department of Statistics
and
Stanford Linear Accelerator Center
Stanford University

Abstract: Predictive learning has been traditionally studied in applied mathematics (function approximation), statistics (nonparametric regression), and engineering (pattern recognition). Recently the fields of artificial intelligence (machine learning) and connectionism (neural networks) have emerged, increasing interest in this problem, both in terms of wider application and methodological advances. This paper reviews the underlying principles of many of the practical approaches developed in these fields, with the goal of placing them in a common perspective and providing a unifying overview.

1 The problem

The predictive learning problem is remarkably simple to state, if difficult to solve in general. One has a system under study characterized by several (possibly many) simultaneously measurable (observable) quantities, called variables. The variables are divided into two groups. The variables in one group are referred to (respectively) as independent variables (applied mathematics), explanatory/predictor variables (statistics), or input variables (neural networks/machine learning). The variables of the other group also have different names depending on the field of study: dependent variables (applied mathematics), responses (statistics), or output variables (neural networks/machine learning). The goal is to develop a computational relationship between the inputs and the outputs (formula/algorithm) for determining/predicting/estimating values for the output variables given only the values of the input variables.

For example, the system under study might be a manufacturing process. The inputs would be the various parameters that control the process such as chemical concentrations, baking time, precision of various machine tools, etc. The outputs would be measures of quality of the final product(s). The goal here would be to forecast the resulting quality(ies) from knowledge of the input parameter values without having to actually run the process. Realizing this goal could eliminate much experimentation with considerable financial benefit. In another example the "system" might be people potentially sick with one of several diseases or maladies. The inputs would consist of the existence/severity of various symptoms and a collection of medical laboratory

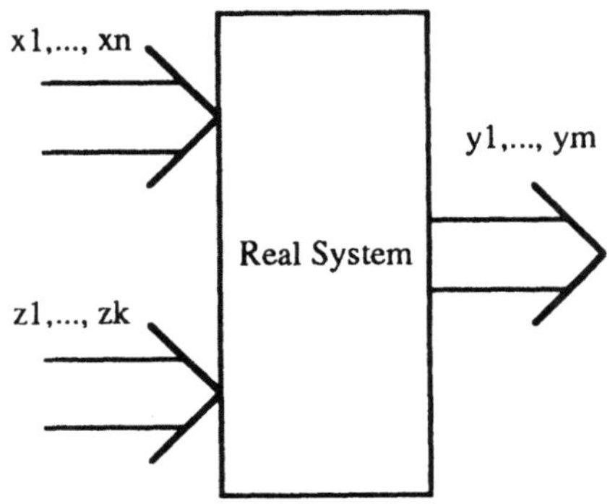

Figure 1. Diagram of the predictive learning problem

measurements. The output(s) would be indicators/severity of the potential diseases.

Figure 1 displays a pictorial representation of the problem. The system is represented by the rectangular box, the inputs as lines on the left side of the box and outputs $\{y_1, \cdots, y_K\}$ as lines on the right. The inputs are grouped into two sets. The first $\{x_1, \cdots, x_n\}$ are the inputs whose values are actually measured or observed. The other set $\{z_1, \cdots, z_L\}$ represent other quantities that relate to (affect) the outputs but whose values are neither observed nor controlled. Sometimes this second set of input variables does not exist ($L = 0$). One might be able to identify and measure all possible input variables that relate to the outputs. Often, however, this is not the case. It is unlikely that all possible things that affect the quality of a manufactured product can be measured, such as operator mood, distractions, etc. In medical diagnosis all symptoms are seldom observed and all possible diagnostic tests are not usually made. This means that a simultaneous set of observed input values $\{x_1, \cdots, x_n\}$ does not uniquely specify the output values. There is some uncertainty in the outputs reflecting the lack of knowledge of the unobserved input values.

By drawing the input lines on the left and outputs on the right (Fig. 1) one is tempted to associate a causal relationship between the values of the inputs and outputs. That is, changing the input values causes a change in the values of the outputs. This is often the case, as in the manufacturing process example. Sometimes, however, the reverse is true. Often it is the existence/severity of a disease that causes the existence/severity of the symptoms. Other times neither is true; changes in values of the inputs and outputs are both reflections of changes in other (unobserved) factors. In many problems all three of these mechanisms exist. The point is that causality is not necessary for a derived relationship between the inputs and outputs to be either accurate, or useful, as in medical diagnosis. The converse is also true; the existence of an accurate input/output relationship need not reflect causality.

1.1 Types of variables

The input and output variables can each be of two different fundamental types: real or categorical. A real valued variable assumes values over a subset of the real line R^1. Examples are height, weight, voltage, course grade (F–A, mapped to 0–4). Values of these variables have an order relation and a distance defined between all pairs of values. Categorical variables have neither. For a categorical variable, two values are either equal or unequal. Examples are brand names, type of disease, nationality, etc. If a categorical variable assumes only two values then one of its values can be mapped to the real value zero and the other to real value one. It can then be treated as a real valued variable with no loss of generality. This is not the case if a categorical variable takes on more than two values.

When a categorical variable assumes more than two (say K) values it can be converted into K (0/1) real valued variables, one real variable for each categorical value. If the categorical variable assumes its kth value, its corresponding (kth) real valued surrogate is set to one and all of the other real surrogates, corresponding to different categorical values, are set to zero. If the categorical variable can assume only one of its values at a time then there is a linear degeneracy among the real variable surrogates and only $K-1$ of them are needed. This technique of mapping a categorical variable to real valued variables is referred to as "dummy variables" in statistics.

The dummy variable technique (trick) can always be used to deal with categorical variables. For categorical inputs it is not always the best way to do so. Methods differ on how well they can accommodate (extract information from) categorical inputs when they exist. (They don't occur for many problems.) Categorical outputs, however, occur often and represent an important class of problems referred to as pattern recognition in engineering, and classification/discriminant analysis in statistics. They are also the main focus of machine learning in artificial intelligence. Medical disease diagnosis is an example. For a categorical output variable the dummy variable trick is nearly always used. A single categorical output variable is converted into its real valued surrogates and the problem becomes a multiple (real-valued) output problem. This is discussed in more detail in Section 6.0. The point here is that it is sufficient to consider only real valued outputs in the supervised learning problem for the present. Translation of real-valued solutions back to the categorical output problem are deferred to Section 6.0.

1.2 Statistical model

The underlying mathematical model associated with the problem (Fig. 1) is

$$y_k = g_k(x_1, \cdots, x_n, z_1, \cdots, z_L), \quad k = 1, K. \tag{1}$$

Here y_k is the kth output value and g_k is a (real) single valued deterministic function of all possible (observed and unobserved) inputs that relate to changing values of y_k. To reflect the uncertainty associated with the nonobserved inputs $\{z_1, \cdots, z_L\}$, this relation (1) is replaced by a statistical model

$$y_k = f_k(x_1, \cdots, x_n) + \varepsilon_k, \quad k = 1, K. \tag{2}$$

Here f_k is a (single-valued deterministic) function of the observed inputs $\{x_1, \cdots, x_n\}$ only, and an additional random (stochastic) component ε_k is added to reflect the fact that simultaneous specification of a set of (observed) input values $\{x_1, \cdots, x_n\}$ does not uniquely specify an output value (unless ε_k is a constant). A specific set of input values specifies a distribution of (random) y_k values, characterized by the distribution of the random variable ε_k.

The fundamental models (1) (2) are represented by separate relationships for each output whose generic form is given by suppressing the k index. This suggests that they can be treated as separate problems without regard to the commonality of their input variable sets. This can be done and sometimes it represents the best way to proceed. Strategies have been proposed, however, that attempt to exploit possible associations among the output values to improve accuracy. Discussion of these strategies and the conditions under which they may (or may not) yield improvement over treating each output independently is deferred to Section 5.0. As noted there, the issue is not yet settled and is still an open topic for research. Until then we will treat the multiple output problem as separate single output problems. In many (most) problems, interest usually focuses on a single output.

In the following we denote

$$\mathbf{x} = \{x_1, \cdots, x_n\} \tag{3}$$

as a simultaneous set of input values. Our statistical model for each output (2) becomes

$$y = f(\mathbf{x}) + \varepsilon, \tag{4}$$

with $f(\mathbf{x})$ being a single valued deterministic function of an n-dimensional argument, and ε a random variable which is presumed to follow some probabilistic law (probability distribution), $\varepsilon \sim F_\varepsilon(\varepsilon)$. That is, $F_\varepsilon(\varepsilon')$ gives the probability of observing a value of $\varepsilon \leq \varepsilon'$. Using statistical notation we will denote with the symbol $E[\cdot]$ the average of a quantity over this distribution, i.e.

$$E_\varepsilon[h] = \int_{-\infty}^{\infty} h(\varepsilon')dF_\varepsilon(\varepsilon').$$

The model (2) is ambiguous since one can add a constant value to ε and subtract the same (constant) value from $f(\boldsymbol{x})$ and leave all values of the output y unchanged. This (definitional) ambiguity is usually resolved by the additional definition

$$E(\varepsilon) = 0 \tag{5}$$

for all values of $\boldsymbol{x}$. In this case one has

$$f(\boldsymbol{x}) = E_\varepsilon[y \mid \boldsymbol{x}]. \tag{6}$$

That is $f(\boldsymbol{x})$ is defined as the (unique) average output value y, for the specified set of input values $\boldsymbol{x}$.

1.3 Supervised learning

The goal of any learning approach is to obtain a useful approximation $\hat{f}(\boldsymbol{x})$, to the true ("target") function $f(x)$ (4) (6) that underlies the predictive relationship between the inputs and output. There are many ways to do this. One could try to derive the fundamental equations corresponding to the physical or chemical laws that control the system. Experts could be consulted as to their knowledge of the system. Supervised learning attempts to learn the input/output relationship by example through a "teacher". This process is depicted in Figure 2. Here one observes the system under study, simultaneously measuring both the (observed) inputs and the corresponding output values. This is done repeatedly, collecting a "training" sample of N simultaneous sets of input/output values

$$\{y_i, x_{i1}, \cdots, x_{in}\}_1^N = \{y_i, \boldsymbol{x}_i\}_1^N. \tag{7}$$

The (observed) input values to the system are also input to an artificial system (learning algorithm – usually a computer program) that also produces outputs $\{\hat{f}(\boldsymbol{x}_i)\}_1^N$ in response to the inputs $\{\boldsymbol{x}_i\}_1^N$. The artificial system has the property that it can modify (under constraints) the input/output relationship $\hat{f}(\boldsymbol{x})$ that it produces in response to differences $\{y_i - \hat{f}(\boldsymbol{x}_i)\}_1^N$ (errors) between the artificial and real system outputs, as provided by a "teacher". This modification process is called learning (by example). Upon completion of the learning process the hope is that the artificial and real outputs will be close enough to be useful for all sets of (simultaneous) values of inputs likely to be encountered.

1.4 Function approximation/estimation

The learning paradigm of the previous section has been the motivation for research into the supervised learning problem in the fields of machine learning (analogies to human reasoning) and neural networks (biological analogies

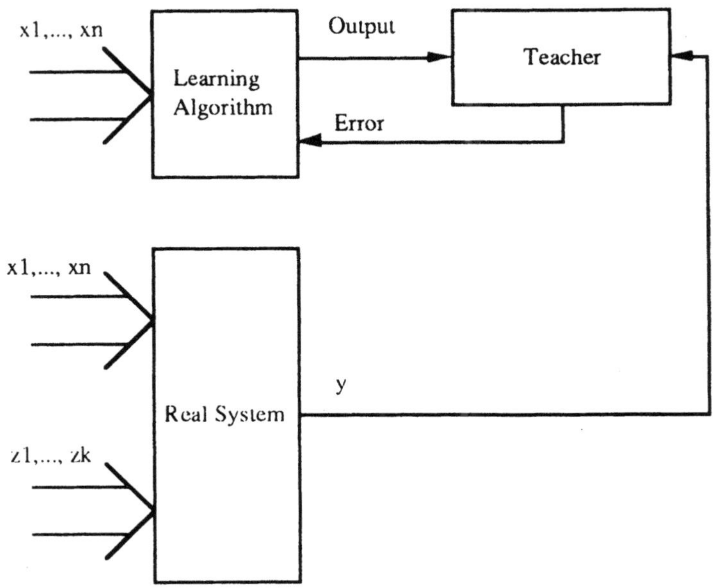

Figure 2. Diagram of supervised learning approach

to the brain). The approach taken in applied mathematics and statistics has been from the perspective of function approximation/estimation. In this view a simultaneous set of input values (3) is regarded as a point in an n-dimensional Euclidean space ($\boldsymbol{x} \in R^n$) and the target function (4) (6) as a function defined on that space. It is thus a surface (manifold) in the $(n + 1)$-dimensional joint input/output space. The training sample (7) represents a point cloud in R^{n+1} related to the surface $[\boldsymbol{x}, f(\boldsymbol{x})] \in R^{n+1}$ by $\{\boldsymbol{x}_i, f(\boldsymbol{x}_i) + \varepsilon_i\}_1^N$ (4). The goal is to obtain a useful approximation to $f(\boldsymbol{x})$ for all $\boldsymbol{x}$ in some region of R^n, given its value (possibly contaminated with noise, $\varepsilon \neq 0$) only at the set of points represented by the training sample. Although somewhat less glamorous than the learning paradigm, treating supervised learning from the point of view of function approximation allows the geometrical concepts of Euclidean spaces and mathematical concepts of probabilistic inference to be applied to the problem. This will be the approach taken here.

Function approximation is often divided into two subjects depending on the existence of an error term ε (4). If it is everywhere equal to zero the problem is referred to as interpolation. In this case there are no unobserved inputs (1), $\{z_i \cdots\}$ = null, and the observed inputs $\boldsymbol{x} = \{x_1 \cdots x_n\}$ are the only ones that relate to changing output y values. In this case specifying a simultaneous set of inputs $\boldsymbol{x}$, uniquely specifies an output value. The interpolations problem is then to approximate true target function $f(\boldsymbol{x})$ everywhere within a region of the input space, given only its value at a finite number of points within the region (training sample). This is the problem treated in applied mathematics (multivariable function approximation).

When unobserved inputs do exist, the error term (4) is not generally zero and the output y becomes a random variable. Specifying a set of (observed) input values $\boldsymbol{x}$, specifies a distribution of output y-values whose mean is the target function $f(\boldsymbol{x})$ (6). This is the problem usually studied in the statistical literature and is referred to as nonparametric (flexible) multivariate regression. One goal is the same as in the interpolation problem; approximate the target function everywhere within a region of the input space given a training sample. The difference is that here the problem is more difficult since the target function is only approximately known at the training (input) points owing to the error term (4). Another (less ambitious) goal often addressed in the statistical literature is to estimate the output values only at the training sample points, given error contaminated values at those points. This is theoretically more tractable but seldom useful in practice.

There are two distinct practical reasons for application of supervised learning/function approximation: prediction and interpretation. In prediction it is expected that in the future new observations will be encountered for which only the input values are known, and the goal is to predict (estimate) a likely output value for each such case. The function estimate $\hat{f}(\boldsymbol{x})$ obtained from the training data through the learning algorithm is to be used for this purpose. In this case the primary goal is accuracy; one would like the estimates $\hat{f}$ to be close to the (unobserved) output y over this future prediction sample. Let $\Delta(y, \hat{f})$ be some measure of distance (error) between the two quantities. Common examples are

$$\Delta[y, \hat{f}] = |y - \hat{f}|, \quad \text{or} \tag{8a}$$

$$\Delta[y, \hat{f}] = (y - \hat{f})^2, \tag{8b}$$

the later being the most popular because its minimization leads to the simplest algorithms. A reasonable measure of (lack of) performance would then be the global prediction error

$$\Delta_P = \frac{1}{N_P} \sum_{i=1}^{N_P} \Delta[y_i, \hat{f}(\boldsymbol{x}_i)]$$

where the sum is over the N_P (future) prediction samples. Generally the precise locations of the prediction sample are not known in advance but can be assumed to be a random sample from some probability density $p(\boldsymbol{x})$, whose values give the relative probabilities of encountering a new observation to be predicted at $\boldsymbol{x}$. The global error then becomes

$$\Delta_P = \int E_\varepsilon \Delta[f(\boldsymbol{x}) + \varepsilon, \hat{f}(\boldsymbol{x})]p(\boldsymbol{x})d\boldsymbol{x}$$

where ε is the noise term (4) and E_ε is the average over its distribution $F_\varepsilon(\varepsilon)$. In particular if (8b) is chosen, then the mean-squared prediction error is given by

$$\begin{aligned} mspe &= \int E_\varepsilon[f(\boldsymbol{x}) + \varepsilon - \hat{f}(\boldsymbol{x})]^2 p(\boldsymbol{x})d\boldsymbol{x} \\ &= \int [f(\boldsymbol{x}) - \hat{f}(\boldsymbol{x})]^2 p(\boldsymbol{x})d\boldsymbol{x} + \int \sigma^2(\boldsymbol{x})p(\boldsymbol{x})d\boldsymbol{x} \end{aligned} \tag{9}$$

where $\sigma^2(\boldsymbol{x}) = E_\varepsilon(\varepsilon^2|\boldsymbol{x})$ is the variance of the noise at $\boldsymbol{x}$. The first term (9) is known simply as the mean-squared-error

$$mse = \int [f(\boldsymbol{x}) - \hat{f}(\boldsymbol{x})]^2 p(\boldsymbol{x})d\boldsymbol{x} \tag{10}$$

and it completely captures the dependence of the prediction error on $\hat{f}(\boldsymbol{x})$. Minimizinig (9) and (10) with respect to $\hat{f}(\boldsymbol{x})$ gives the same result. In particular, these results show that the target function $f(\boldsymbol{x})$ (4) (6) is the best (mean-squared-error) predictor of future outputs and accurate approximation and future prediction are equivalent goals.

Another reason for applying supervised learning is interpretation. The goal here is to use the structural form of the approximating function $\hat{f}(\boldsymbol{x})$ to try to gain insight and understanding concerning the mechanism that produced the data. In this context no future data is necessarily envisioned. The approximation is intended to serve primarily as a descriptive statistic for illuminating the properties of the input/output relationship. Some properties of interest might include identification of those input variables that are most relevant to (associated with) the variation in the output, the nature of the dependence of the output on the most relevant inputs, and how that changes with changing values of still other input values. Such information can be quite useful for understanding how the system works and perhaps how to improve it. Also, nearly all scientific research is based on understanding from data rather than (the narrow goal of) future prediction.

Accuracy (10) has some importance to this application since its not very useful to interpret an approximation that bears little resemblance to the true input/output relationship $f(\boldsymbol{x})$. However it is not the only goal. The informal criterion (to be optimized) is the amount of (correct) information learned about the system. Human engineering considerations are involved in determining the best ways to summarize and present the approximating equation/algorithm in the best form (graphical and tabular) for human interpretation. As will be seen below, the major successful methods for supervised learning differ greatly in the extent to which they can be adapted to this interpretational goal. These differences tend to be much larger than their differences in prediction accuracy, and only a few provide highly interpretable output.

2 Difficulty of the problem

Although the problem addressed by supervised learning is straight forward to state it has (so far) been difficult to provide a completely general (useful) solution. This difficulty, coupled with the broad range of important applications, has motivated much research activity in this area producing a large number of diverse learning algorithms. In this section we address reasons for the difficulty and in following sections many of the proposed solutions are presented, compared and contrasted.

All the disparate difficulties stem from one common origin – the finite size of the training sample. If the training sample were infinite in size (and one had an infinitely fast computer) one could directly compute the target function from (6) at any point $\boldsymbol{x}$ (or more precisely its average value over an infinitesimal volume centered at $\boldsymbol{x}$, in the limit that the volume approaches zero). The problem is well posed and the solution (6) unique. For example, (6) uniquely minimizes (9) and (10).

In the case of a training sample (7) of size N, the solution to the analog of (9)

$$\hat{f}(\boldsymbol{x}) = \underset{g(\boldsymbol{x})}{\operatorname{argmin}} \sum_{i=1}^{N} [y_i - g(\boldsymbol{x}_i)]^2 \tag{11}$$

is not unique. There are a large (infinite) number of functions that can interpolate the data points yielding the minimum value (zero) for the criterion (11). In the case of no noise, $\varepsilon = 0$ everywhere (4), one of these functions will be the target $f(\boldsymbol{x})$. In the noisy case, $\varepsilon \neq 0$, none of them will be $f(\boldsymbol{x})$, or perhaps even close to it. Thus (11) represents an ill-posed problem. In both the noiseless and noisy cases solving (11) does not solve the problem for finite training samples.

In order to obtain useful results for finite N, one must restrict the eligible solutions to (11) to a smaller set then all possible functions. The nature of this restriction is decided by the user based on considerations outside the data. This is usually done by a choice of learning method. The restrictions imposed (explicitly or implicitly) by many popular learning algorithms is the topic of Sections 4.0–4.4. It is clear, however, that this restrictive approach does not really remove the ambiguity caused by the multiplicity of possible solutions. Imposing a particular restriction may result in a unique solution to (11), but there are an infinite number of possible restrictions, each of which can lead to a different (unique) solution to (11); the multiplicity has simply been transferred to a different mechanism (constraint choice).

All learning methods impose some type of smoothness constraint on solutions to (11). This does not completely remove the ambiguity since there are a wide variety of possible ways to define and impose smoothness. However all (reasonable) definitions require some type of regular behavior in small neighborhoods of the input space. That is, for all input points x that lie close enough to each other, $\hat{f}(x)$ exhibits some special structure (e.g. nearly constant, linear, or close to a polynomial of low degree). The strength of the constraint is controlled by the size of the neighborhood; choosing a larger neighborhood imposes a stronger constraint. Imposing a stronger constraint in turn makes solutions to (11) more sensitive to the particular type of constraint chosen, thereby increasing the variability of solutions to differing smoothness definitions.

Minimal neighborhood size is dictated by the training sample size or, more precisely, by the density with which the input space is sampled. Clearly, if a particular neighborhood contains no training data then all information concerning the target function $f(x)$ in that neighborhood must be inferred from sample points outside the neighborhood through the smoothness constraint alone. The more densely the input space is sampled the smaller such regions become thereby placing less reliance on the constraint to approximate the target function. This in turn makes the approximation less sensitive to the particular type of constraint chosen. In the limit of infinite training sample size ($N \rightarrow \infty$) all regions of the input space are sampled with infinite density, the size of the constraint neighborhoods can become arbitrarily small (thereby effectively removing the constraints), and the solution to (11) is uniquely defined by (6), which is, in fact, the true target function.

2.1 Curse-of-dimensionality

The discussion of the previous section implies that there are two ways to obtain an accurate estimate of the target function $f(x)$ (4) (6). One way would be to place a very restrictive set of constraints on the approximation $\hat{f}(x)$ defining a small set (class) of eligible solutions to (11). This will be effective to the extent that the target function $f(x)$ is a member of this class or sufficiently close to one of its members. A good choice of constraints would in turn require knowledge (outside the data) concerning the properties of the target function. In absence of such knowledge one must appeal to the second alternative for obtaining a good approximation: a large enough training sample to densely pack the input space. Although this is often feasible for input variable spaces of low dimension (few input variables), it is not possible for high dimensional spaces, even with very large training samples. This fact is often referred to as the "curse-of-dimensionality" (Bellman, 1961).

There are many manifestations of this curse, all of which tend to render geometrical intuition gained from low dimensional settings inapplicable to higher dimensional problems. As above, let n be the dimensionality of the input space ($x \in R^n$) and N be the training sample size. One problem is that sampling density is proportional to $N^{\frac{1}{n}}$. Thus, if $N_1 = 100$ represents a dense sample for a single input problem ($x \in R^1$), then $N_{10} = N_1^{10} = 10^{20}$ is the sample size required for the same sampling density with ten inputs ($x \in R^{10}$). Thus, in high dimensions all (feasible) training samples very sparsely populate the input space.

This sparse sampling property complicates geometric intuition in a number of ways. One is that in a high dimensional space interpoint distances between sample points are all large and approximately equal. This is because the volume of a sphere in an n-dimensional space is proportional to its radius to the nth power. Therefore neighborhoods that contain even only a few sample points have large radii. Consider a random set of training points sampled from a uniform distribution in the n-dimensional unit hypercube, $x \sim U^n[0,1]$. The average (expected) edge length of a hypercubical neighborhood containing a fraction p of the training points (volume) is $e_n(p) = p^{\frac{1}{n}}$. In ten dimensions, $e_{10}(.01) = 0.63$ and $e_{10}(0.1) = 0.80$. The edge length corresponding to the entire training sample is 1.0, so that to capture 1% or 10% respectively of the data points one must include over 63% or 80% (respectively) of the range of each input variable. Such neighborhoods are not very "local".

Another consequence of the sparsity of sampling in high dimensions is that all sample points are close to an edge of the sample. Again consider $x \sim U^n[0,1]$. In a sample of size N the expected L_∞ distance to any data points is

$$d(n, N) = \frac{1}{2}\left(\frac{1}{N}\right)^{\frac{1}{n}}.$$

for $n = 10$, $d(10, 1000) \simeq 0.5$ and $d(10, 10000) \simeq 0.4$. The maximum possible distance to any edge is 0.5 (the point located at the very center in each dimension). Thus, almost every point will be closer to an edge or boundary of the sample than to its closet sample point. Note that using L_∞ distance represents the most favorable choice since an L_∞ ball (hypercube) has the largest volume for a given radius. The situation would be much worse for say L_2 (Euclidean) distance. The reason that this represents a problem is that prediction (estimation) is much more difficult near the edges of the training sample. One must extrapolate (using the smoothness constraints) from neighboring sample points rather than interpolating between them.

This edge effect problem is not peculiar to uniform sampling in bounded (hypercubical) regions. Consider a training and prediction sample drawn from a (standard) normal distribution (unbounded), in the input space $x \sim N(0, I_n)$ where I_n is the n-dimensional identity matrix. The distance squared from the origin to any point follows a χ_n^2-distribution on n degrees of freedom. The expected distance is then $\sqrt{n - 1/2}$ and its standard deviation is $1/\sqrt{2}$. Consider a unit vector $a = x/|x|$ in the direction defined by a prediction point $\boldsymbol{x}$ and the origin, and project $\boldsymbol{x}$ and the training data $\{\boldsymbol{x}_i\}_1^n$ onto this direction. That is the projected points are

$$z = \boldsymbol{a}^T \boldsymbol{x}, \quad \{z_i = \boldsymbol{a}^T \boldsymbol{x}_i\}_1^N.$$

From the χ_n^2 distribution the expected location of the prediction point in this projection is $\sqrt{n - 1/2}$ with standard deviation of $1/\sqrt{2}$. However, since the training sample is unrelated to the direction $\boldsymbol{a} = \boldsymbol{x}/|\boldsymbol{x}|$, the projected training data points will follow a standard normal distribution $z_i \sim N(0, 1)$. For $n = 10$, the expected location of a test point $\boldsymbol{x}$ is 3.1 standard deviations from the center of the training data (origin) in its own projection $a = \boldsymbol{x}/|\boldsymbol{x}|$. For $n = 20$ it is 4.4 standard deviations away. Thus, (nearly) every prediction point sees itself lying at the edge of the training sample with all of the training points clumped to one side near the origin. This effect is clearly aggravated by increasing the dimension of the input space.

The above discussion indicates that the curse-of-dimensionality represents a formidable obstacle to accurate function approximation in high dimensions (many inputs). There are also arguments to the contrary; the curse-of-dimensionality is a fiction that does not really exist. One such argument is based on Kolmogorov's solution to Hilbert's 13th problem (Kolmogorov, 1957). Kolmogorov's theorem states than any continuous function of n-variables can be completely specified by a function of a single argument,

$$f(x_1, \cdots, x_n) = \sum_{j=1}^{2n+1} g_f \left[\sum_{i=1}^{n} \lambda_i \, \varphi_j(x_i) \right]. \tag{12}$$

The constants $\{\lambda_i\}_1^n$ are universal in the sense that their values do not depend on $f(\boldsymbol{x})$. The functions $\{\varphi_j(u)\}_1^{2n+1}$ are functions of a single argument and also universal in the same sense; they do not depend on $f(\boldsymbol{x})$. The single argument (continuous) function $g_f(z)$ does depend on $f(\boldsymbol{x})$ and thus completely specifies it through (12). Therefore, there exists a continuous function of one variable $g_f(z)$ that completely characterizes any continuous function $f(\boldsymbol{x})$ of n variables. From this one can draw the conclusion that, fundamentally, functions of more than one variable do not exist; expressing them in that way is simply a matter of choice of representation. Thus, the curse-of-dimensionality is also simply a matter of representation and not a fundamental aspect of the problem.

Although the premise of the preceding paragraph is clearly correct, the conclusion is not. The reason is that representing $f(\boldsymbol{x})$ by $g_f(z)$ does not change its complexity. Even very mild functions of n variables result in very "wild" corresponding functions $g_f(z)$ (12). Thus, the density of training sample points $\{z_i\} \in R^1$ must be much greater than $\{\boldsymbol{x}_i\} \in R^n$, leading to the requirement of comparable training sample sizes. Hilbert conjectured that a result like (12) was not true; "bad" (high dimensional) functions cannot be represented in a simple way by "good" (low dimensional) functions. His intuition was correct. Quoting G. G. Lorentz (1986) "Kolmogorov's theorem shows only that the number of variables n is not a satisfactory characteristic of badness." The fundamental issue is the complexity of $f(\boldsymbol{x})$, and common functions of many variables tend (have greater opportunity) to be more complex that those of a lower dimensional argument.

Another argument against the fundamentality of the curse-of-dimensionality is that is can be overcome in many situations. Consider the case (most) often studied in statistics. The model is given by (4) with the target function linear in its arguments.

$$f(\boldsymbol{x}) = \sum_{j=1}^{n} \alpha_j x_j. \tag{13}$$

The errors (ε) are taken to be homoscedastic [variance of ε is constant (σ^2) independent of $\boldsymbol{x}$], and one restricts the approximation to also be linear

$$\hat{f}(\boldsymbol{x}) = \sum_{j=1}^{n} \hat{a}_j x_j, \tag{14}$$

with the coefficients $\{\hat{a}_j\}_1^n$ estimated by least squares

$$\{\hat{a}_j\}_1^n = \underset{\{a_j\}_1^n}{\operatorname{argmin}} \sum_{i=1}^{N} \left[y_i - \sum_{j=1}^{n} a_j x_{ij} \right]^2. \tag{15}$$

It is easily shown that in this case

$$E_\varepsilon[f(\boldsymbol{x}) - \hat{f}(\boldsymbol{x})]^2 = n\sigma^2/N \tag{16}$$

which increases only linearly with the number of input variables n, not exponentially as the curse-of-dimensionality would suggest.

More generally, suppose

$$f(\boldsymbol{x}) = \sum_{m=1}^{M} \alpha_m B_m(\boldsymbol{x}) \tag{17}$$

where $\{B_m(\boldsymbol{x})\}_1^M$ are fixed prespecified functions of n variables, and we restrict the approximation to

$$\hat{f}(\boldsymbol{x}) = \sum_{m=1}^{M} \hat{a}_m B_m(\boldsymbol{x}), \tag{18}$$

again using least squares to estimate the coefficients

$$\{\hat{a}_m\}_1^M = \operatorname{argmin} \sum_{i=1}^{N} \left[y_i - \sum_{m=1}^{M} a_m B_m(\boldsymbol{x}_i) \right]^2.$$

In this case

$$E_\epsilon[f(\boldsymbol{x}) - \hat{f}(\boldsymbol{x})]^2 = M\sigma^2/N \tag{19}$$

which is independent of the input dimensionality n.

In both cases (16) (19) the curse-of-dimensionality was overcome by the fact that the target function $f(\mathbf{x})$ (13) (17) was a member of a restricted class of functions and we chose an approximation method (14) (18) especially appropriate for that class. Either we knew the class in advance or were very lucky. In the context of the discussion in Section 2.0, we have restricted the eligible solutions to (11) to be a small subset of all possible functions, and the target function happened to a be member of that subset.

As another illustration that complexity rather than dimensionality is the fundamental issue consider two target functions

$$f_n(\boldsymbol{x}) = \sum_{j=1}^{n} \alpha_j x_j,$$

$$f_1(x_1) = \sum_{j=1}^{n} \beta_j g_j(x_1).$$

The first $f_n(\boldsymbol{x})$ is a simple (linear) function of n variables and the second $f_1(x_1)$ is a more complicated function of a single variable ($\{g_j(x_1)\}_1^n$ nonlinear). If we choose the most appropriate respective approximators

$$\hat{f}_n(\boldsymbol{x}) = \sum_{j=1}^{n} \hat{a}_j x_j \quad \text{and} \quad \hat{f}_1(x_1) = \sum_{j=1}^{n} \hat{b}_j g_j(x_1)$$

then the approximation difficulty is the same in both cases (16) (19) even though the number of input variables for the first can be much larger than the second.

The basic reason for the curse-of-dimensionality is that functions of a high dimensional argument have the potential to be much more complex that lower dimensional ones and those complications are harder to discern. For a problem with a single input one can make a scatter plot of $\{y_i, x_i\}_1^N$ and graphically view the (approximate) relationship. For two-inputs one can use advanced data visualization techniques to view the resulting three dimensional point cloud. Problems involving many inputs result in correspondingly higher dimensional point clouds that are difficult to visualize.

Since it is impossible to densely populate high dimensional spaces with feasible training samples the only way to overcome the curse-of-dimensionality and be successful is to incorporate knowledge from outside the training data (assumptions) concerning the target function $f(\boldsymbol{x})$. As discussed below, choosing a particular approximation method either explicitly or implicitly does this. The degree of success depends on how closely the actual target function (in any particular situation) matches the assumptions associated with the chosen method. This was illustrated (in very simple settings) with the above examples. The various available approximation methods differ in the particular nature of the "knowledge" they impose, the strength of that imposition, and their robustness to violations of those assumptions. No method dominates all others over all situations (potential target functions). Also, as noted in Section 1.4, methods differ widely on the interpretability of the approximations they produce.

3 Penalization

One way to restrict solutions to (11) is to add a penalty to the criterion to be optimized

$$\hat{f}(\boldsymbol{x}) = \underset{g(\boldsymbol{x})}{\operatorname{argmin}} \left\{ \sum_{i=1}^{N} [y_i - g(\boldsymbol{x}_i)]^2 + \lambda \phi[g(\boldsymbol{x})] \right\}. \tag{20}$$

Here $g(\boldsymbol{x})$ ranges over all possible functions and $\phi[g(\boldsymbol{x})]$ is (non-negative) number (functional) associated with each one. The quantity $\lambda > 0$ ("regularization parameter") is inserted so that the strength of the penalty can be conveniently adjusted separately from its form $\phi[g(\boldsymbol{x})]$. For example, restricting $f(\boldsymbol{x})$ to be member of a particular class of functions [as in (14) or (18)] can be accomplished by setting $\phi[g(\boldsymbol{x})] = \infty$ for all $g(\boldsymbol{x})$ not in that class. Additionally, if some functions within the class were to be favored more than others, they would be assigned relatively smaller values of the penalty.

3.1 Bayesian formulation

Choice of a penalty (20) is equivalent to supplying external (outside the data) information concerning the target function $f(\boldsymbol{x})$. This is most easily seen in a Bayesian formulation. Bayes theorem states that the probability of a model (approximation) given the training data is proportional to the probability of seeing the data given the model, times the a priori probability of the model. In our notation this becomes

$$\Pr\,[g(\boldsymbol{x}) | \{y_i, \boldsymbol{x}_i\}_1^N] \sim \Pr\,[\{y_i, \boldsymbol{x}_i\}_1^N | g(\boldsymbol{x})] \cdot \Pr\,[g(\boldsymbol{x})]. \tag{21}$$

A natural choice for $\hat{f}(\boldsymbol{x})$ would be the function that is most probable given the training data

$$\hat{f}(\boldsymbol{x}) = \underset{g(\boldsymbol{x})}{\operatorname{argmax}}\ \Pr\,[g(\boldsymbol{x}) | \{y_i, \boldsymbol{x}_i\}_1^N]. \tag{22}$$

This is known as the maximum aposteriori probability (MAP) estimate. The first factor on the right side of (21) is called the likelihood of the data (given the model $g(\boldsymbol{x})$) and is thus a model for the error mechanism $\varepsilon(4)$. Suppose that the errors have a Gaussian distribution with constant variance $\sigma^2, \varepsilon \sim N(0, \sigma^2)$. Then from (4) the likelihood becomes

$$\Pr\left[\{y_i, \boldsymbol{x}_i\}_1^N | g(\boldsymbol{x})\right] = \Pr\left[\{\boldsymbol{x}_i\}_1^N\right] \prod_{i=1}^{N} \frac{1}{2\pi\sigma} e^{-\varepsilon_i^2/2\sigma^2}$$

with $\varepsilon_i = y_i - g(\boldsymbol{x}_i)$. Substituting this into (21), taking the logarithm of both sides, and discarding terms that do not involve $g(\boldsymbol{x})$ gives an equivalent to (22)

$$\hat{f}(\boldsymbol{x}) = \underset{g(\boldsymbol{x})}{\operatorname{argmin}} \left\{ \frac{1}{\sigma^2} \sum_{i=1}^{N} [y_i - g(\boldsymbol{x}_i)]^2 - 2 \log \Pr\left[g(\boldsymbol{x})\right] \right\}. \tag{23}$$

The solution to (23) is the same as that for (20) provided one makes the association

$$\lambda\phi[g(\boldsymbol{x})] = -2\sigma^2 \log \Pr\left[g(\boldsymbol{x})\right]. \tag{24}$$

Thus, in this setting the penalty in (20) has a direct interpretation involving the a priori probability ("prior") of $g(\boldsymbol{x})$ occurring, which (by definition) can only be determined from information outside the training data.

As the error variance σ^2 increases, (23) shows that the influence of the data on the MAP solution decreases relative to that of the prior probability. In the limit $\sigma^2 \to \infty$, there is no information in the training data and the a priori knowledge incorporated into the prior completely determines the solution (perhaps not uniquely). As the error variance σ^2 decreases the training data receives increasing weight relative to the prior $Pr[g(\boldsymbol{x})]$ in determining the MAP solution. In the limit $\sigma^2 \to 0$ (interpolation problem) only functions that interpolate the training data points are eligible solutions (data term zero). The MAP procedure then chooses the particular one among them with the highest a priori probability as determined by the chosen prior $\Pr[g(\boldsymbol{x})]$, unless all functions $g(\boldsymbol{x})$ that interpolate the data have zero probability (infinite penalty) under that prior. In this case the MAP solution may not be defined (for the interpolation problem) since there is no allowed (nonzero prior probability) function that could have (exactly) produced the observed training sample. This implies that the assumed prior cannot be (completely) correct (reflect reality). However, even in this situation it may be possible to express $\Pr[g(\boldsymbol{x})]$ as a limiting case of a more inclusive prior (permitting functions that interpolate the data) and adjust the limiting rates as that prior approaches $\Pr[g(\boldsymbol{x})]$ so that as $\sigma^2 \to 0$ the corresponding limit of the right hand side of (23) exists. In any case (20) is always well defined and $\lambda\phi[g(\boldsymbol{x})]$ retains the interpretation as representing (user supplied) external information.

One should not interpret the above discussion to imply that in the noiseless case ($\sigma^2 = 0$) an approximation that interpolates the training data is necessarily superior to one that does not. This point is illustrated in Figure

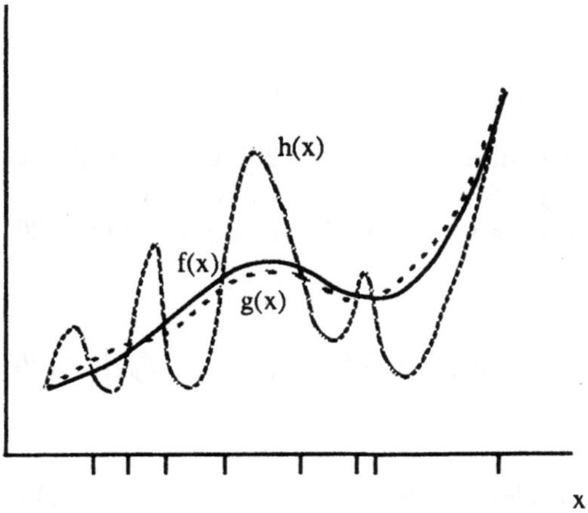

Figure 3. Illustration that interpolators are not necessarily the best approximators

3. The target function is represented by $f(x)$, $h(x)$ represents a solution from (20) obtained by a penalty that was finite (non zero prior probability) for some functions that interpolate the training data points, and $g(x)$ is a solution using another penalty (prior) that precludes data interpolation. As illustrated, the second solution $g(x)$ is superior by almost any reasonable error measure (e.g. *mse* (10)). In this case neither penalty corresponded to a prior (24) that correctly reflected the (relative) probability of realizing the actual target function $f(x)$. The second penalty corresponded to a prior probability that, while giving zero chance to the true target, gave high probability to functions close to it (small *mse* (10)).

3.2 Parametric penalties

Many of the well known learning (function approximation) methods restrict their solutions to a particular functional form, that is, $\hat{f}(x)$ (20) is a member of a class of functions characterized by a set of parameters $\{\theta_1 \cdots \theta_p\}$

$$\hat{f}(x) \in \{h(x|\theta_1, \cdots, \theta_p)\} \tag{25}$$

(Many examples are provided in the following sections.) This implies that

$$\hat{f}(x) = h(x|\hat{\theta}_1, \cdots \hat{\theta}_p)$$

for some particular set of parameter values $\{\hat{\theta}_1 \cdots \hat{\theta}_p\}$. This can be accomplished by setting $\varphi[g(x)]$ to be infinitely large for all functions not of that particular parametric family

$$g(\mathbf{x}) \notin \{h(\mathbf{x}|\theta_1, \cdots \theta_p)\} \Rightarrow \varphi[g(\mathbf{x})] = \infty.$$

This is equivalent to restricting the minimization in (20) to be only over functions in that family (finite penalty). Since each function in the parametric family is uniquely specified by a simultaneous set of parameter values, (20) becomes a parameter estimation problem

$$\{\hat{\theta}_1, \cdots, \hat{\theta}_p\} = \underset{\theta_1, \cdots, \theta_p}{\operatorname{argmin}}\}\{\sum_{i=1}^{N}[y_i - h(\mathbf{x}_i|\theta_1, \cdots \theta_p)]^2 + \lambda\eta(\theta_1, \cdots, \theta_p)\} \quad (26)$$

with

$$\hat{f}(\mathbf{x}) = h(\mathbf{x}|\hat{\theta}_1, \cdots, \hat{\theta}_p). \quad (27)$$

Because of the one-to-one mapping between sets of parameter values and functions in the parametric family, the (finite) penalty functional $\varphi[h(\mathbf{x}|\theta_1, \cdots, \theta_p)]$ becomes a (simple corresponding) function of the parameters $\eta(\theta_1, \cdots, \theta_p)$ as indicated in (27).

If all functions $h(\mathbf{x}|\theta_1, \cdots \theta_p)$ are taken to have equal a priori probability then the (least restrictive) parameter penalty function $\eta(\theta_1, \cdots \theta_p)$ would be a constant independent of the parameter values. If one has a prior preference for certain functions among this class then this would translate into a non-constant penalty with smaller values for (those parameter values corresponding to) the more (a priori) highly favored functions. Two such penalties that are very popular are

$$\eta_r(\theta_1, \cdots, \theta_p) = \sum_{j=1}^{p} \theta_j^2 \quad \text{(ridge)} \quad (28)$$

and

$$\eta_s(\theta_1, \cdots, \theta_p) = \sum_{j=1}^{p} I(\theta_j \neq 0) \quad \text{(subset selection)}. \quad (29)$$

The ridge penalty (28) favors approximations corresponding to small values of the parameters and causes a preference for solutions with many small values over those with a wide variation of parameter values. It corresponds to a Gaussian prior probability distribution on the parameters centered at zero (for all parameters) with covariance matrix proportional to the identity matrix. The strength parameter λ (26) characterizes the (common) variance under this prior for each parameter.

The subset selection penalty (29) simply counts the number of non zero parameter values. That is

$$I(\theta_j \neq 0) = \begin{cases} 1 & \text{if } \theta_j \neq 0 \\ 0 & \text{if } \theta_j = 0 \end{cases} \quad (30)$$

It clearly favors approximations with a large number of the parameters set to zero, but does not specify which ones. The strength parameter λ (26) in this case can be viewed as a charge or cost for each parameter that is allowed to enter (non zero value). This penalty (29) (30) can take on only $p+1$ distinct (integer) values from zero (all parameters equal to zero) to λp (all non zero). For each distinct value λk ($k = 1, p$) minimizing (26) is equivalent to minimizing the data term

$$\hat{f}_k(\mathbf{x}) = \underset{\#\{\theta_j \neq 0\}_1^p = k}{\operatorname{argmin}} \sum_{i=1}^{N} [y_i - h(\mathbf{x}_i | \theta_1, \cdots, \theta_p)]^2 \tag{31}$$

under the constraint that the number of non zero parameter values $\#\{\theta_j \neq 0\}_1^p$ is equal to k. It (31) thus selects the best subset of k (out of p) nonzero parameters (and their optimal values). For a given value of $\lambda \geq 0$ one of these k subset solutions will minimize (26). Thus, as the value of λ is increased from zero (all parameters potentially nonzero) to infinity (all parameters equal to zero), each of the k subset solutions (31) in turn becomes the solution to (26) and there are there therefore only $p+1$ distinct solutions. Thus one could equivalently regard k as the regularization parameter.

If both $\eta(\theta_1, \cdots, \theta_p)$ and $h(\mathbf{x}|\theta_1, \cdots, \theta_p)$ are continuous functions of the parameters, and the parameters themselves take on continuous real values, then the solution to (26) can be obtained by numerical optimization techniques. The ridge penalty (28) is such a continuous penalty function. However, the subset selection penalty is not a continuous function of its arguments owing to the discontinuous indicator function (30). Therefore, combinatorial optimization is required to obtain a solution to (26) (29) (30). Basically this reduces to minimizing (31) over all possible $\binom{p}{k}$ subsets of size k, for $k = 1, p$. This is generally too expensive computationally. For some especially simple parameterizations, e.g. linear

$$h(\mathbf{x}|\theta_1, \cdots, \theta_p) = \sum_{k=1}^{p} \theta_k B_k(\mathbf{x}) \tag{32}$$

"branch and bound" techniques can be derived (Furnival and Wilson, 1974) to greatly speed up the combinatorial optimization making it feasible for $p \leq 30$. Otherwise, fast (combinatorial) techniques for obtaining approximate solutions are used based on greedy (stepwise) strategies or random search (genetic) algorithms (Holland, 1975).

Another approach is to approximate the discontinuous penalty (30) by a close continuous one, thereby enabling the use of numerical optimization. This is motivated by the observation that both (28) and (29) (30) can be viewed as two points on a continuum of penalties, such as

$$\eta_q(\theta_1, \cdots, \theta_p) = \sum_{j=1}^{p} |\theta_j|^q \quad (\text{“bridge”}) \tag{33}$$

(Frank and Friedman, 1993), or

$$\eta_w(\theta_1, \cdots, \theta_p) = \sum_{j=1}^{p} \frac{(\theta_j/w)^2}{1+(\theta_j/w)^2} \quad (\text{"weight decay"}) \tag{34}$$

(Weigend, Huberman and Rumelhart, 1991). With the "bridge" penalty (33) $q = 2$ yields the ridge penalty (28), whereas subset selection (29) (30) is approached in the limit as $q \to 0$. For "weight decay" (34) the ridge penalty (28) is approached as $w \to \infty$, while subset selection is approached in the opposite extreme $w \to 0$. Both penalties are continuous functions of the parameters $\{\theta_1, \cdots, \theta_p\}$ for $(q, w) > 0$, and the smaller their values the more (33) (34) encourage diverse parameter values, behaving more like the subset selection penalty (29) (30). Care must be taken, however, not to approach subset selection too closely (q, w too small) since as q, w become smaller, an increasing number of local minima are included in the objective function (26), (33) or (34), making the numerical optimization more difficult. In the limit $q, w = 0$, there are so many local minima the optimization effectively becomes combinatorial.

A particular parametric form (25) characterizes a parametric family of functions, but that characterization may not be unique. There may be a wide variety of parameterizations that specify the same parametric family. Consider, for example, the linear case (32). In this case the parameterization is in terms of a linear expansion in a set of (basis) functions $\{B_k(\boldsymbol{x})\}_1^p$ with the parameters $\{\theta_1, \cdots, \theta_p\}$ being the expansion coefficients. Clearly one could obtain an equivalent representation

$$h(\boldsymbol{x}|\alpha_1, \cdots, \alpha_p) = \sum_{l=1}^{p} \alpha_l C_l(\boldsymbol{x}) \tag{35}$$

where each

$$C_l(\boldsymbol{x}) = \sum_{k=1}^{p} \beta_{lk} B_k(\boldsymbol{x}), \quad l = 1, p$$

is a (specified) linear combination of $\{B_k(\boldsymbol{x})\}_1^p$ and

$$\theta_k = \sum_{l=1}^{p} \alpha_l \beta_{lk}, \quad k = 1, p.$$

Although (32) and (35) have a different form they both specify the same family of functions.

If all members of the parametric family are taken to be equally likely (constant penalty function in (26), or $\lambda = 0$) then the particular form of its representation does not matter. Different representations will yield different solutions for the parameter values in (26) but they will correspond (uniquely) to the same function (27). This continues to be true if a penalty is applied that depends on the actual function, i.e. $\varphi[h(\boldsymbol{x}|\theta_1,\cdots,\theta_p)]$, and not on its representation (32) (35). However, this is not the case for (generic) penalties that are expressed purely in terms of parameter values such as (28), (29), (33) or (34). Changing the representation (e.g. (32) to (35)) changes the function penalty $\phi[g(\boldsymbol{x})]$ giving rise to different solutions to (26) (27). Therefore, specifying a penalty of this type only specifies a function penalty in the context of a particular representation of the parametric family, and changing the representation changes which functions are favored within the family. Although obvious, this point is often overlooked.

The ridge penalty (28) can be viewed as the Euclidean distance (squared) from the origin to a point $\boldsymbol{\theta} = \{\theta_1,\cdots,\theta_p\}$ in the p-dimensional parameter space. It thus places highest prior probability on the function $h(\boldsymbol{x}|\theta_1,\cdots,\theta_p)$ corresponding to all parameters set to zero. There is clearly nothing fundamental about the origin; a similar ridge penalty could be defined in term of Euclidean distance squared from any prespecified point $\boldsymbol{\theta}_0 = \{\theta_1^{(0)},\cdots,\theta_p^{(0)}\}$

$$\eta_r(\theta_1,\cdots,\theta_p) = \sum_{j=1}^{p}(\theta_j - \theta_j^{(0)})^2. \tag{36}$$

There is also nothing special about simple Euclidean distance; one could, for example, multiply each of the squares in (36) by a scale factor w_j making some parameters more important than others in defining the penalty.

One method of defining a distance penalty that is very popular in the neural network community consists of defining a particular (one-dimensional) path ("curve") through the p-dimensional parameter space, and restricting solutions to those that lie on the specified path. The penalty is taken to be the distance along the path (arc-length) from some prespecified point $\boldsymbol{\theta}_0$ also lying on the path. A one dimensional locus of points ("curve") in the p-dimensional parameter space can be defined by specifying a set of p functions

$$\theta_j = \Theta_j(s), \quad j = 1, p, \tag{37}$$

each of the same (one-dimensional) argument s. Changing the value of s changes the point $\boldsymbol{\theta} = \{\theta_1,\cdots,\theta_p\}$ in the parameter space, and the locus of all such points, corresponding to all values of s $(-\infty < s < \infty)$, maps out a one-dimensional manifold (curve) in the parameter space. The nature or topology of such a curve is determined by the particular functions $\{\Theta_j(s)\}_1^p$ (37) used to define it.

One (but not the only) way to specify these functions is through a set of differential equations

$$\frac{d\Theta_j(s)}{ds} = \frac{\partial U}{\partial \theta_j} \tag{38a}$$

where $U(\theta_1, \cdots, \theta_p)$ is (yet another) specified function of the parameters. The solutions are

$$\Theta_j(s) = \int_{s_0}^{s} \frac{d\Theta_j}{ds}(s')ds' + \theta_j^{(0)} \tag{38b}$$

with the derivatives defined in (38a), and $\{\theta_j^{(0)} = \Theta_j(s_0)\}_1^p$ represents and arbitrary starting point (on the curve). Here (38) the path is defined by picking a starting point $\{\theta_j^{(0)}\}_1^p$ and then taking repeated (infinitesimal) steps in the direction of the gradient (38a) of the chosen function $U(\theta_1, \cdots, \theta_p)$ in the parameter space. The penalty $\eta(\theta_1, \cdots, \theta_p)$ (26) is taken to be infinite for points $\{\theta_1, \cdots, \theta_p\}$ not lying on the path and proportional to distance along the path from the starting point $\{\theta_1^{(0)}, \cdots, \theta_p^{(0)}\}$ otherwise.

Defining a penalty in this framework requires the specification of a starting point $\{\theta_1^{(0)}, \cdots,$
$\theta_p^{(0)}\}$ and a function $U(\theta_1, \cdots, \theta_p)$ whose gradient determines the particular path. A particularly convenient choice for the latter is

$$U(\theta_1, \cdots, \theta_p) = \sum_{i=1}^{N} [y_i - h(\boldsymbol{x}_i | \theta_1, \cdots, \theta_p)]^2 \tag{39}$$

This is just the data part of the combined (penalized) criterion (26) whose minimum defines the solution approximation $\hat{f}(\boldsymbol{x})$ (27). Common choices for a starting point are all parameters set to zero (or nearly so if the gradient happens to be zero at that point) or a point chosen at random in the parameter space. Beginning there, a small step is taken in the direction of the gradient (38a) (39). The gradient is evaluated at the new point so obtained, and the next step is taken along this new gradient direction. These steps are continued until the gradient becomes zero, indicating a (local) minimum of (39).

The (numerical) procedure for obtaining the path (37) – (39) is just the steepest descent procedure for minimizing (39) and thereby providing the solution to (26) for $\lambda = 0$. This is the solution approximation $\hat{f}(\boldsymbol{x})$ under a prior that considers all functions $h(\boldsymbol{x} | \theta_1, \cdots, \theta_p)$ equally likely. For positive values of the strength parameter, $\lambda > 0$, a penalty is incurred proportional to the path length along the steepest-descent trajectory from the starting point. If the step lengths are equal this is proportional to the number of steps taken, and even when they are not equal, the number of steps is most often used

$$\eta(\theta_1, \cdots, \theta_p) = \#\,[\text{gradient descent steps}]. \tag{40}$$

This ($\lambda > 0$) will cause the solution approximation (26) (40) to be another point on the steepest descent path uphill from the minimum of (39) (or (26) with $\lambda = 0$). One can view the value of λ as a charge or cost associated with each step and increasing its value will reduce the number of steps associated with the solution approximation. This one-to-one correspondence between a λ value and the number of allowed steps implies that the latter could equally serve as the regulating strength parameter.

There is nothing inherently fundamental in choosing (39) to characterize the path of solutions to be considered. It corresponds to a prior belief that the target function is likely to be close to one of those on the path, preferably closer to the starting point. This may or may not be true and there may well be another path, defined by another $U(\theta_1, \cdots, \theta_p)$, that serves this purpose better in terms of coming closer to the target function (earlier). Any such path, however, should include the point that minimizes (39) (data part of (26)) so that there is not a discontinuity in the criterion (26) at $\lambda = 0$. Another important property that should apply to any path selected for this purpose is that (39) be a monotonically decreasing function of the number of steps taken along the path. That is, each step should be in a descent direction of (39) (data part of (26)). Since the penalty (26) (40) is monotonically increasing, this insures a unique minimum of (26) along the path and a one-to-one correspondence between λ-values and the number of resulting steps associated with the solution. Choosing (39) to define the path meets all of these criteria but there are other paths that also meet them. For example, a trajectory generated by any other numerical optimization algorithm (such as conjugate gradients, Gauss-Newton, etc.) shares these properties.

Like those defined by (28) (29) (33) (34), penalties defined in this manner (39) (40) depend on the particular parametric family chosen as well as the choice of a particular representation (e.g. (32) or (35)) of the functions in that family. In addition they depend on the particular one-dimensional path of eligible solutions chosen in the parameter space. If this path depends on the training data (as in (39)) it will not even be known in advance. As a result it is difficult to interpret such a penalty in terms of the actual functions it tends to favor as solutions to (26) (27), making the incorporation of actual a priori knowledge difficult. In fact, this data dependence clouds the interpretation connecting the penalty to such prior knowledge through the Bayesian framework (24). It is clear, however, that penalties of this type do favor certain solutions over others and those that are favored depend on (the definition of) the particular path that is chosen.

3.3 Nonparametric penalties

Constraining an approximating function $\hat{f}(\boldsymbol{x})$ to be a member of a specified parametric family (25) is one way an approximation method can require its solutions to be smooth. In all applications of this approach the parametric form $h(\boldsymbol{x}|\theta_1, \cdots, \theta_p)$ is a smooth function of $\boldsymbol{x}$ for all (allowable) values of the parameters $\{\theta_1, \cdots, \theta_p\}$. As noted in Section 2.0, it is the smoothness property that is basically used to infer function values in $\boldsymbol{x}$-regions where data is sparse, which is everywhere in high dimensional $\boldsymbol{x}$-spaces. However, the parametric constraint (25) imposes more than just smoothness, since a large number of parametric families produce a smooth function (of $\boldsymbol{x}$) and the constraint restricts the solution to be in just one of them. This has motivated the formulation of smoothness penalties based on differential operators, that do not (explicitly) involve parametric restrictions. These penalties have the form

$$\varphi[g(\boldsymbol{x})] = \int_{R^n} |Dg(\boldsymbol{x})|^2 d\boldsymbol{x}, \tag{41}$$

where $Dg(\boldsymbol{x})$ is a differential operator. Examples of such differential operators are the (norm of the) gradient

$$|Dg(\boldsymbol{x})|^2 = \sum_{j=1}^{n} (\frac{\partial g}{\partial x_j})^2 \tag{42a}$$

or the Laplacian

$$|Dg(\boldsymbol{x})|^2 = \sum_{j=1}^{n}\sum_{k=1}^{n} (\frac{\partial^2 g}{\partial x_j \partial x_k})^2. \tag{42b}$$

Embodied in these (and other) definitions is the notion that wigglyness is the opposite of smoothness and ought to be penalized; the penalties (41) (42a,b) clearly get larger as $g(\boldsymbol{x})$ oscillates more.

These nonparametric penalties (41 – 42) seem more general than their parametric counterparts (25) in that they appear to directly enforce smoothness without any parametric constraints. However this is not necessarily the case. Solutions to (20) involving penalties of the form (41) generally are members of particular parametric families with parameter penalties similar to (28). The number of parameters p, however is usually equal to the training sample size N. For example, solutions to (20) with penalty (41) (42) lead to basis function expansions (32) with $p = N$ and

$$B_k(\boldsymbol{x}) = \begin{cases} r_k^{2n+1}, & n = \text{odd} \\ r_k^{2n} \log r_k, & n = \text{even} \end{cases} \tag{42a}$$

with $r_k = [(\boldsymbol{x} - \boldsymbol{x}_k)^T(\boldsymbol{x} - \boldsymbol{x}_k)]^{1/2}$ being the Euclidean distance from $\boldsymbol{x}$ to each sample point $\boldsymbol{x}_k$. Wahba (1990) and Girosi, Jones and Poggio (1993) establish similar relationships for a wide variety of other penalties based on differential operators and their corresponding parametric representations in terms of basis function expansions (32).

3.4 Model selection

For a given training data set (7), choice of a penalty $\lambda\varphi[g(\boldsymbol{x})]$ (20) determines the solution approximation $\hat{f}(\boldsymbol{x})$. The preceding sections discussed the relationships among several popular (broad classes of) choices for such penalties.

Specific choices are associated with particular procedures (discussed below). Thus (given the data) the accuracy (10) of the approximation will depend on penalty choice. Clearly, the best penalty $\varphi[g(\boldsymbol{x})]$ for a particular target function $f(\boldsymbol{x})$ will be one that has small values for $g(\boldsymbol{x}) \approx f(\boldsymbol{x})$ and large values otherwise. This is why the penalty should incorporate as much (prior) information about $f(\boldsymbol{x})$ that is known to the user. This knowledge (by definition) cannot completely determine target $f(\boldsymbol{x})$, otherwise there is no need for supervised learning. It is the purpose of the data (first) part of the criterion (20) to use information from the training data to complement the prior information incorporated into the penalty to produce a usable approximation $\hat{f}(\boldsymbol{x})$ in terms of acceptably small values of *mse* (10).

Strict application of the Bayesian paradigm (21) (22) forbids the use of the training data in formulation of a prior probability model leading to a specific penalty term (20). The likelihood $\Pr[g(\boldsymbol{x})|\,\text{data}]$ captures the data information and the prior $\Pr[g(\boldsymbol{x})]$ captures all information outside the data. A problem with this approach that it presumes a correctly specified prior. This is difficult is practice. First, it is not always easy to accurately incorporate one's knowledge in terms of a mathematical formula for a penalty, and second, one may in fact posses very little knowledge concerning the nature of the target function. On the other hand a penalty is required to make (20) a well posed problem. In such cases, the pure Bayesian philosophy requires one to choose a prior (penalty) and simply hope that (if incorrect) it does not overwhelm the (information contained in) the training data.

The "empirical" Bayesian paradigm attempts to mitigate this problem. In this approach one incorporates prior knowledge into a penalty $\varphi[g(\boldsymbol{x})]$ (20) but allows the training data to choose the values of the "strength" parameter λ. This parameter is viewed as regulating the degree-of-belief in the corresponding prior information. If the training data appear highly compatible with the prior penalty, λ is given a larger value than would be the case if the data seemed to contradict the prior information (i.e. a surprise). In this way one "hedges one's bet" on the reliability of the chosen penalty to favor functions close to the true (but unknown) target function (low penalty value) and discourage competing functions far from it (high penalty value). If the penalty is deemed to be good in this sense an appropriately large value of λ is used, resulting in a substantial increase of accuracy, whereas if not, a small value is selected thereby controlling the corresponding damage. Thus, one wins big with a good penalty choice (method) but does not encounter a catastrophe with a bad choice.

A penalty with a corresponding strength parameter value $\lambda\varphi[g(\boldsymbol{x})]$ is deemed to be good to the extent that its use (20) yields an accurate estimate of the target function (10). This implies that for a given penalty $\varphi[g(\boldsymbol{x})]$ we want to choose the strength parameter to minimize *mse* (10) or equivalently the *mspe* (9)

$$mspe(\lambda) = \int E_{\epsilon}[y - \hat{f}(\boldsymbol{x} \mid \lambda)]^2 p(\boldsymbol{x}) d\boldsymbol{x} \tag{43}$$

with y given by (4). Here (43), the dependence of the solution to (20) on the strength parameter λ (given $\varphi[g(\boldsymbol{x})]$) is explicitly identified. An optimal value for λ, λ^*, would minimize (43),

$$\lambda^* = \underset{\lambda}{\operatorname{argmin}}\, mspe(\lambda). \tag{44}$$

Unfortunately, the target $f(\boldsymbol{x})$ is unknown so that (43) (or equivalently (10)) cannot be explicitly evaluated (for each λ-value) and minimized (44).

If we have a data sample presumed to have been generated by the same (probability) model (4) (6), we can estimate (43) by

$$\widehat{mspe}(\lambda) = \frac{1}{N_T} \sum_{i=1}^{N_T} [y_i - \hat{f}(\boldsymbol{x}_i|\lambda)]^2 \tag{45}$$

and

$$\hat{\lambda} = \underset{\lambda}{\operatorname{argmin}}\, \widehat{mspe}(\lambda). \tag{46}$$

Here (45) N_T is the sample size. The training data (7) is just such a sample. However, it is clear from the definition of $\hat{f}$ (20) that (45) (46) will always yield $\hat{\lambda} = 0$ as a solution. By definition the unpenalized solution provides the best fit to the training data, but this is generally not the case for (future) data to be predicted. Thus, (45) (46) must be evaluated for such future data, which (again by definition) we don't have.

A common approach to this dilemma is to divide the training sample (7) into two (disjoint) parts, a "learning" sample

$$\{y_i, \boldsymbol{x}_i\}_1^{N_L} \tag{47}$$

and a "test" or "prediction" sample

$$\{y_i, \boldsymbol{x}_i\}_1^{N_T} \tag{48}$$

where $N_L + N_T = N$, the training sample size. The presumption here is that the test sample (48) is representative of future data to be predicted, which will be the case if the training sample is so representative and the division (47) (48) is done randomly. The learning sample (47) is used in (20) to obtain the approximations $\hat{f}(\boldsymbol{x}|\lambda)$ and the test sample is used to evaluate (45) for each of them. Then (46) is used to estimate the optimal value $\hat{\lambda}$ of the strength parameter λ. This approach is usually referred to as "cross-validation," and is often very effective.

One problem with this form of cross-validation is that the resulting estimate $\hat{\lambda}$ depends on the detailed manner in which the training sample is partitioned into learning and test samples, in terms of both their relative sizes and which particular observations are assigned to the respective samples. If the training sample is very large, so that both the learning and test samples can also be large, then this does not represent a major difficulty; both will give reliable estimates of the corresponding predictive squared errors (20) (45). If this is not the case then this indeterminancy translates into increased inaccuracy in both $\hat{f}(\boldsymbol{x} \mid \lambda)$ (20) and the estimate $\hat{\lambda}$ (45) (46). This has motivated modifications to this simple method of cross-validation.

Given the sizes of the respective (learning and test) samples (N_L and N_T) the ambiguity associated with the particular assignments to each can be eliminated by computing (20) (45) for all $\binom{N}{N_L}$ possible assignments and then minimizing the average of (45) over these replications. This is of course not feasible for even moderately small values of N, so it can be approximated by many repeated random divisions and averaging the results. Even this can represent too much of a computational burden when the evaluation of (20) is computationally intensive, so generally only a few replications are performed. In this case the procedure is often approximated by "K-fold" cross-validation. Here the training sample is divided into K disjoint subsamples of (approximately) equal size. Each is used in turn as a test sample (48) with the complement sample serving as the learning sample (47). This is like the random division approach except the sampling is done without replacement and repeated K-times. Thus, each training observation appears in one and only one of the test samples and is used exactly once to evaluate (the average of) (45). This can be expressed as

$$\widehat{mspe}(\lambda) = \frac{1}{N}\sum_{i=1}^{N}[y_i - \hat{f}_{\backslash i}(\boldsymbol{x}_i|\lambda)]^2 \tag{49}$$

where $\hat{f}_{\backslash i}(\boldsymbol{x}_i|\lambda)$ indicates the solution to (20) for that learning sample in which the ith observation does not appear. This approach does not remove the ambiguity associated with observation assignment to each of the K test samples; that is which observations are assigned together in each individual group. It does however insure that each and every training observation is used to estimate the *mspe* (λ) (49) the same number of times (once).

None of these cross-validation methods (so far) removes the ambiguity in the relative sizes N_L, N_T of the learning and test samples. This can be done in the context of K-fold cross-validation by setting $K = N$; that is each test subsample consists of one of the training observations ($N_T = 1$) and the corresponding learning sample consists of the remining observations ($N_L = N - 1$). This is the well known (in statistics) "leave-one-out" estimate of *mspe* (λ) (49). In fact, $K < N$ fold cross-validation is often motivated as being a computationally faster approximation to the leave-one-out estimate, since it requires only $K < N$ solutions to (20). However, there is evidence that setting $K = N$ is not necessarily the best choice, and that more accurate estimates of $\hat{\lambda}$ can be derived for smaller values [Efron (1983), Breiman and Spector (1989)].

Criteria such as (45) (48) or (49) that are used to select a penalty strength parameter value are known as "model selection" criteria. Although easiest to motivate, criteria based on cross-validation are not the only ones used for model selection. Most model selection criteria are based on trying to approximate *mspe* (λ) (43) from the training data and then minimizing it with respect to λ (44). Cross-validation is one way to attempt this but there are others such as AIC (Akaike, 1974), C_p (Mallows, 1973), PSE (Barron, 1984), GCV (Caven and Wahba, 1979), and Moody (1992). Notable exceptions to this paradigm for model selection are MDL (Rissanen, 1983) and BIC (Schwartz, 1978). Model selection is still a very active research topic and there is no universal agreement as to which methods are best. Complete treatment of this subject is beyond the scope of this article.

Once a model selection criterion is chosen, solutions to (20) (26) $\hat{f}(\boldsymbol{x}|\lambda)$ are obtained for a sequence of λ-values. Each are evaluated, (45) (48) or (49), and the (estimated) best one is chosen (46). One could also employ various directed single parameter optimization strategies such as repeated bisections or "golden" searches (see Gill, Murray, and Wright, 1981). These can reduce the number of required solutions to (20) (26) which can be especially beneficial if obtaining those solutions is computationally intensive.

In the special case where solutions are restricted to the steepest-descent path (38) (39) (40), and a single learning-test division (47) (48) is employed for cross-validation, one can minimize (26) and (45) simultaneously in a single operation. Beginning with the starting parameter values $\{\theta_1^{(0)}, \cdots, \theta_p^{(0)}\}$, steepest descent steps are taken in the parameter space until a (local) minimum of (39) is reached. This local minimum represents a solution of (26) for $\lambda = 0$. Each set of parameter values corresponding to all earlier steps along the path represents a solution to (26) for (all) larger values of λ. Therefore, beginning at the starting point, the approximation (27) corresponding to each set of parameter values $\{\theta_1, \cdots, \theta_p\}$, associated with each successive step, are evaluated on the left-out test sample (27) (45) as the gradient search proceeds (to the minimum) of (39). The set with the smallest value for (45) is selected (46). Therefore, only one minimization (steepest descent) provides all the approximations corresponding to all λ-values, as opposed to a separate minimization of (20) or (26) (27) to obtain $\hat{f}(\boldsymbol{x}|\lambda)$ for each λ-value. This implementational convenience is the principal motivation for this approach to model selection, rather than any belief that approximations corresponding to points along the steepest-descent path are especially likely to be close to the target function $f(\boldsymbol{x})$. A major computational disadvantage is that steepest-descent is used for the numerical optimization, which is generally one of the least efficient methods. For many $g(\boldsymbol{x})$ (20) or $h(\boldsymbol{x}|\theta_1, \cdots, \theta_p)$ (26) and penalties $\varphi[g(\boldsymbol{x})]$ or $\eta(\theta_1, \cdots, \theta_p)$, the minima can be found by direct linear algebra or more sophisticated numerical techniques such as conjugate gradient or Gauss-Newton methods (see Gill, Murray, and Wright, 1981).

Model selection criteria (based on estimating *mspe*) such as cross-validation (49) can be used to obtain an estimate of *mspe* for any approximation $\hat{f}(\boldsymbol{x})$. In particular, one can compare solutions to (20) for different types of penalties $\varphi[g(\boldsymbol{x})]$ as well as for relative strengths λ for a given type. Since the penalty type is usually dictated by the method used, approximations derived from different methods can be compared, in any given problem, by cross-validation. This can be a quite useful way to choose (estimate) the best method for the problem at hand (training sample (7) and target function $f(\boldsymbol{x})$ (4) (6)). If some (or all) of the methods being compared themselves intrinsically involve model selection (for a strength parameter λ (45) (48) or (49)) then such comparisons must be done with care. One cannot use the minimized criterion value (with respect to the strength parameter) directly for comparison since it tends to provide an over optimistic (too small) estimate owing to the minimization. The degree of over optimism depends on the particular method. An "honest" (unbiased) estimate of *mspe* for a given method can be obtained by first (randomly) dividing the data sample into a training sample and a prediction sample. The training sample is used for all estimation including the strength parameter (perhaps by dividing it into learning and test samples) and the left out prediction sample is used only to estimate *mspe* for the complete procedure. This is known as "double" cross-validation if cross-validation (45) (48) or (49) is used to estimate the strength parameter. Although this "double" procedure provides an unbiased estimate, it still can be highly variable owing to the ambiguities associated with choice of a prediction sample discussed above. One can *estimate* which procedure is best, but not *determine* it, in any given situation.

3.5 Bias-variance trade-off

Model selection was motivated in the previous section through the empirical Bayes paradigm. It can also be motivated from another ("frequentist") perspective involving the so called "bias-variance trade-off." This involves the identification of two distinct mechanisms that contribute to approximation error (10); these are the bias and the variance.

The variance contribution is a result of the random nature of the training data (7). Training data sets sampled from the same system at different times will generally not be identical. This can be expressed in terms of an (unknown) probability (density) model $p(\boldsymbol{x})$ associated with the system, that gives the relative probability of observing a particular input vector $\boldsymbol{x}$ from that system. In addition, there is the randomness associated with the error ε (4) representing the effect of the unobserved inputs $\{z_1, \cdots, z_L\}$ (1) (if any) which is also expressed in terms of a probability distribution $F_\varepsilon(\varepsilon)$. A particular training data set (7) is presumed to be a random sample drawn according to these probability distributions with the outputs y (4) being the (deterministic) target function $f(\boldsymbol{x})$ evaluated at the random $\boldsymbol{x}$-points with random noise ε added to it.

The criterion (20) to be minimized depends on the training data through its first term. Therefore its value for a given argument $g(\boldsymbol{x})$ will be random as a consequence of the randomness associated with the training data. Thus the location of its minimum $\hat{f}(\boldsymbol{x})$ will also be random; different training samples from the same system will give rise to different (estimated) approximations $\hat{f}(\boldsymbol{x})$. This is the source of the variance component of the approximation error. It can be quantified by the definition

$$var[\hat{f}(\boldsymbol{x})] = E[\{\hat{f}(\boldsymbol{x}) - E[\hat{f}(\boldsymbol{x})]\}^2] \tag{50}$$

at each point $\boldsymbol{x}$ in the input variable space. Here (50), the expected value $E[\cdot]$ represents an average over all training samples (7) (of size N) that could be realized from the system with probabilities governed by $p(\boldsymbol{x})$ and $F_\varepsilon(\varepsilon)$; $E[\hat{f}(\boldsymbol{x})]$ is the average approximation value at $\boldsymbol{x}$ (over all such training samples). The var $[\hat{f}(\boldsymbol{x})]$ characterizes the (square of the) dispersion of $\hat{f}(\boldsymbol{x})$ values about its mean. The variance of the whole approximation is characterized as the point-wise variance (50) averaged over all points

$$var\hat{f} = \int var[\hat{f}(\boldsymbol{x})]p(\boldsymbol{x})d\boldsymbol{x}. \tag{51}$$

Since the randomness of the training data gives rise to a variety (distribution) of different approximations $\hat{f}(\boldsymbol{x})$, and since some of these will be more accurate than others (10), the variance will contribute to approximation error (10). This can be quantified by the well know identity

$$E[\{f(\boldsymbol{x}) - \hat{f}(\boldsymbol{x})\}^2] = var[\hat{f}(\boldsymbol{x})] + \{f(\boldsymbol{x}) - E[\hat{f}(\boldsymbol{x})]\}^2 \tag{52}$$

with var$[\hat{f}(\boldsymbol{x})]$ given by (50). As in (50) the $E[\cdot]$ operation in (52) represents an average over all $\hat{f}(\boldsymbol{x})$ that can be obtained from (20) for all possible different training data sets that can be realized from the system with appropriate probabilities. Thus, the left hand side of (52) represents the average mean-squared-error (at each point $\boldsymbol{x}$) for a particular method characterized by a penalty $\varphi[g(\boldsymbol{x})]$ and a given strength parameter value λ (20). This is equal to the corresponding variance of $\hat{f}(\boldsymbol{x})$ plus the last term in (52). This last term is the difference (squared) between the target function $f(\boldsymbol{x})$ and the average approximation value $E[\hat{f}(\boldsymbol{x})]$ (at the point $\boldsymbol{x}$). This difference is called the "bias" of the $\hat{f}(\boldsymbol{x})$ values (at $\boldsymbol{x}$).

$$bias[\hat{f}(\boldsymbol{x})] = f(\boldsymbol{x}) - E[\hat{f}(\boldsymbol{x})]. \tag{53}$$

Defining the mean-squared-error (at $\boldsymbol{x}$)

$$mse[\hat{f}(\boldsymbol{x})] = E[\{f(\boldsymbol{x}) - \hat{f}(\boldsymbol{x})\}^2] \tag{54}$$

one has from (52)

$$mse[\hat{f}(\boldsymbol{x})] = var[\hat{f}(\boldsymbol{x})] + bias^2[\hat{f}(\boldsymbol{x})], \tag{55}$$

and for the corresponding global averages

$$mse\hat{f} = \int mse[\hat{f}(\boldsymbol{x})]p(\boldsymbol{x})d\boldsymbol{x} \tag{56a}$$

$$bias^2\hat{f} = \int bias^2[\hat{f}(\boldsymbol{x})]p(\boldsymbol{x})d\boldsymbol{x}, \tag{56b}$$

one has from (55)

$$mse\hat{f} = var\hat{f} + bias^2\hat{f}. \tag{56c}$$

The random mechanism (probability distributions) associated with the training data $(\boldsymbol{x}, \varepsilon)$ are presumed to be a property of the system producing the data and not under the user's control. This is referred to as an "observational" setting. In a "designed experiment" the user can choose the set of $\boldsymbol{x}$-values $\{\boldsymbol{x}_i\}_1^N$ but the errors ε (4) are still random. In both cases the user has control over the choice of penalty $\varphi[g(\boldsymbol{x})]$ (20) and its strength λ, with the goal of minimizing the mean-squared error (56). For a given penalty $\varphi[g(\boldsymbol{x})]$, increasing the value of $\lambda > 0$ reduces the variance (50) (51) because it increases the importance of the penalty part of (20) relative to the (random) data contribution (first term) of the criterion. If the penalty part does not depend on the training data [e.g. (28) (29) (33) (34)], then it is a deterministic quantity (functional) and has no random component; it contributes nothing to the variation of the criterion (20) and thus to the variation in the location of its minimum $\hat{f}(\boldsymbol{x})$. As the relative importance to the criterion (20) of the (random) data term is diminished by increasing the value of λ, the criterion variation itself is diminished, thereby decreasing the variation in the location of its minimum. In the limit $\lambda \to \infty$, the criterion becomes deterministic as does its minimum and $var\ \hat{f} = 0$ (51) (provided the minimum of $\varphi[g(\boldsymbol{x})]$ is unique).

By altering the value of the strength parameter λ the user has control over the variance of the approximation $\hat{f}(\boldsymbol{x})$; it can be reduced at will. However, decreasing the variance (51) does not necessarily decrease prediction error (56) owing to the bias contribution. Increasing the value of λ may increase the bias-squared, and that increase may more than offset the resulting decrease in variance, resulting in increased $mse\hat{f}$ (56). The rate of increase of $bias^2\hat{f}$ with increasing λ-values depends on the true target function and the chosen penalty $\varphi[g(\boldsymbol{x})]$ (20). As $\lambda \to \infty$ the bias-squared approaches the limit.

$$\lim_{\lambda \to \infty} bias^2\hat{f}(\boldsymbol{x}|\lambda) \to \int [f(\boldsymbol{x}) - g^*(\boldsymbol{x})]^2 p(\boldsymbol{x})d\boldsymbol{x} \tag{57}$$

where $g^*(\boldsymbol{x})$ is a function that minimizes the penalty

$$g^*(\boldsymbol{x}) = \operatorname*{argmin}_{g(\boldsymbol{x})} \varphi[g(\boldsymbol{x})]. \tag{58}$$

(If the minimum (58) is not unique, then the one closest to the target $f(\boldsymbol{x})$ is used in (57)). This (57) is the mean-squared-error associated with the function(s) most favored by the chosen penalty (20) (58). If the target $f(\boldsymbol{x})$ happens to a minimizer of the penalty $f(\boldsymbol{x}) = g^*(\boldsymbol{x})$, then no bias increase is incurred by increasing the value of λ and the optimal choice would be $\lambda = \infty$ (minimum variance).

If the target $f(\boldsymbol{x})$ is not a minimizer of the chosen penalty (the usual case) then the dependence of the bias-squared on λ-value can be quite complicated in general. However, in some specific cases it can be determined. Suppose, for example that the approximation is restricted to lie in a parametric family (25) (the penalty $\varphi[g(\boldsymbol{x})] = \infty$ for functions not in that family) so that the estimate is obtained from (26) (27). Suppose further that the parameterization is linear (32); that is, the approximation is taken to be an expansion in a set $\{B_k(\boldsymbol{x})\}_1^p$ of predetermined (basis) functions. If the true target function happens to also be a member of the same parametric family

$$f(\boldsymbol{x}) = \sum_{k=1}^{p} \theta_k^* B_k(\boldsymbol{x}) \tag{59}$$

(for some $\{\theta_1^*, \cdots, \theta_p^*\}$) then one can show that the solution to (26) (27) for $\lambda = 0$ is unbiased (Gauss-Markov theorem)

$$bias^2 \hat{f}(\boldsymbol{x}|\lambda = 0) = 0.$$

(In fact, it is the unbiased estimator with minimum variance (50)(51) and thus minimum mean-squared-error (56).) In this case, the bias-squared will increase (monotonically) with increasing values of λ (26) (except in the unlikely case that $\{\theta_1^*, \cdots, \theta_p^*\}$ minimize the penalty $\eta(\theta_1, \cdots, \theta_p)$). If the true target function is not a member of the (linear) parametric family (25) (32) characterizing the approximation ((59) is not true) then the bias-squared will also monotonically increase with increasing λ-values but the minimum bias (for $\lambda = 0$) will not be zero

$$bias^2 \hat{f}(\boldsymbol{x}|\lambda = 0) = \underset{g(\boldsymbol{x}) \in \{h(\boldsymbol{x}|\theta_1, \cdots, \theta_p)\}}{\operatorname{argmin}} \int [f(\boldsymbol{x}) - g(\boldsymbol{x})]^2 p(\boldsymbol{x}) d\boldsymbol{x}.$$

This is the distance squared between the target $f(\boldsymbol{x})$ and the closest function in the (restricted) approximating family (25) (32) to it.

The variance decreases with increasing values of the strength parameter λ. In the special case (25) (32) the bias-squared increases with increasing λ-values. The mean-squared-error (56) is sum of these two effects. Thus, in increasing the value of λ one trades increasing bias-squared for decreasing variance. For some value $0 \leq \lambda \leq \infty$ this trade-off will be optimal in the sense of minimizing mean-squared-error. The optimal value will depend upon the true target function $f(\boldsymbol{x})$, the detailed properties of the randomness of the training data $p(\boldsymbol{x})$ and $F_\varepsilon(\varepsilon)$, all of which are unknown, and the training sample size N, and choice of penalty $\varphi[g(\boldsymbol{x})]$ (method) which are both known.

This analysis of the bias-variance trade off presumed that the penalty $\varphi[g(\boldsymbol{x})]$ (20) was chosen independently of the training data, thereby not contributing to the random variation of of the criterion and its solution $\hat{f}(\boldsymbol{x})$. This is not the case for the penalty (40), or any such penalty where the data is used to define the path through the parameter space (37) - (39). In these cases the analysis is a bit more complicated but a similar result obtains. Clearly the results for the variance are the same at the two extremes ($\lambda = \infty$ and $\lambda = 0$). For $\lambda = \infty$ the solution to (26) (27) is given by

$$\hat{f}(\boldsymbol{x}) = h(\boldsymbol{x}|\theta_1^{(0)}, \cdots, \theta_p^{(0)})$$

where $\{\theta_1^{(0)}, \cdots, \theta_p^{(0)}\}$ represents the (user defined) starting point. It thus has zero variance. The solution for $\lambda = 0$ is the (unpenalized) least-squares solution which as maximal variance. At points along the path in-between these extremes the solution is constrained to lie closer to the starting point (as measured along the path) so that its ability to react to changes in the training sample is thereby limited. The larger the value for λ the more the solution is constrained to lie close to the starting point so the variance is smaller. Thus the variance tends to decrease with increasing values of λ.

The behavior of the bias in this case (40) as a function of λ-value can be more complicated. Clearly if the target function is a member of the approximating (linear) parametric family (59) then the bias-squared achieves its minimal value (zero) at $\lambda = 0$. However, even in this case, there is no guarantee that the bias increases monotonically with increasing λ-value or even that it achieves its maximum value for $\lambda = \infty$ (starting point). When the $\lambda = 0$ solution is biased (target not a member of the parametric family) then it may not even be the one corresponding to minimum bias. Therefore, this type of regularization (40) provides variance control through choice of λ-value but very little control over the corresponding bias that is produced in its place.

The bias-variance trade-off characteristic was developed above strictly for the case of linear parameterizations (25) (32). Many popular approximation methods are of this form. For nonlinear parameterizations (25) things become more complicated. For example, even when the target $f(\boldsymbol{x})$ is a member of the same parametric family characterizing the approximations, the bias-squared may be nonzero for $\lambda = 0$. It is even possible for the bias-squared to decrease with increasing λ-values. (The variance always decreases with increasing λ-values.) However, the same general trend, established for the linear case above, seems to obtain in nearly all applications involving nonlinear parameterizations as well. The bias-squared tends to increase as the value of λ is increased (with the exception of (40)). This is due to the fact that most nonlinear methods used in practice are not too far from being linear so they share many of the characteristics of linear approximations. Considering approximations from parametric families (25) is not a severe restriction since nearly all approaches reduce to (25) however they are implemented. For example, nonparametrically motivated penalties such as (41) (42) involve solutions that are members of parametric families (see Girosi, Jones and Poggio, 1993)

Since the optimal bias-variance trade-off (λ-value) is unknown, it must be estimated from the training data. This is, of course, the same model selection problem discussed in Section 3.4. The reason for discussing it in this framework is to show that model selection can be motivated from non-Bayesian ("frequentist") principles without appeal to prior probability distributions, or empirical Bayesian degree-of-belief ideas. Applying a penalty $\lambda\varphi[g(\boldsymbol{x})]$ (20) to a (least-squares) criterion is known in this setting as the "method-of-regulation" and λ (20) is referred to as the "regularization parameter".

In whatever way model selection is motivated, its degree of success depends on the relationship between the target function $f(\boldsymbol{x})$ and the penalty $\varphi[g(\boldsymbol{x})]$. The more influence the penalty term has, relative to the data term (20), the smaller the variance. The degree-of-influence is determined by the model selection process which, if successful, will allow such influence to increase to the extent that not too much bias is produced. The bias is bounded by the distance-squared (57) between the target and the function that minimizes the penalty (58), or the closest such minimizer if there is more than one. Therefore, the closer the penalty matches the target function in this sense, the more benefit is realized from the regulation process in terms of smaller mean-squared-error.

The ability of the penalty $\varphi[g(\boldsymbol{x})]$ to influence the resulting approximation $\hat{f}(\boldsymbol{x})$ (20) is also related to its specificity, which is (inversely) related to the multiplicity of its minimizing functions (58). Such multiple solution degeneracy can only be resolved by the training data through the least squares term in (20) giving it more influence, thereby reducing the relative influence of the penalty, and thus increasing the variance. For example, a penalty that restricts approximations to be in a parametric family (25) characterized by small number of parameters is generally more specific than one characterized by a larger number, since more (a larger class of) functions minimize the latter. Therefore, for the same value of λ (20), the former penalty will have more influence than the latter on the solution, thereby producing less variance but perhaps more bias. Penalties such as (28) (29) (33) (34) or (36) are the most specific (within a parametric family) since they usually have unique minimizing functions (58).

Regularization produces the greatest accuracy (lowest mean-squared-error) when the penalty is the most specific and most closely matched to the target function (57). If it is highly specific but not well matched then model selection will tend to diminish its influence by choosing a small value of λ

(20) and variance is not significantly reduced. If it is well matched but non specific, then even with large λ-values it has little effect on the approximation again resulting low variance reduction. Knowing how well a chosen penalty $\varphi[g(\boldsymbol{x})]$ matches the target function $f(\boldsymbol{x})$ depends on knowledge about the target function itself. The more knowledge, the more specific a well matched penalty can be made, thereby achieving more accuracy. One thus returns to the Bayesian notion of the relation of the penalty to a priori knowledge about the target (24).

With most approximation methods the penalty $\varphi[g(\boldsymbol{x})]$ is implicitly or explicitly incorporated into the method itself and not directly adjustable. Therefore, the user controls penalty choice through choice of method. It is the goal of the next section to review some of the more popular methods for supervised learning/function approximation from this point of view. That is, what are the nature of the penalties they impose, or equivalently, for what types of target functions will they tend to be most successful. No method dominates all others, or even can be successful, over all situations (target functions).

4 Selected methods

In this section several popular methods for predictive learning / function approximation are reviewed from the perspective of the preceding discussion. This review is incomplete and necessarily brief. The purpose is to highlight their commonality and expose their differences.

All of the methods discussed here can be viewed as "dictionary" methods. Each establishes a set of predefined functions (dictionary)

$$\{b(\mathbf{x}|\gamma)\}_{\gamma} \tag{60}$$

where

$$\gamma = \{\gamma_1, \cdots, \gamma_q\} \tag{61}$$

are a set of parameters that characterize the functions and thus index each member ("entry") of the dictionary. As the joint set of parameters (61) range over all of their allowed values, the entire dictionary of functions (60) is created. The goal is to select a subset of entries characterized by specific sets of parameter values (61)

$$\{b(\mathbf{x}|\gamma_m)\}_{m=1}^{M} \subseteq \{b(\mathbf{x}|\gamma)\}_{\gamma} \tag{62}$$

whose linear combination

$$\hat{f}(\mathbf{x}) = \sum_{m=1}^{M} a_m b(\mathbf{x}|\gamma_m) \tag{63}$$

best (most accurately) approximate the target function $f(\mathbf{x})$. This approximator (63) lies within a subspace of the space of all functions, namely that subset of functions that can be exactly represented by (63). As the values of $\{a_m, \gamma_m\}_1^M$ range over all of their allowed values, all functions (approximators) in the subspace are generated. The number of entries M that comprise the approximation (63) is either fixed (prespecified) in advance or is taken to be a model selection parameter (Section 3.4).

A dictionary is said to be "complete" with respect to a set (class) of target functions if any target function in that class can be exactly represented by the entire dictionary

$$f(\mathbf{x}) = \sum_{m=1}^{\infty} a_m^* b(\mathbf{x}|\gamma_m) \tag{64}$$

for some set of expansion coefficient $\{a_m^*\}_1^\infty$ values. The corresponding method is said to be a "universal" approximator for that class. The methods reviewed below are all universal approximators for the class of all continuous target functions.

The finite size N of the training sample (7) does not permit the use of the entire dictionary. As entries are added to (62) the approximation (63) is better able to fit the (random) training data and variance is thereby increased. However the bias squared

$$\text{bias}^2\left[\hat{f}(\mathbf{x})\right] = \arg \min_{\{a_m, \gamma_m\}_1^M} \int \left[f(\mathbf{x}) - \sum_{m=1}^{M} a_m b(\mathbf{x}|\gamma_m)\right]^2 p(\mathbf{x}) d\mathbf{x} \tag{65}$$

is decreased since adding entries enlarges the function space spanned by the approximation. The approximating subspace can be defined as the set of all functions for which the squared bias (65) is zero. The goal is to choose a dictionary that best matches the target function in the sense that the bias squared (65) is kept low for small M so that the variance is also kept small, thereby producing small mean squared error (56).

For finite M (62) (63), this dictionary approach can be viewed as a penalized method (20) where the penalty functional $\phi[g(\mathbf{x})]$ is taken to be zero for all functions in the subspace spanned by the (basis) functions (62), and infinity for all other functions,

$$\phi[g(\mathbf{x})] = H\{bias^2[g(\mathbf{x})]\} \tag{66}$$

(65), where

$$H(\eta) = \begin{cases} 0 & \text{if } \eta = 0 \\ \infty & \text{otherwise} . \end{cases}$$

Under this constraint (66) the (learning) problem reduces to that of parametric learning (26) (27) with the parameters being

$$\boldsymbol{\theta} = \{\theta_m\}_1^p = \{a_m, \gamma_{1m}, \cdots, \gamma_{qm}\}_1^M . \tag{67}$$

An (additional) parametric penalty $\eta(\theta)$ (26) (if present, $\lambda > 0$) further restricts solutions in the approximation subspace to those functions characterized by parameter values that are favored by that particular penalty. Ridge (28), subset selection (29), weight decay (34), and the gradient descent penalty (40), along with no additional penalty at all ($\lambda = 0$), are among the most popular choices. If a penalty is involved ($\lambda > 0$) the value for λ is (also) determined through model selection (Section 3.4).

The various methods for predictive learning / function approximation described below (along with nearly all others) are primarily differentiated by their (often implied) choice of a particular dictionary (60). Thus, each is especially effective for those target functions that can be accurately approximated by a relatively small number of entries from its dictionary, and less effective when this is not the case. The methods discussed below employ distinctly different dictionaries so that if success is possible ($f(\mathbf{x}) >> \varepsilon$ (4)), there is a chance that at least one of them will be successful. No method is universally superior to all others over all target functions. Each is most appropriate for the particular classes of target functions that most closely match its dictionary in the above sense.

4.1 Projection pursuit and feed-forward neural networks

These are among the most popular and highly promoted class of methods (especially neural networks). Their dictionaries are comprised of functions of the form

$$\left\{ b(\mathbf{x}|\boldsymbol{\gamma},\gamma_0) = s(\gamma_0 + \boldsymbol{\gamma}^t\mathbf{x}) \right\}_{\boldsymbol{\gamma},\gamma_0} \tag{68}$$

where

$$\boldsymbol{\gamma}^t\mathbf{x} = \sum_{j=1}^{n} \gamma_j x_j \tag{69}$$

is a linear combination of the input variables. In the case of neural networks (Rumelhart, Hinton, and Williams, 1986) the single variable ("activation") function $s(z)$, $z = \gamma_0 + \boldsymbol{\gamma}^t\mathbf{x}$ (68), takes the form of a "sigmoid"; that is, it is an S-shaped function that assumes monotonically increasing values between zero and one, as the value of its argument z goes from $z = -\infty$ to $z = \infty$. The most popular choice is the "logistic" function

$$s(z) = \frac{1}{1 + e^{-z}}. \tag{70}$$

The arctangent function

$$s(z) = \frac{1}{\pi} \tan^{-1} z + \frac{1}{2} \tag{71}$$

is also popular. A particular choice (among the many possible S-shaped functions) is seldom crucial.

In the case of projection pursuit (Friedman and Stuetzle, 1981) the single argument function $s(z)$ is given some flexibility by (for example) expressing it in a parameterized form

$$s_{\alpha}(z) = s(z|\alpha) \tag{72}$$

where $\alpha = \{\alpha_1, \cdots, \alpha_p\}$ are additional parameters that characterize a wide class of (single argument) functions, not necessarily S-shaped. These parameters α are fit to the training data simultaneously with those of the linear combination (γ, γ_0), permitting the individual activation functions to adapt to the target function as well. This approach (72) basically enlarges the dictionary to include a wide variety of activation functions for each different linear combination (69) associated with the dictionary (68). This increased generality is achieved at the expense of introducing additional parameters (72). Therefore, for the same number of entries into the approximation (63) projection pursuit has less bias but more variance than neural networks. Whether this trade-off is beneficial or not will depend on the nature of the target function $f(\mathbf{x})$.

Neural networks as described above (63), (68) – (71), are known as "three-layer" networks. The first layer is comprised of the inputs $\mathbf{x} = \{x_1, \cdots, x_n\}$, the second "hidden" layer is the set of dictionary entries (63) (68), and the output $\hat{f}(\mathbf{x})$ is the third layer. Three layer networks are universal (64) for all continuous target functions, and are most often used in practice. Four layer networks can be constructed by introducing another hidden layer. This is accomplished by using the values of the individual dictionary entries in (63) as inputs to another set of functions taken from the same dictionary, rather than simply taking their linear combination to form the output $\hat{f}(\mathbf{x})$, as in (63). The resulting approximation takes the form

$$\hat{f}(\mathbf{x}) = \sum_{m=1}^{M_2} a_m^{(2)} b(a_{0m}^{(1)} + \sum_{k=1}^{M_1} a_{km}^{(1)} b(\gamma_{0k} + \sum_{j=1}^{n} \gamma_{jk} x_j)) \tag{73}$$

where M_1 and M_2 are respectively the number of entries ("units") in the two hidden layers. This (73) is an expansion of the same form as (63) but with a different dictionary. This dictionary is represented by the collection of functions

$$\left\{ b(\alpha_0 + \sum_{k=1}^{K} a_k b(\gamma_0 + \sum_{j=1}^{n} \gamma_{jk} x_j)) \right\}_{\alpha,\gamma}$$

as the (nonlinear) parameters (α, γ) range over their allowed values. The value of K is usually prespecified.

One can define networks of more than four layers in direct analogy with (73). In all such cases the dictionary is comprised of functions represented by the final hidden layer, as the parameters associated with all previous layers range over their allowed values. Whether adding such layers improves performance will depend on how well the resulting dictionary matches the target function in the sense discussed above. Adding a layer to an existing network enlarges the dictionary by involving more parameters and thereby increases the variance while reducing the bias. For a given number of parameters (comparable variance) the resulting bias-squared (65) for a particular network architecture, and thus its accuracy (56), will depend on the particular target function encountered.

4.2 Radial basis functions

The dictionary for this approach is comprised of the functions

$$\left\{r[((\mathbf{x}-\mathbf{t})^t H(\mathbf{x}-\mathbf{t}))^{\frac{1}{2}}]\right\}_{\mathbf{t},H} \tag{74}$$

characterized by the n parameters $\mathbf{t} \in R^n$, and the $\frac{n(n+1)}{2}$ parameters associated with the nonnegative definite matrix $H \in R^{n \times n}$. There are many popular choices for the single-argument functions $r(z)$, the most common being the Gaussian

$$r(z) = e^{-z^2}. \tag{75}$$

This dictionary is very large ($\frac{n(n+3)}{2}$ parameters) and its size is often reduced by placing constraints on the matrix H, thereby reducing the number of parameters. Requiring H to be diagonal

$$H = \mathrm{diag}(h_1, \cdots, h_n) \tag{76}$$

reduces the parameter count to $2n$, whereas requiring it to be a multiple of the $n \times n$ identity matrix

$$H = \rho^2 I_n \tag{77}$$

further reduces it to $n+1$. This (77) is the most popular choice in practice. Parameter count is also often further reduced by constraining all of the selected entries from (74) into (63) to involve the same matrix H.

As with the other methods, there is a bias-variance trade-off associated with the richness of the dictionary (as characterized by the number of parameters), and the number of entries in the expansion M (63). For the same variance, a smaller dictionary (fewer parameters) can include more entries. Whether the associated bias-squared (65) will be less than that of a small expansion from a richer dictionary (similar variance) will depend on the target function $f(\mathbf{x})$.

4.3 Recursive partitioning tree-structured methods

There are a wide variety of methods of this type. The dictionary for all of them takes the form

$$\{I(\mathbf{x} \in R)\}_R \tag{78}$$

where $I(\eta)$ is an indicator function of the truth of its (logical) argument η

$$I(\eta) = \begin{cases} 1 & \text{if } \eta \text{ is true,} \\ 0 & \text{otherwise .} \end{cases}$$

The symbol R in (78) represents subregions of the space of all possible values of $\mathbf{x} \in R^n$

$$R \subseteq R^n. \tag{79}$$

It is characterized by a set of parameters that define the subregion. For example, if the subregions are constrained to be axis oriented hyper-rectangles (the usual case) one has

$$I(\mathbf{x} \in R) = \prod_{j=1}^{n} I(u_j \le x_j < v_j) \tag{80}$$

where the $2n$ parameters $\{u_j, v_j\}_1^n$ are the respective lower and upper limits of the region on each input axis.

Recursive partitioning methods (78) nearly always restrict the entries into (63) to represent disjoint regions so that for any set of input values $\mathbf{x}$, only one entry (indicator function (78)) will be nonzero. Thus, in this case (63) can be equivalently expressed as

$$\mathbf{x} \in R_m \Longrightarrow \hat{f}(\mathbf{x}) = a_m \tag{81}$$

where $\{R_m\}_1^M$ represent the chosen entries in (63). This (81) is a piecewise-constant function; all values of $\mathbf{x}$ in the same region R_m have the same approximation value a_m.

Even with the axis-oriented simplification (80) the corresponding optimization problem (20) (66) is combinatorial (rather than numerical) and represents a formidable problem for M (63) not small. For this reason, approximate solutions using greedy optimization strategies are employed based on recursive partitioning. The various approaches associated with methods of this type differ on the particular details of how the partitioning is carried out. Described here is the technique employed by CART (Breiman, et. al., 1984). Most of the other methods use fairly similar strategies. An initial region R_0 consisting of the entire input space is considered first. This region is optimally divided into two regions R_1 and R_2 by a split on one of the input variables v at a split point t. Such a split is defined by:

if $\mathbf{x} \in R_0$ **then**
  if $x_v \le t$ **then** $\mathbf{x} \in R_1$
  else $\mathbf{x} \in R_2$
end if

The values for v and t are jointly chosen so that when the "parent" entry $I(\mathbf{x} \in R_0)$ is replaced by its two "daughters" $I(\mathbf{x} \in R_1)$ and $I(\mathbf{x} \in R_2)$ in (63) the best fit to the training data is achieved. Each of these newly created daughter regions (R_1 and R_2) is then optimally split in turn by replacing R_0 by R_1 (respectively R_2), and by replacing R_1 and R_2 by their respective daughters, in the above split definition. As each region is successively split, its corresponding entry in (63) is replaced by its two newly created daughter regions.

This recursive application of optimal splitting is continued until a large number of regions are created giving rise to a relatively large expansion (M big) in (63). These regions are then optimally recombined through their unions with other adjacent regions to form a smaller set of (larger) regions to be used in the final approximation. Optimality for this recombination process is based on an estimate of future prediction error using some model selection criterion such as cross-validation (Section 3.4). This strategy of producing a large number of regions which are then recombined to form a smaller optimal subset ("pruning") helps overcome some of the limitations associated with the greedy top-down recursive partitioning approach used for their formation.

The discontinuous piecewise-constant nature of approximations based on recursive partitioning (81) limits their accuracy on continuous (smooth) target functions, especially near the region boundaries. This limitation is mitigated however by other attractive properties of the procedure. One such property is input variable subset selection. Each split chooses the best input variable to divide an existing region (parent) into its two daughter subregions. Thus, input variables that have little or no effect on the variation of the target function are less likely to be chosen for splitting. In this way the resulting approximation tends to include only input variables that are "relevant" to target function variation. The corresponding limits (80) on such nonrelevant variables x_j include their entire range ($u_j = -\infty$, $v_j = \infty$) so that

$$I(-\infty \le x_j \le \infty) = 1 \tag{82}$$

for all values of x_j. This effectively removes each such variable from (80) and thus (63). Moreover, this subset selection strategy extends to local regions of the input variable space as well. As the initial (top down) partitioning proceeds, the corresponding regions include smaller and smaller subregions of the input space thereby becoming more and more local. Since the split of any parent region only involves the training data in the subvolume of the input space which it spans, the input variables most relevant in that local subvolume are most likely to be chosen for its split, and the splits of its daughters and further grandchildren. A particular target function $f(\mathbf{x})$ may (globally) have a strong dependence on many of the input variables, but it may depend on only a (different) few of them in different (local) regions of the input space. If so, then this approach can take advantage of this "local relevance" property due to its recursive nature. Approximations derived by the methods discussed above (Sections 4.1 - 4.2) involve all of the input variables everywhere in the input space and thus are less able to take advantage of this property (if it exists).

The one area where recursive partitioning strategies tend to dominate all others is in interpretability. Owing to the recursive (nested) nature of the partitioning it can be represented graphically as a binary tree. Each node of the tree represents a subregion of the input space. The root node represents the entire space. The two edges connecting an interior node to its two daughter nodes represent the split of that region. The daughter nodes represent the subregions produced by the split of that region. The terminal nodes of the tree represent the regions (63) (80) associated with the final partition. Each interior node is labeled by the splitting variable v and split point t that divided it into its two daughters. The terminal nodes are labeled with the approximation value a_m (81) associated with its region. The boundaries (80) of any terminal region can simply be obtained by traversing the tree from the root node to that region, updating the boundaries with the split points on the splitting variables, at each nonterminal node visited in the traversal. Thus, the binary tree contains all of the information (parameter values) associated with the approximation (63) (80) in a single easily interpreted graphic. [See Breiman et al. (1984) for many such examples.] The binary tree associated with recursive partitioning methods is considered an integral part of the methodology, and such methods are usually referred to as "tree-structured" methods.

4.4 Tensor product methods

The dictionary for methods of this type are the functions

$$\left\{\prod_{j=1}^{n} \phi(x_j|\gamma_j)\right\}_{(\gamma_1,\cdots,\gamma_n)} . \tag{83}$$

Each of these functions (83) is a (tensor) product of functions of a single variable. Each factor $\phi(x_j|\gamma_j)$ in (83) is a function of one of the inputs x_j and is characterized by one or more parameters γ_j. All implementations of tensor product methods allow the constant function

$$\phi(x_j|\gamma_0) = 1 \tag{84}$$

to appear as a factor associated with one or more of the variables in (83) so that the dictionary can be equivalently expressed as

$$\left\{\prod_{k=1}^{K} \phi(x_{v(k)}|\gamma_k)\right\}_{(K,\{v(k),\gamma_k\}_1^K)} \tag{85}$$

where the number of (nonconstant) factors K, the input variables associated with each of these factor $\{v(k)\}_1^K$, and $\{\gamma_k\}_1^K$, are parameters characterizing each dictionary entry, with $0 \le K \le n$ and $1 \le v(k) \le n$. By definition $K = 0$ produces the constant function with value always equal to one.

The goal of tensor product methods is generally to favor entries (85) into the approximation (63) with relatively small number of factors K, $K << n$, by judiciously choosing the input variable set $\{v(k)\}_{k=1}^K$ and corresponding parameter values $\{\gamma_k\}_1^K$ associated with each one. This incorporates both the global and local input variable subset selection capabilities associated with recursive partitioning methods (Section 4.3). In fact from (80) one sees that axis oriented recursive partitioning results in tensor product approximations where each factor (85) is an indicator function

$$\phi(x_j|u_j,v_j) = I(u_j \le x_j < v_j) \tag{86}$$

and $\{v(k)\}_1^K$ are the factors for which $u_j > -\infty$ and $v_j < \infty$ [see (82)].

More refined tensor product methods use a paradigm similar to recursive partitioning but employ continuous and more flexible functions for each of the factors $\phi(x_{v(k)}|\gamma_k)$ appearing in the products (83) (85). This permits more accurate approximation of target functions that are continuous (no sharp approximation discontinuity at the region boundaries), and of a wider class of target functions. For example, multivariate adaptive regression splines ("MARS", Friedman, 1991) uses (two-sided truncated power) spline functions

$$\phi(x_j|s_j,t_j) = [s_j(x_j - t_j)]_+ \tag{87}$$

where the subscript "+" indicates the positive part of the argument,

$$\eta_+ = \max(\eta, 0). \tag{88}$$

The parameter $s_j = \pm 1$ indicates the (left / right) sense of the truncation, and t_j is the "knot" location of the spline.

As with recursive partitioning, optimizing the approximation (63) (85) over all possible parameter values is not computationally feasible. The MARS strategy (Friedman, 1991) approximates this with a forward stepwise procedure (in analogy with recursive partitioning) that attempts to incrementally add entries to (63), and factors (85) (87) to the products that enter, simultaneously. The approximation is initialized with the constant entry

$$b(\mathbf{x}|\gamma_0) = 1. \tag{89}$$

At each successive step (iteration) two additional entries of the form

$$b(\mathbf{x}|\gamma_l)\,\phi(x_v|1,t) \quad \text{and} \quad b(x|\gamma_l)\,\phi(x_v|-1,t) \tag{90}$$

are incorporated into (63). Here (90) the $\phi(x_v|s,t)$ are the spline factors (87) and $b(\mathbf{x}|\gamma_l)$ is one of the entries (products) already in the approximation that was entered at an earlier step. The particular choices for l, v, and t are taken to be the ones that provide the best fit to the training data of the resulting (incremented) approximation. The values of the parameters associated with the selected previously entered term γ_l are not refit. This forward stepwise procedure is iterated until a large number of entries are incorporated into (63). Entries are then selectively deleted in a backward stepwise strategy, to find the best subset of entries, using a cross-validation criterion (49).

The MARS approach reduces to that of recursive partitioning if the factors (86) are used in place of (87) and the "parent" entry $b(\mathbf{x}|\gamma_l)$ is removed from the approximation (63) when its two "daughters" (90) are included. As noted above, using continuous functions (87) allows more accurate approximation of continuous target functions. Not removing the parent increases the generality of the procedure by widening the class of approximators (increasing the size of the dictionary). The MARS approach thereby retains all of the advantages of recursive partitioning while overcoming its principal disadvantages. Although not as interpretable as those of recursive partitioning (binary tree), MARS approximations retain a high degree of interpretability through a technique known as the ANOVA decomposition. See Friedman (1991) for many examples. For another tensor product approach see Breiman (1991).

With the tensor product approach (83) (85) (86) there is no requirement the individual factors $\varphi(x_j|\gamma_j)$ be functions from the same parametric family. Different families could be associated with different input variables x_j. In particular, different parametric families could be employed for input variables of different type (Section 1.1). This enables tensor product methods (including tree-structured recursive partitioning – Section 4.3) to handle categorical input variables, and input variables with missing values, in a much more natural way than other methods [Breiman et al. (1984) and Friedman (1993)]. Methods designed for real valued inputs (projection pursuit, neural networks, radial basis functions, etc.) are generally forced to use "dummy variables" (Section 1.1) to represent categorically valued inputs, thereby reducing their generality and effectiveness when such variables are present. Missing valued inputs also present more difficulty for these methods than for those based on tensor products.

4.5 Discussion

Five methods (projection pursuit, feed-forward neural networks, radial basis functions, recursive partitioning decision trees, and tensor product methods) were presented (Sections 4.1 – 4.4). The first two (projection pursuit and neural networks) shared some similar properties whereas the last three were fairly different from the first two and from each other. They were primarily discussed and compared in terms of the types (properties) of the target functions for which each is most appropriate in terms of the dictionaries they employ. As pointed out repeatedly, none of these methods dominate any of the others, over all possible target function, in terms of accuracy. These methods were also compared in terms of the interpretability of (the structure of) the approximations each produces. Some were seen to be much more interpretable than others.

There are other properties associated with approximation methods that, while very important, were not emphasized here. These properties include training speed (computation), and ease of use. The latter property involves the expertise and experience with the method required on the part of the user to make it perform to its potential in situations (target functions) for which it is most appropriate. Specific implementations of each of these methods involve procedural ("tuning") parameters, that can be adjusted by a user, to increase performance in a particular situation. Judicious choices for the values of such parameters can often greatly improve accuracy whereas poor choices can severely degrade performance. Thus a particular technique can be quite powerful (in a particular situation) in the hands of an expert with that method, and ineffectual when used by a novice. There is no way to separate the power of a method from the expertise of the person applying it. Some methods, however, are less sensitive than others to variations in the values of their tuning parameters and thus more robust against suboptimal choices. For such robust methods, default tuning parameter values can often be provided that provide acceptable performance over a wide variety of situations. In this context, the tree structured methods (Section 4.3), adaptive splines (Section 4.4), and to a somewhat lesser extent, projection pursuit (Section 4.1) are the more robust of the methods discussed here. This is likely due to the fact that these methods were originally developed in the field of statistics where ease of use (and interpretability) are often regarded as being equally important as accuracy.

The inability to separate the performance of a method from the expertise of the person that applies it complicates the interpretation of empirical performance comparisons between methods. The author(s) performing a comparison may have differential skills in their ability (and perhaps motivation) to tune the respective methods being compared. This can especially be the case when the purpose of the comparison is to validate a particular procedure, often one developed by the author(s). The developer of a particular method generally has the most skill (and motivation) to tune it well, in comparison to the other procedures, and this should be taken into account when interpreting the corresponding results. In addition, when a comparison (contest) involves data from a specific field (domain of application) then the relative domain specific knowledge of the user can greatly affect the outcome. Clever use of such knowledge can often be far more important in determining the outcome (approximation accuracy), than choice of a particular approximation method used in the context of such knowledge. Purely methodological comparisons are most easily interpreted when the same person(s) apply all of the respective methods to the same sets of data and have no differential skills among the methods, nor preferential interest in the outcome.

The computational resources required to obtain a solution approximation (training speed) can be an important consideration, especially when there are (multiple) tuning parameters to be adjusted. Exploration to obtain a good set of values may require repeated training runs using different values in each one. Restricted computational resources can limit the number of such runs, and thereby the potential accuracy of the result. Again the methods originating from statistics (recursive partitioning, adaptive splines, and to a lesser extent projection pursuit) tend to allow (much) faster training owing to the (perhaps excessive) regard in that field for rapid computability.

The methods discussed here (Sections 4.1 - 4.4) far from exhaust all of those that have been proposed for function approximation (supervised learning). Although these are among the more popular, there exist a plethora of other competitive proposals in the respective literatures that study this problem. Many of these can be regarded as variations on the methods discussed here. For example, most methods that employ interpoint distances in the input variable space bear a strong similarity to radial basis functions (Section 4.2). There are also a great many adaptations of both the feed-forward neural network (Section 4.1), and tree-structured (Section 4.3) paradigms. As noted, a few variations on the tensor product approach have also been proposed. The goal here was to choose a particular method from each distinctive class of methods as being representative of its class in terms of the types of target functions for which that class of methods is appropriate, as dictated by its dictionary.

5 Multiple outputs

All of the discussion so far has concerned the approximation of a single target function $f(\boldsymbol{x})$ (4) from a training sample (7). Most applications of supervised learning only involve a single output quantity of interest. Sometimes however the system under study produces several output variables (2), such as the quality control example mentioned in Section 1.0. The problem then becomes one of approximating several target functions $\{f_k(\boldsymbol{x})\}_1^K$ (2) of the same set of input variables $\boldsymbol{x}$, using the same input training data $\{\boldsymbol{x}_i\}_1^N$ with different outputs $\{y_{i1}\}_1^N, \cdots, \{y_{iK}\}_1^N$.

Multiple outputs ($K > 1$) (2) do not fundamentally change the approximation problem. One could approach this in a straightforward way by simply treating the approximation of each separate target function $f_k(\boldsymbol{x})$

$(1 \le k \le K)$ as a different (unrelated) problem. With this strategy one would develop a separate approximation $\hat{f}_k(\boldsymbol{x})$ for each output using separate training sets $\{y_{i1}, \boldsymbol{x}_i\}_1^N, \cdots, \{y_{iK}, \boldsymbol{x}_i\}_1^N$, without regard to the commonality of their input variables $\boldsymbol{x}$, nor to the fact the same system gives rise to all of them. If the respective target functions $\{f_k(\boldsymbol{x})\}_1^K$ have very different properties in terms of their dependencies on the inputs $\boldsymbol{x}$ then this is the best strategy. In fact, one might even envision using different methods for approximating different targets in this case, if one's a priori knowledge concerning the respective target functions suggested that this might be appropriate.

One's priori knowledge might however indicate that all of the target functions should have a similar dependence on the input variables. This would dictate that the same (appropriate) method be used for approximating all of them. In addition, if the target functions were sufficiently similar, there may be gains to be made by limiting the dissimilarity of the resulting approximations $\{\hat{f}_k(\boldsymbol{x})\}_1^K$, perhaps by imposing a penalty for the degree of such dissimilarity. As with all such constraining penalties, bias (53) (56b) will tend to be increased and the variance (50) (51) will decrease. If there is sufficient similarity among the target functions, the increase in bias may be small enough so that the resulting decrease in variance gives rise to smaller mean-squared error (54) (56c). If not, mean-squared error will increase and the exercise will be counter productive. One might even envision associating a strength parameter λ with such a dissimilarity penalty and using (an additional level of) model selection to try to estimate its value. There has been however very little work in this area and the development of such approaches remains an open research topic.

Another motivation for attempting to connect or combine the approximations of different target functions, associated with the same inputs, is computational. If the method being employed is sufficiently computationally intensive (e.g. feed-forward neural networks or adaptive radial basis functions) there may not be sufficient computing resources available to separately approximate several target functions in a reasonable time. With most (nonlinear) function approximation methods the dominant part of the computation is concerned with minimizing the objective criterion (26) with respect to the nonlinear parameters $\{\gamma_m\}_1^M$ (63) associated with choosing each of the dictionary entries $\{b(\boldsymbol{x}|\gamma_m)\}_1^M$ (62). This suggests that considerable computation can be saved in the multiple output problem by sharing a single set of dictionary entries among all of the corresponding approximations,

$$\hat{f}_k(\boldsymbol{x}) = \sum_{m=1}^{M} \hat{a}_{km} b(\boldsymbol{x}|\hat{\gamma}_m) \qquad (91)$$

Here (91) each target function $f_k(\boldsymbol{x})$ is approximated by (different) linear combinations of the same set of dictionary entries. All of the (linear) expansion coefficient $\{\hat{a}_{km}\}_{m=1}^{M}{}_{,k=1}^{K}$ and the nonlinear parameters $\{\hat{\gamma}_m\}_1^M$ associated with the (common) set of dictionary entries are obtained by

$$(\hat{A},\hat{\Gamma}) = \underset{A,\Gamma}{\operatorname{argmin}} \sum_{k=1}^{K}\sum_{i=1}^{N}[y_{ki} - \sum_{m=1}^{M} a_{km} b(\boldsymbol{x}_i|\gamma_m)]^2 + \lambda \cdot \eta(A,\Gamma). \tag{92}$$

Here (92) matrix notation is used to represent the respective collections of parameters

$$A = [a_{km}],\ \Gamma = (\gamma_1, \cdots, \gamma_M). \tag{93}$$

This (91) (92) constrains all the approximations $\{\hat{f}_k(\boldsymbol{x})\}_1^K$ to lie in the same function subspace spanned by the (commonly) chosen dictionary functions. Implementations of projection pursuit (Friedman, 1985), feed-forward neural networks (Rumelhart, Hinton, and Williams, 1986), recursive partitioning (CART-Breiman, Friedman, Olshen, and Stone, 1984), and MARS (Hastie, Tibshirani, Buja, 1992) all use this approach (91–93) for multiple outputs. The value of the single (common) strength parameter λ is chosen by optimizing a common collective model selection criterion. For example, this analog for cross-validation (49) would be

$$\hat{\lambda} = \underset{\lambda}{\operatorname{argmin}} \sum_{k=1}^{K}\sum_{i=1}^{N}[y_{ki} - \hat{f}_{k\backslash i}(\boldsymbol{x}_i|\lambda)]^2, \tag{94}$$

Here (94), $\hat{f}_{k\backslash i}(\boldsymbol{x}|\lambda)$ is the solution to (91–93) for a given value of λ, with the ith training observation removed.

In addition to reducing computation, this approach to multiple outputs imposes a similarity constraint on the respective approximations (91); they are all expansions in the same set of dictionary entries and they are all regularized by the same value for the strength parameter $\hat{\lambda}$ (94). For example, if subset selection (29) were used, the value of $\hat{\lambda}$ would regulate the (same) number M of (identical) dictionary entries appearing in each approximation (91). If the respective target functions $\{f_k(\boldsymbol{x})\}_1^K$ happen to exhibit a great deal of common structure then this may be a virtue (as discussed above) by reducing the variance component (50) of the approximation mean-squared error (54) (56c), for each approximation (91). This is however by no means assured since the (compromise) value of λ chosen by (94) can be considerably larger that[1 n some (or all) of the separate strength parameters associated with completely separate (unrelated) approximations $\{\hat{f}_k(\boldsymbol{x})\}_1^K$.

The imposition of such a similarity constraint is also often used to (heuristically) motivate this strategy for multiple outputs, by arguing that it "takes advantage" of possible similarities among the target functions associated with the respective outputs. Although these motivations are plausible, this procedure has serious flaws that can cause considerable degradation of accuracy as compared to independently approximating each target function separately. First, (91) (92) is a "natural" generalization of the single output case (20) only in a very restrictive setting. Even when the respective errors $\boldsymbol{\varepsilon} = \{\varepsilon_1, \cdots, \varepsilon_K\}$ (2) are assumed to have a (joint) Gaussian distribution

$$\Pr[\varepsilon_1, \cdots, \varepsilon_K | \boldsymbol{x}] \sim e^{-\frac{1}{2}\boldsymbol{\varepsilon}^T \Sigma^{-1} \boldsymbol{\varepsilon}} \tag{95}$$

with $(K \times K)$ covariance matrix Σ, the multiple output generalization of the maximum a posteriori probability (MAP) criterion (23) (24) reduces to (92) (assuming (91)) only if Σ is a multiple of the identity matrix

$$\Sigma = \sigma^2 I_K. \tag{96}$$

This (96) requires all of the respective response errors ε_k (2) to have the same variance and to be completely uncorrelated with each other. This is not likely to be (even approximately) true in general. The correct multiple output generalization of the MAP procedure under these assumptions (91) (95) and Σ known is

$$(\hat{A}, \hat{\Gamma}) = \underset{A,\Gamma}{\operatorname{argmin}} \sum_{i=1}^{N} (\boldsymbol{y}_i - \hat{\boldsymbol{f}}(\boldsymbol{x}_i))^T \Sigma^{-1} (\boldsymbol{y}_i - \hat{\boldsymbol{f}}(\boldsymbol{x}_i)) + \lambda \cdot \eta(A, \Gamma) \tag{97}$$

where vector notation is used to represent the output variables and their corresponding approximations in the K-dimensional output space

$$\boldsymbol{y} = \{y_k\}_1^K \quad \text{and} \quad \hat{\boldsymbol{f}}(\boldsymbol{x}) = \{\hat{f}_k(\boldsymbol{x})\}_1^K \tag{98}$$

with $\hat{f}_k(\boldsymbol{x})$ given by (91). If Σ (95) is unknown (the usual case) it can be estimated by

$$\hat{\Sigma} = \frac{1}{N} \sum_{i=1}^{N} (\boldsymbol{y}_i - \hat{\boldsymbol{f}}(\boldsymbol{x}_i))\,(\boldsymbol{y}_i - \hat{\boldsymbol{f}}(\boldsymbol{x}_i))^T \tag{99}$$

and this estimate (99) substituted in (97). However this estimate (99) depends on the parameters (A, Γ) through (91) so that the process would have to be iterated. Starting with an initial guess for Σ (say $\Sigma = I_K$) the solution to (97) is found. The resulting estimates (91) are then used to re-estimate Σ (99) for the next iteration, and so on. This iterative procedure is equivalent (Bates and Watts, 1988) to solving

$$(\hat{A}, \hat{\Gamma}) = \underset{A,\Gamma}{\operatorname{argmin}} \log \; det \; \hat{\Sigma}(A, \Gamma) + \lambda \cdot \eta(A, \Gamma) \tag{100}$$

where $\hat{\Sigma}(A, \Gamma)$ is a function of the parameters through (91) (99). Using (99) (100) in place of (92) would overcome the limitation (96) and probably produce superior results in most cases. Of course this (99) (100) is a computationally much more complex criterion than (92). For example, all of the fast updating tricks used to speed up least-squares minimization (92) do not work for (99) (100). Simple numerical optimization methods such as steepest descent ("back propagation") can still be applied (as is routine with feed-forward neural networks using (92)) with this criterion (99) (100), but there may be more of a problem with local (suboptimal) minima owing to its increased complexity.

Examination of (97) (99) elucidates the major problem associated with using the usual approach (92) to multiple outputs. By the inclusion of $\hat{\Sigma}^{-1}$ (99) the proper criterion (97) gives more relative weight to those target functions that can be most accurately approximated by the chosen method. This may be due to a smaller associated (irreducible error) ε_k (2) or to the fact that the method is better matched to those particular target functions (57) (58). This relative weighting gives each target function its proper influence in determining the parameters associated with the (common) dictionary entries. Using (92), by contrast, allows those targets that are difficult to approximate to overly influence (and perhaps dominate) entry (parameter) selection. This can (and often does) cause severe degradation in (relative) approximation accuracy for those outputs for which high accuracy is possible, in exchange for modest (relative) gain for those that cannot be reasonably approximated under any circumstance. This effect is aggravated further by the use of an (unweighted) model selection criterion, such as (94), to estimate the common strength parameter value $\hat{\lambda}$. Here again the poorly approximated target functions will dominate the model selection giving rise to possibly highly suboptimal λ-values for those target functions that could have been accurately approximated separately.

If one had a priori knowledge of which target functions are the ones most likely to be accurately approximated, the criterion (92) could be modified so as to give more influence to the corresponding outputs. This knowledge could be incorporated into a conjecture for an appropriate matrix Σ (97). For example, setting it to the diagonal matrix

$$\Sigma = diag(\sigma_1^2, \cdots, \sigma_K^2)$$

would assign a relative influence (weight) of $1/\sigma_k^2$ to each corresponding output y_k in determining the common set of dictionary entries (91). The model selection criterion (94) could be similarly weighted to emphasize the importance of the outputs in estimating the value $\hat{\lambda}$ of the (common) strength parameter. However, such a priori knowledge is seldom available so that (92) (94) is usually the default choice.

Even if the proper criterion (100) is utilized, and the model selection criterion (94) is appropriately modified, one still has the restrictions of a common set of dictionary entries (91), and a common strength parameter value λ, associated with this multiple output strategy. It is easy to imagine a great many situations where the target functions $\{f_k(\boldsymbol{x})\}_1^K$ (2) are sufficiently different so that these restrictions impede performance, perhaps on all of them, compared to separate independent approximations.

Although the multiple output strategy characterized by (91) (92) (94) is the one most commonly advocated, the above discussion indicates that it should be used with caution. If sufficient computing resources are available a more robust strategy is to treat the approximation of each target function $f_k(\mathbf{x})$, associated with each output y_k (2), as a separate independent problem. Only when all the respective target functions $f_k(\mathbf{x})$, and the corresponding noise ε_k (2), have highly similar structure will the collective strategy (91) (92) (94) produce superior results. The degree of improvement in such favorable settings however is not likely to be sufficient to overcome the risk associated with the (possibly) severe loss in accuracy incurred in settings unfavorable to this approach. Alternative methods for dealing with multiple outputs are currently under investigation (Breiman and Friedman, 1994). These can take advantage of target function similarity (irrespective of the noise structure) to improve accuracy when such similarity exists, but do not sacrifice performance (compared to separate independent approximations) when it does not.

6 Classification (categorical outputs)

As noted in Section 1.1, situations in which the output variable takes on unorderable categorical values constitute an important (often occurring) class of problems. These types of problems dominate in the fields of engineering, pattern recognition, and machine learning. The categorical output value can be viewed as a label that classifies an object (observation) i, characterized by input variable values $\mathbf{x}_i$, to one of K groups. Each group is identified by one of the K (categorical) values y can assume

$$y \in \{a_1, \cdots, a_K\}. \tag{101}$$

Labeling these groups as $G_1, \cdots, G_K$ we can define classification group (class) membership as

$$y_i = a_k \Rightarrow i \in G_k. \tag{102}$$

Since we assume (define) that an output y_i must take on one (and only one) of its categorical values (101) for each observation, the assignment rule (102) implies that object i must belong to one (and only one) of the groups (classes) in $\{G_k\}_1^K$. The classification problem can thus be viewed as deriving a procedure (rule) for assigning each observation to its correct group or class. Supervised learning in this setting consists of using a training sample (7) whose correct classifications $\{y_i = a_k\}_1^N$ (101) are known, to obtain a good classification (prediction) rule $r(\mathbf{x})$ for assigning future observations (of unknown class) to their correct groups (102), given only their input values $\mathbf{x}$.

In order to derive a good classification rule degree-of-goodness (accuracy) must be defined. Since the output variable is categorically valued, error (lack-of-accuracy) measures like (8a), (8b), or (10) have no meaning, since (continuous) distances (differences) do not exist between categorical values; two categorical values are either equal, or they are not equal. A natural measure of error would therefore be the fraction of times that the prediction rule assigns (future) objects to an incorrect group

$$\Delta[r(\mathbf{x})] = \frac{1}{N_T}\sum_{i=1}^{N_T} I(r(\mathbf{x}_i) \neq y_i). \tag{103}$$

Here (103), $\{y_i, \mathbf{x}_i\}_1^{N_T}$ are a (test) sample of observations not used (in any way) in the training of $r(\mathbf{x})$.

Just as with real valued outputs (4), a given set of measured input variable values $\mathbf{x}$ may not uniquely specify a categorical output value. There may be other unobserved inputs $\{z_j\}$ (1) whose values affect the output (class membership), but are not in any way controlled. Therefore specifying a particular set of input values $\mathbf{x}$ determines a probability distribution of the output values

$$\{\Pr(y = a_k|\mathbf{x})\}_1^K \tag{104}$$

induced by the varying values of the unobserved inputs $\{z_j\}$ (1). In the case of a real valued output this effect is accounted for by the statistical model (4). Introducing the probability distribution (104) for the value of y, at each set of input values $\mathbf{x}$, represents the corresponding statistical model for a categorical output. As with all probability distributions, one has

$$\sum_{k=1}^{K} \Pr(y = a_k|\mathbf{x}) = 1 \tag{105}$$

for all values of $\mathbf{x}$. At each $\mathbf{x}$, the (categorical) output takes on a random value according to a multinomial distribution with respective probabilities given by (104).

At each $\mathbf{x}$-value, the derived decision rule $r(\mathbf{x})$ assigns a unique predicted (categorical) value. The probability that this prediction will be incorrect is the sum of the probabilities (104) for those categorical values (101) not equal to the predicted value

$$\Pr[y \neq r(\mathbf{x})] = \sum_{k=1}^{K} I(r(\mathbf{x}) \neq a_k)\Pr(y = a_k|\mathbf{x}) \tag{106}$$

so that the population ($N_T \to \infty$) analog of (103) is

$$\Delta[r(\mathbf{x})] = \int [\sum_{k=1}^{K} I(r(\mathbf{x}) \neq a_k)\Pr(y = a_k|\mathbf{x})]p(\mathbf{x})d\mathbf{x}. \tag{107}$$

Thus (107) is the analogous error measure, for categorical outputs, to (9) for real valued outputs.

The error measures (103) (107) assume that all misclassification errors $y \neq r(\boldsymbol{x})$ are equally costly, irregardless of the values of y and $r(\boldsymbol{x})$. This is not always the case. For example, in medical diagnosis the cost (or "loss") associated with misclassifying someone as being well, when they are actually severely ill, is generally greater than the converse misclassification. This can be accommodated by specificing a "loss"

$$L(r(\boldsymbol{x}), y) \tag{108}$$

associated with assigning the (categorical) value $r(\boldsymbol{x})$ when the true value is actually y. By convention the loss (108) associated with a correct assignment is defined to be zero, and to be positive for incorrect assignment. The expected (average) loss of assigning $r(\boldsymbol{x})$ to an object with input values $\boldsymbol{x}$ is

$$R(\boldsymbol{x}) = \sum_{k=1}^{K} L(r(\boldsymbol{x}), a_k) \Pr(y = a_k|\boldsymbol{x}). \tag{109}$$

Thus (109) is called the misclassification "risk" at $\boldsymbol{x}$, and this quantity averaged over all $\boldsymbol{x}$-values

$$R = \int [\sum_{k=1}^{K} L(r(\boldsymbol{x}), a_k) \Pr(y = a_k|\boldsymbol{x})] p(\boldsymbol{x}) d\boldsymbol{x} \tag{110}$$

becomes the (generalized) lack-of-accuracy measure analogous to (107). If all assignment errors are deemed to be equally costly then this is specified by

$$L(r(\boldsymbol{x}), a_k) = I(r(\boldsymbol{x}) \neq a_k) \tag{111}$$

and (110) reduces to (107), which simply counts the proportion of incorrect assignments. In any case the loss matrix (108) is dictated by the nature of the problem and specified by the user.

If the respective conditional probabilities (104) were know for all values of $\boldsymbol{x}$ then (109) (110) is minimized by the classification assignment rule

$$r^*(\boldsymbol{x}) = \underset{r}{\operatorname{argmin}} \sum_{k=1}^{K} L(r, a_k) \Pr(y = a_k|\boldsymbol{x}). \tag{112}$$

This (112) is known as the "Bayes" rule and it achieves the lowest value of misclassification risk (109) (110) among all possible assignment rules for the particular problem at hand. The corresponding minimizing (average) risk R^* is obtained by substituting $r^*(\boldsymbol{x})$ (112) for $r(\boldsymbol{x})$ in (110), and is called the "Bayes risk" for that problem. The Bayes risk characterizes the irreducible error associated with the problem in analogy with the irreducible mean-squared prediction error (9)

$$\int \sigma^2(\boldsymbol{x}) p(\boldsymbol{x}) d\boldsymbol{x}.$$

for real valued outputs.

Knowing the true class probabilities (104) (for all $\boldsymbol{x}$) is analogous to knowing the true target function $f(\boldsymbol{x})$ (4) in the real valued output case. In practice they are never known and it is the goal of supervised learning to obtain approximations (estimates) for them using the training data (7). One way to do this is to use the "dummy variable" technique described in Section 1.1. the K-valued categorical output variable y is mapped to K real valued variables $\{d_1, \cdots, d_k\}$ each one of which assumes only two values ($d_k = 0$ or $d_k = 1$) through the definition

$$d_k = \begin{cases} 1 & \text{if } y = a_k \\ 0 & \text{otherwise.} \end{cases} \tag{113}$$

For a given categorical value $y = a_k$ all of the dummy variables but one (d_k) have the value zero, and

$$\sum_{k=1}^{k} d_k = 1. \tag{114}$$

The collective values $\{d_k\}_1^K$ (113) clearly contain the same information as the single (categorical value) of y (101), and predicting their values for given input $\boldsymbol{x}$ is equivalent to predicting the value of y. The linear degeneracy (114) implies that it is sufficient to predict only $K-1$ of them. The value of introducing the (real-valued) dummy variables (113) stems from the relation

$$\Pr(y = a_k|\boldsymbol{x}) = \Pr(d_k = 1|\boldsymbol{x}) = E(d_k|\boldsymbol{x}). \tag{115}$$

The right most quantity in (115) has the defining form (6) of a real-valued target function $f_k(\boldsymbol{x})$ based on a real valued output d_k,

$$\{f_k(\boldsymbol{x}) = E(d_k|\boldsymbol{x})\}_1^K. \tag{116}$$

If these target functions (116) were known they could be used (115) to derive the optimal (Bayes) prediction rule (112). Since they are unknown, supervised learning is used to obtain approximations

$$\{\hat{f}_k(\boldsymbol{x})\}_1^K \tag{117}$$

for them using training data (7) (113). Thus, the supervised learning problem for a (single) K-valued categorical output y (101) is equivalent to the corresponding problem of (multiple) function approximation (116) (117) involving K real-valued outputs (113). The training data for obtaining each approximation (117) is

$$\{d_{ki}, \boldsymbol{x}_i\}_1^N, \quad k = 1, K, \tag{118}$$

with d_{ki} derived from (categorical) y_i (7) through (113).

The dummy variable trick converts a classification problem (102) to that of multiple output function approximation (Section 5.0). All of the function approximation methods discussed herein (and elsewhere) are eligible candidates to be used for this purpose. The one that is most appropriate for any given problem will depend (as always) on the (properties of) the (true) target functions (116) encountered.

The multiple output problem associated with classification (116) (117) has special characteristics that are not usually present in the general problem of multiple outputs (Section 5.0). These stem from the constraints

$$\{0 \leq f_k(\boldsymbol{x}) \leq 1\}_1^K \text{ and } \sum_{k=1}^{K} f_k(\boldsymbol{x}) = 1 \tag{119}$$

on the true target functions (116). It is reasonable to expect that imposing the corresponding constraints (119) on the resulting approximations (117) should improve accuracy since information (outside the training data) is being incorporated, that is known to be true from the nature of the problem. Some function approximation methods (117) when used in the classification context (116) automatically produce estimates (117) that satisfy (119). An example of this is recursive partitioning, using a common set of dictionary entries (regions) for each (dummy) output (113) (116). Most methods however do not produce approximations (117) that satisfy these constraints (119) when applied in this context.

The second constraint in (119) can be met by replacing each derived approximation by

$$\hat{h}_k(\boldsymbol{x}) = \hat{f}_k(\boldsymbol{x}) / \sum_{l=1}^{K} \hat{f}_l(\boldsymbol{x}) \tag{120}$$

where $\{\hat{f}_k(\boldsymbol{x})\}_1^K$ are the (unconstrained) approximations produced by the chosen method. The first constraint in (119) is more difficult to enforce. One proposal (Denker and LeCun, 1991) is to make the replacement

$$h_k(\boldsymbol{x}) = \frac{e^{g_k(\boldsymbol{x})}}{\sum_{l=1}^{K} e^{g_l(\boldsymbol{x})}} \tag{121}$$

during training (20). That is,

$$\{\hat{g}_k(\boldsymbol{x})\}_1^K = \underset{\{g_k(\boldsymbol{x})\}_1^K}{\operatorname{argmin}} \sum_{k=1}^{K} \sum_{i=1}^{N} [d_{ki} - \frac{e^{g_k(\boldsymbol{x})}}{\sum_{l=1}^{K} e^{g_l(\boldsymbol{x})}}]^2 + \lambda \cdot \varphi(\{g_k(\boldsymbol{x})\}_1^K), \tag{122}$$

$$\{\hat{f}_k(\boldsymbol{x}) = e^{\hat{g}_k(\boldsymbol{x})} / \sum_{l=1}^{K} e^{\hat{g}_l(\boldsymbol{x})}\}_1^K. \tag{123}$$

The penalty in (122) is dictated by the function approximation method used and specifies the form of each $\hat{g}_k(\mathbf{x})$, that is the particular set of dictionary entries (60) (62). This approach (122) (123) is called the "softmax" method. It (usually) requires the use of a common basis function set (91), with common regularization (94). Also fast least-squares optimization tricks used by some of the function approximation methods are not valid for (122), so that relatively slow optimization methods (such as steepest-descent) must be used. Even when this is done the minimization of (122) is often more difficult than its function approximation analog (20).

Requiring the constraints (119) on the derived approximations (117) is generally not necessary and in fact can be counter productive if their enforcement (say by softmax (122)) leads to implementation difficulties. First, conforming to these constraints (119) is neither a necessary nor sufficient condition for accuracy. A set of approximations (117) that violate them may in fact be more accurate than another set that obeys them. Second, the goal of the classification exercise is an accurate decision rule

$$\hat{r}(\mathbf{x}) = \underset{r}{\operatorname{argmin}} \sum_{k=1}^{K} L(r, a_k) \hat{f}_k(\mathbf{x}) \tag{124}$$

based on the approximators (117), and not necessarily the accurate approximation of the target functions (116) themselves (10). It is true that if the approximators are able to achieve perfect accuracy ($mse = 0$ (10)), then the resulting rule (124) will achieve the minimum (Bayes) risk (110) (112). This need not imply however that an imperfect set of approximations (117) ($mse > 0$ (10)) necessarily produce a more accurate decision rule (124) than an even less perfect set (greater mse (10)).

This lack of a direct (one-of-one) connection between approximation error (10) on the target functions (116) and misclassification risk

$$\hat{R} = \int \hat{r}(\mathbf{x}) p(\mathbf{x}) d\mathbf{x} \tag{125}$$

of the resulting decision rule (124) can be easily illustrated by considering the simple loss function (111). In this case the Bayes (minimum misclassification rate) rule (112) (115) (116) becomes

$$r^*(\mathbf{x}) = a_{k^*(\mathbf{x})}, \tag{126}$$

$$k^*(\mathbf{x}) = \underset{1 \le k \le K}{\operatorname{argmax}} f_k(\mathbf{x}),$$

where $a_{k^*(\mathbf{x})}$ is one of the categorical output values (101). The corresponding rule derived from the training data is

$$\hat{r}(\mathbf{x}) = a_{\hat{k}(\mathbf{x})}, \tag{127}$$

$$\hat{k}(\boldsymbol{x}) = \underset{1 \le k \le K}{\operatorname{argmax}} \hat{f}_k(\boldsymbol{x}).$$

Comparing (126) and (127) one sees that the only requirement for obtaining the optimal decision at $\boldsymbol{x}$ is that the approximation, corresponding to the target function (116) with greatest value there, be the largest valued among all the respective approximations (117) at $\boldsymbol{x}$; that is $k^*(\boldsymbol{x}) = \hat{k}(\boldsymbol{x})$. The actual values of all of the approximations (117) could be very far from their respective targets (116), and need not even have the same ordering. As long as the right one has the largest (approximated) value, the optimal decision will be made. Although illustrated here (126) (127) for the simple loss function (111), a similar effect clearly obtains for more general loss structures (108).

The fact that function approximation accuracy (10) does not necessarily directly translate into classification accuracy (125) (and conversely) implies that in any given situation the best method for approximating the target probabilities (115) (116) may not necessarily be the best one for use in constructing a decision rule (124). Sometimes the probabilities (115) (116) are themselves of direct interest and other times only a decision rule is required. Therefore, even in the same situation different methods may be appropriate for the two different goals. Also, certain methods that have generally limited success in function approximation (10) can be quite effective when used in the classification context solely to construct a decision rule (124). An example of this is tree-structured recursive partitioning methods (Section 4.3) and nearest neighbor methods (Duda and Hart, 1973) not discussed here.

Owing to the discontinuous piecewise-constant nature of their approximations, recursive partitioning is seldom competitive with other methods (in terms of accuracy) for function approximation. Even though it tends to provide inaccurate estimates of the target probabilities (115) (116), it generally has better success at estimating which one is the largest (127) at a given point $\boldsymbol{x}$ in the input space. Therefore, recursive partitioning methods tend to be more competitive when used for classification than in the function (or probability) approximation context, particularly when the simple loss structure (111) is used. The same tends to be true for nearest neighbor techniques.

The dummy variable approach (113) (115) (116) (117) (124) provides a connection between the classification problem (101) (102) and (real valued) function approximation. It thereby allows all of the methodology developed for function approximation to be brought to bear on the classification problem. With this dummy variable – function approximation approach, the construction of the decision rule (124) can be considered a "post-process" applied to the approximations (117) after they are obtained from the function approximation procedure that was used. Generally the procedure attempts to obtain accurate approximations using a criterion like (9) (10) to assess accuracy, without regard to the fact that the ultimate goal is classification accuracy of the resulting decision rule (124). Unfortunately, directly using misclassification risk (110) (124) as a criterion for (joint) function approximation is generally not feasible since unlike (20) it does not vary continuously as the approximations (117) change. As was noted above, the approximating functions (117) can change (dramatically) without effecting the decision rule (124) (127) (and thus misclassification risk) at all. This rules out the use of numerical optimization methods for training, requiring instead more costly combinatorial optimization techniques if misclassification risk were to be used directly as the criterion to be minimized.

Another way to try to improve the use of function approximation on classification problems is to implement more elaborate "post-processors" than simply directly inserting the approximations (117) into (124) to construct the decision rule. The idea is to regard the function approximation part of the combined procedure as a "pre-processor" for transforming the original input variables $\boldsymbol{x} = \{x_j\}_1^n$ to a new set

$$\boldsymbol{z} = \{z_k = \hat{f}_k(\boldsymbol{x})\}_1^K \tag{128}$$

(117) which are then used as inputs to a (traditional) classification procedure. Nearest neighbor classification (Lippmann, 1989) and linear discriminant analysis (Hastie, Tibshirani and Buja, 1992), and (Ripley, 1994), have been suggested for this latter classification on the transformed inputs $\boldsymbol{z}$ (128). An attractive feature of this approach is that the constraints (119) are irrelevant to the function approximation preprocess since they are automatically enforced by the post classification part of the combined procedure. The approximating functions (117) are simply regarded as new "features" (128) and the function approximation preprocess is viewed as an (automatic) feature selection mechanism for the (post) classifier employed.

To the extent that the approximations (117) accurately represent their corresponding targets (115) (116) they ought to provide a good set of features (128) for separating the individual classes (102). Using the true target functions (115) (116) for the transformations (128) would cause the n-dimensional input space to be mapped onto a $K-1$ dimensional simplex imbedded in the K-dimensional Euclidean space of the transformed variables (probabilities) $\boldsymbol{z}$. The K vertices of this simplex are points in the positive direction along each z_k-axis at unit distance from the origin. Each such vertex can be identified with one of the classes $y = a_k$ (102) since it corresponds to the point for which the probability for that class (115) (116) is one, and those for all the other classes $y \neq a_k$ are zero. The optimal "post-process" in this case (Bayes decision rule (126) with equal losses (111)) would be to assign each point $\boldsymbol{z}$ to the class associated with the vertex closest to it in Euclidean distance

$$k^*(\boldsymbol{z}) = \underset{1 \leq k \leq K}{\operatorname{argmin}} \sum_{l=1}^{K} [\delta(k,l) - z_l]^2 \tag{129}$$

with

$$\delta(k,l) = \begin{cases} 1 & \text{if } k = l \\ 0 & \text{otherwise.} \end{cases}$$

Therefore, if the approximations (117) provided perfectly accurate representations of their corresponding targets (115) (116) then (126) (129) represents the optimal post-processor. Any other post-processor would yield suboptimal performance to the extend that its resulting decision rule differed from (126).

In practice, however, the chosen function approximation method ("preprocess") will not provide perfect approximations to the true target probabilities (115) (116). It is therefore possible that a (suboptimal) post-processor, different from (126) (129), will yield superior performance when used in conjunction with these suboptimal function approximations. This will tend to be the case as the approximations tend towards lesser accuracy. Heuristic arguments and some empirical evidence (Hastie, Tibshirani, and Buja, 1992, and Ripley, 1993) indicate that this is sometimes (but not always) the case. The connections between (suboptimal) function approximators (preprocess), and various possible classification post-processors to be used in conjunction with them, is as yet not well understood. As usual, it will no doubt depend on the particular problem at hand, as characterized by the true target function probabilities (115) (116), as well as the particular function approximation method used.

Because accurate function approximations (117) are not (necessarily) required to produce accurate classification decision rules (124), there tends to be less difference (in terms of accuracy) among the various methods for classification than there is for (direct) function approximation. Nevertheless, substantial classification accuracy differences can (and sometimes do) exist between chosen methods in particular problems. As with the function approximation problem, method choice should reflect one's (a priori) knowledge concerning the (true) nature of the class probabilities (115) (116).

As is the case with function approximation, classification methods differ widely on the interpretive value of the decision rule they produce, in terms of the usable information provided concerning the relationships between the probability distributions of the respective classes in the input space. As might be expected, the relative merits of the respective classification methods follow those of their corresponding function approximation counterparts. Classification methods based on tree-structured recursive partitioning (Section 4.3) and tensor product splines (Section 4.4) tend to have more interpretive value than those based on projection pursuit (Section 4.1), and especially more than those based on feed-forward neural networks (Section 4.1), radial basis functions (Section 4.2) and nearest-neighbor methods (Duda and Hart, 1973).

Bibliography

Akaike, H. (1974). A new look at statistical model identification. *IEEE Trans. Auto. Control* **19** 716–723.

Barron, A. (1984) Predicted squared error: a criterion for automatic model selection. In *Self-Organizing Methods in Modeling*. S. Farrow, ed., Marcel Dekker, New York.

Bates, D. M. and Watts, D. G. (1988). *Nonlinear Regression Analysis and its Applications*. Wiley, New York, NY.

Bellman, R. E. (1961). *Adaptive Control Proceses*. Princeton University Press.

Breiman, L. (1991). The Π-method for estimating multivariate functions from noisy data. *Technometrics* **33** 125–160.

Breiman, L., Friedman, J. H., Olshen, R. A. and Stone, C. J. (1984). *Classification and Regression Trees*. Wadsworth, Belmont, CA.

Breiman L. and Friedman, J. H. (1994). A new approach to multiple outputs through stacking. Stanford University, Department of Statistics, Technical Report LCS114.

Breiman, L. and Spector, P. (1989). Submodel selection and evaluation in regression X random case. *Internat. Statist. Rev.* (to appear).

Craven, P. and Wahba, G. (1979). Smoothing noisy data with spline functions. Estimating the correct degree of smoothing by the method of generalized cross-validation. *Numer. Math.* **31** 317–403.

Denker, J. S. and LeCun, Y. (1991). Transforming neural-net output levels to probability distributions. In *Advances in Neural Information Processing Systems 3*. Lippmann, Moody, and Touretzky eds. Morgan Kaufman, San Mateo, CA.

Duda, R. O. and Hart, P. E. (1973). *Pattern Classification and Scene Analysis*. Wiley, New York, NY.

Efron, B. (1983). Estimating the error rate of a prediction rule. *J. Amer. Statist. Assoc.* **78** 316–333.

Frank, I. E. and Friedman, J. H. (1993). A statistical view of some chemometrics regression tools (with discussion). *Technometrics* **35** 109–148.

Friedman, J. H. (1985). Classification and multiple response regression through projection pursuit. Stanford University, Department of Statistics, Technical Report LCS012.

Friedman, J. H. (1991). Multivariate adaptive regression splines (with discussion). *Ann. Statist.* **19** 1–141.

Friedman, J. H. (1993). Estimating functions of mixed ordinal and categorical variables using adaptive splines. In: *New Directions in Statistical Data Analysis and Robustness*, Morgenthaler, Ronchetti, and Stahel, eds. Birkhauser

Friedman, J. H. and Stuetzle, W. (1981). Projection pursuit regression. *J. Amer. Statist. Assoc.* **76** 817–823.

Furnival, G. M. and Wilson, R. M. (1974). Regression by leaps and bounds. *Technometrics* **16** 499–512.

Gill, P. E., Murray, W. and Wright, M. H. (1981). *Practical Optimization*. Academic Press.

Girosi, F., Jones, M. and Poggio, T (1993). Priors, stabilizers and basis functions: from regularization to radial, tensor, and additive splines. Massachusetts Institute of Technology Artificial Intelligence Laboratory Technical Report A. I. 1430.

Hastie, T., Buja, A., and Tibshirani, R. (1992). Flexible discriminant analysis. *J. Amer. Statist. Assoc.* (to appear).

Holland, J. (1975). *Adaptation in Artificial and Neural Systems*. University of Michigan Press. Ann Arbor, MI.

Kolmogorov, A. N. (1957). On the representation of continuous functions of many variables by superposition of continuous functions of one variable and addition. *Dokl. Akad. Nauk. USSR* **114** 953–956 (In Russian).

Lippmann, R. (1989). Pattern classification using neural networks. *IEEE Communications Magazine* **11** 47–64.

Lorentz, G. G. (1986). *Approximation of Functions*. Chelsea, New York, NY.

Mallows, C. L. (1973). Some comments on C_p. *Technometrics* **15** 661–675.

Moody, J. E. (1992) . The *effective* number of parameters: an analysis of generalization and regularization in nonlinear learning systems. In *Advances in Neural Information Processing Systems 4*, Moody, Hanson, and Lippmann, eds., Morgan Kaufmann Publishers, San Mateo, CA.

Ripley, B. D. (1994). Neural networks and related methods for classification (with discussion). *J. Roy. Statist. Soc. B* **56** (to appear).

Rissanen, Y. (1983). A universal prior for integers and estimation by minimum description length. *Ann. Statist.* **6** 416–431.

Rumelhart, D., Hinton, G., and Williams, R. (1986). Learning internal representations by error propagation. In *Parallel Distributed Processing: Explorations in the Microstructure of Cognition*. Rumelhart, McClelland, eds. MIT Press, Cambridge, MA.

Schwartz, G. (1978). Estimating the dimension of a model. *Ann. Statist.* **6** 461–464.

Wahba, G. (1990). *Spline Models for Observational Data*. SIAM, Philadelphia.

Weigend, A. S., Huberman, B. A. and Rumelhart, D. (1991). Predicting the future: a connectionist approach. *Intl. J. Neural Syst.* **1** 193–209.

Nonparametric Regression and Classification
Part I—Nonparametric Regression

T. J. Hastie[1] and R. J. Tibshirani[2]

[1] Statistics and Data Analysis Research Department, AT&T Bell Laboratories
Room 2C-261, AT&T Bell Laboratories, 600 Mountain Avenue, Murray Hill, NJ 07974.
trevor@research.att.com

[2] Department of Preventive Medicine and Biostatistics and Department of Statistics, University of Toronto
Department of Preventive Medicine & Biostatistics, University of Toronto, Toronto, Canada
M5S 1A8. tibs@utstat.toronto.edu

Abstract. In classical statistics, regression means linear regression. Recently, more flexible regression tools have been developed, that exploit the dramatic increase in computing power and speed. In this paper we describe some of these developments. The main background reference is Hastie and Tibshirani (1990).

1 Introduction

One of the most popular and useful tools in data analysis is the linear regression model. In the simplest case, we have n measurements of a response (or dependent) variable Y and a single predictor (or independent) variable X. Our goal is to describe the dependence of the mean of Y as a function of X. For this purpose we assume that the mean of Y is a linear function of X,

$$\mathrm{E}(Y|X) = \alpha + X\beta. \tag{1}$$

The parameters α and β are usually estimated by least-squares, that is, by finding the values $\hat{\alpha}$ and $\hat{\beta}$ that minimize the residual sum of squares. If the dependence of the mean of Y on X is linear or almost linear, the linear regression model is very useful. It is simple to compute and provides a concise description of the data.

It is easy to envisage data for which the linear regression model is inappropriate. If the dependence of $\mathrm{E}(Y)$ on X is far from linear, we wouldn't want to summarize it with a straight line. We can generalize the straight line regression very simply by adding terms like X^2 to the model but often it is difficult to guess the most appropriate functional form just from looking at the data. The point of view that we take here is: *let the data show us the appropriate functional form*. That is the idea behind a *scatterplot smoother*. It tries to expose the functional dependence without imposing a rigid parametric assumption about that dependence.

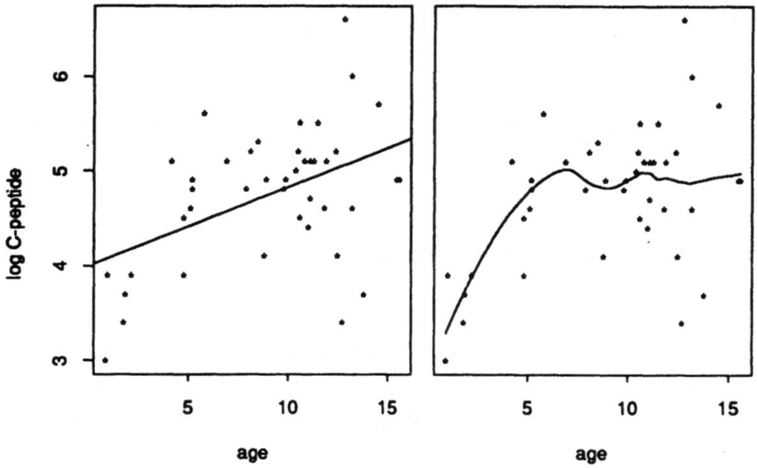

Fig. 1. *Left figure shows a scatterplot of* `log(C-peptide)` *versus* `age` *for the diabetes data, together with the least-squares regression line. The right figure shows the locally-weighted running mean smooth of* `log(C-peptide)`. *It summarizes the relationship with* `age`, *and can be regarded as a nonparametric estimate of the regression of* `log(C-peptide)` *on* `age`.

To make the ideas more concrete, let's look at some data. Figure 1 shows a plot of a response variable `log(C-peptide)` versus a predictor `age`, two variables from some diabetes data. It is quite clear from the graph that we wouldn't want to fit a straight line to these data. Instead let's apply a simple scatterplot smoother, the *locally-weighted running-mean*. Consider some fixed data point (X_0, Y_0). We find the 11 data points closest in X-value to (X_0, Y_0), and assign weights to them according to their distance in X from X_0. We compute the weighted average of the Y-values of these 11 data points to produce $\hat{Y}_0$, our estimate of the mean of Y at X_0. Doing this for all the data points produces the curve in Fig. 1. The curve is smooth and follows the trend of the data fairly well. The underlying assumption that we have made here is that the dependence of the mean of Y on X should not change much if X doesn't change much. This assumption is very often reasonable. We call the output of a scatterplot smoother a *scatterplot smooth* or simply a *smooth*.

Some basic scatterplot smoothers include the running mean, locally-weighted running-line, kernel and cubic-spline smoothers,

An important issue is how to choose the smoothing parameters (like the "11" above) for a given smoother, and how to make inferences about the fitted curve. One can use a fixed "degrees of freedom" approach, or use an adaptive method such as cross-validation.

We can think of a smooth as simply a description of the dependence of Y on X but if one is interested in building models, as we are here, a slightly more formal definition is in order. If we generalize the linear regression model (1) to

$$E(Y|X) = f(X)$$

where $f(X)$ is an arbitrary unspecified function, then a smooth may be defined as an estimate of $f(X)$.

2 Multiple predictors and additive models

More often than not, we have more than one predictor variable at our disposal. How we approach multi-predictor regression depends on whether our objective is inference or prediction. In the first case we seek a relatively simple model that allows us to describe and assess the role played by the predictors. In the second case, we are solely interested in predicting Y for a given set of inputs; simplicity of the model is only important if it makes our predictions more accurate.

In the diabetes example, our goal is inference. We will discuss this problem first and then discuss methods that are more aimed at the prediction problem. There are five predictors and 43 observations. Let's consider just two of them; `age` (X_1) and `base deficit` (X_2). The usual way to model the dependence of Y on both X_1 and X_2 is through the multiple linear regression model

$$E(Y|X_1, X_2) = \alpha + X_1\beta_1 + X_2\beta_2.$$

The three parameters α, β_1 and β_2 are usually estimated by least-squares.

The multiple linear regression model will be inappropriate if the regression surface $E(Y|X_1, X_2)$ is not well approximated by a plane. As in the single-predictor case we can add polynomial terms to the model but it will be difficult to guess which terms will be appropriate, and even more so if there are many predictors in the model.

There is a heuristic way to apply a scatterplot smoother to the multiple predictor case. The model that we envision is

$$E(Y|X_1, X_2) = f_1(X_1) + f_2(X_2) \tag{2}$$

Given an estimate $\hat{f}_1(X_1)$, an intuitive way to estimate $f_2(X_2)$ is to smooth the residual $Y - \hat{f}_1(X_1)$ on X_2. With this estimate $\hat{f}_2(X_2)$ we can get an improved estimate of $\hat{f}_1(X_1)$ by smoothing $Y - \hat{f}_2(X_2)$ on X_1. We continue this process until our estimates $f_1(X_1)$ and $f_2(X_2)$ are such that the smooth of $Y - \hat{f}_1(X_1)$ on X_2 is $\hat{f}_2(X_2)$ and the smooth of $Y - \hat{f}_2(X_2)$ on X_1 is $\hat{f}_1(X_1)$. Applying this algorithm to the diabetes data produces the curves in Fig. 2. The curves are far from linear (as a linear regression model would force on the data) and the shapes can help to discover important facts about the underlying phenomena. In this instance, the shape of the age estimate confirmed a prior belief of the investigators.

The model (2) is an example of an *additive model*. The iterative smoothing process described above is an example of *backfitting*, the main tool used for estimating additive models. The term *additive* means that the model is a sum of terms, but such

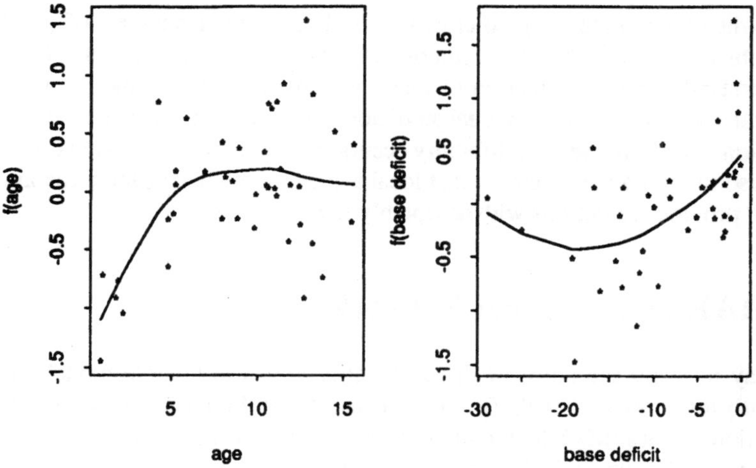

Fig. 2. *The fitted functions for* `age` *and* `base deficit` *in the additive model with response* `log(C-peptide)`. *The functions are fitted jointly by iteratively smoothing partial residuals, also known as backfitting.*

models can in fact be quite general. For example, some terms may be nonparametric, others linear, and others even a function of more than one predictor variable. Thus a product interaction like X_1X_2 may be incorporated into a model simply by defining a new predictor $X_3 = X_1X_2$ and including the term $X_3\beta_3$. More generally, one may allow terms like $f(X_1, X_2)$ where $f(\cdot, \cdot)$ is an unspecified function, estimated by a bivariate smoother.

In Hastie and Tibshirani (1990, chapter 9) we describe an adaptive backfitting procedure called "BRUTO". In this procedure, cubic smoothing splines are used to estimate each of the functions f_j, and the smoothing parameters are simultaneously estimated using a GCV (generalized cross-validation) criterion.

Additive models can also used with other kinds of response variables, for example, binary data for which the response takes on only two values such as survived or died. Such a model is an example of a *generalized additive model*. The idea is the same as in the usual regression setting: in this case, the *linear predictor* is replaced by an *additive predictor*. The estimation procedure for these models uses the backfitting idea in a procedure similar to the standard Fisher scoring method; more details are given in part II.

3 Surface smoothers

A more direct way of estimating the regression surface $E(Y|X_1, \ldots X_p)$ would be to use a multidimensional (or "surface") smoother. Most smoothers such as kernels, locally weighted lines and splines have multidimensional analogues and these are useful when the number of predictors is 2 or 3. For larger numbers of predictors, two problems occur with surface smoothers. The first problem is that it is difficult to understand a general function of many variables. For example, how can one assess the contribution of individual predictors? This is not a drawback if the goal is prediction. But then a second difficulty occurs: the "curse of dimensionality". Data are sparse in high dimensions, so that local averaging methods cannot remain local and still provide predictions with acceptably low variance.

4 MARS and Neural Networks

One way to avoid the curse of dimensionality is to use flexible models that are inherently lower dimensional. Two prime examples of this are Multivariate Adaptive Regression Splines (MARS) and multilayer perceptrons (neural networks). MARS, introduced by Friedman (1991). estimates a model of the form

$$f(\mathbf{x}) = \beta_0 + \sum_{m=1}^{M} \beta_m \prod_{k=1}^{K_m} b_{km}(x_{v(k,m)}) \tag{3}$$

Here $x_1, x_2, \ldots x_p$ are predictors, and $v(k, m)$ is the predictor used in the kth term of the mth product. The basis functions b_{km} are defined in pairs:

$$\begin{aligned} b_{km}(x) &= [x - t_{km}]_+ \\ b_{k,m+1}(x) &= [t_{km} - x]_+ \end{aligned} \tag{4}$$

for m an odd integer, where the knot value t_{km} is one of the unique values of $x_{v(k,m)}$. This model is a sum of products of piecewise linear basis functions of the form (4). The model is built up in a forward stepwise hierarchical manner, adding into the model at each stage a product of a model term times a term of the form $[x - t_{km}]_+$. MARS is a powerful predictive tool, because it automatically builds in product interactions where they are needed. The order of the products can also be restricted, allowing the possibility of interpreting the fitted model as well.

The single layer neural network model operates instead on linear combinations of the predictors:

$$f(\mathbf{x}) = \alpha + \sum_{j=1}^{M} f_j(\mathbf{a}_j^T \mathbf{x}) \tag{5}$$

Here the f_j are nonlinear functions, typically sigmoids $1/(1 + \exp(-x))$. The vectors $\mathbf{a}_j$ are called weights. The linear combinations $z_j = \mathbf{a}_j^T \mathbf{x}$ can be thought of as features of the inputs, so that the neural network is fitting an additive model to features z_j. By fitting the model to data ("learning"), we try to find the best set of features for prediction. The fitted neural networks is difficult to interpret, since each predictor enters into each term of the model. Some fitting methods try to increase interpretability by setting small weights to zero. A good general reference for neural networks is Hertz, Krogh & Palmer (1991). The single layer perceptron is also called the projection pursuit regression model in statistics: see Friedman & Stuetzle (1981).

5 Comparison of different approaches

There is not sufficient space here for a thorough comparison the different techniques mentioned above; this topic is open-ended and an important one for future research. We will touch however on some on the main points below:

- *prediction/classification (test set) performance.* In some situations prediction error is the "bottom line". The relative performance of additive models, MARS and neural networks is clearly situation-dependent. Each model assumes an underlying structure, and will work well if that structure is a good approximation in the given problem. Thus additive models and MARS will tend to work well when the structure is additive or has at most lower order product interactions, while neural networks will be appropriate when the structure is a function of a few linear combinations of the inputs.

- *computational requirements—both speed and memory.* Neural networks seem to require the most training time, but this has not been investigated thoroughly.

- *interpretability of results.* Additive models and MARS have an advantage here, due to the simple way in which the inputs appear in the model. Thus the contribution of individual inputs can be assessed relatively easily. Neural networks use linear combinations of inputs and hence each input can appear many times in the model; interpretation is therefore difficult.

- *ability to be trained online.* Neural networks can be trained as the observations are added sequentially, an essential feature for very large training sets. Online training has typically not been explored for the other procedures

- *amount of problem-specific fine-tuning required.* The adaptive backfitting and MARS procedures are fully automatic, while neural network procedures seem to require problem-specific choices such as number of hidden units, learning rates etc.

A number of other factors are potentially important. A thorough comparison of the models with respect to these factors would be valuable:

- *generalizability to different test conditions*

- *flexibility in incorporating prior knowledge about the domain*

- *ability to make effective use of correlated inputs such as the pixels in diagnostic image*

- *size of training set required*
- *ability to incorporate large numbers of input features*

6 Some recent statistical books

We conclude by giving a brief annotated bibliography of some recent statistical books that may be of interest to researchers in neural networks and artificial intelligence.

Statistical models in S (1991), by J. Chambers, J. and T.J. Hastie. (eds) Wadsworth, Belmont, CA.

An overview of the modelling software in the new S/Splus statistical languages. Includes a description of generalized linear models, generalized additive models, tree-based models and locally weighted regression methods.

An Introduction to the bootstrap (1993) by B. Efron. and R. Tibshirani. Chapman and Hall, London and New York.

Surveys the bootstrap, jackknife, cross-validation and other methods for assessing statistical accuracy.

Applied Non-parametric Regression (1990) by W. Härdle. Oxford University Press.

A thorough introduction to scatterplot smoothing, with a special emphasis on kernel methods.

Generalized additive models (1990) by T. Hastie and R. Tibshirani. Chapman and Hall, London and New York.

Gives an introduction to scatterplot smoothing, additive modelling and other flexible nonparametric regression methods. The main source for this article.

Discriminant analysis and statistical pattern recognition (1992) by G.J MacLachlan. Wiley, New York.

Gives an up-to-date survey of discriminant analysis and classification from a statistician's viewpoint.

Multivariate density estimation: theory, practice and visualization (1992) by David Scott. Wiley, New York. An overview of modern developments in density estimation in one and more dimensions.

Density Estimation for Statistics and Data Analysis(1986) by B.W. Silverman. Chapman and Hall, London.

A concise overview of density estimation techniques.

Spline Functions for Observational Data (1990), by G. Wahba. CBMS-NSF Regional Conference series, SIAM. Philadelphia.

A mathematical treatment of spline and regularization methods in statistics.

References

Friedman, J. (1991), 'Multivariate adaptive regression splines (with discussion)', *Annals of Statistics* **19**(1), 1–141.

Friedman, J. & Stuetzle, W. (1981), 'Projection pursuit regression', *Journal of the American Statistical Association* **76**, 817–823.

Hastie, T. & Tibshirani, R. (1990), *Generalized Additive Models*, Chapman and Hall.

Hertz, J., Krogh, A. & Palmer, R. (1991), *Introduction to the theory of neural computation*, Addison Wesley, Redwood City.

Nonparametric Regression and Classification Part II—Nonparametric Classification

T. J. Hastie[1] and R. J. Tibshirani[2]

[1] Statistics and Data Analysis Research Department, AT&T Bell Laboratories
Room 2C-261, AT&T Bell Laboratories, 600 Mountain Avenue, Murray Hill, NJ 07974.
trevor@research.att.com

[2] Department of Preventive Medicine and Biostatistics and Department of Statistics, University of Toronto
Department of Preventive Medicine & Biostatistics, University of Toronto, Toronto, Canada M5S 1A8. tibs@utstat.toronto.edu

Abstract. The traditional statistical approach to pattern recognition is a natural application of Bayesian decision theory. In order to classify well, we require either the posterior class probability distributions or the class densities. This distinction captures two branches of techniques: 1) those that model the class densities, such as kernel methods and classical linear discriminant analysis, and 2) those that model the posterior probabilities directly, such as classification trees, linear and nonparametric logistic regression.

In this paper we focus on an example from each class. The theme of the paper is modular generalization: taking classical linear methods and enriching them using nonparametric regression.

1 Bayes optimal classification rules

Suppose objects in a population can be classified into one of J groups or classes: $\mathcal{G} = \{1, 2, \ldots, J\}$, with $G \in \mathcal{G}$ denoting this class membership. In addition objects are characterized by a vector of measurements or features $X \in \mathcal{X}$. Suppose only X is available and we wish to know G. A classifier is a decision rule $d(X) : \mathcal{X} \mapsto \mathcal{G}$ that assigns a class label to an object with feature X. The goal of statistical pattern recognition is to produce a good rule of this kind, based on a sample of training examples (x_i, g_i), $i = 1, \ldots, n$ from the population.

Examples come from all branches of science, technology and medicine, and in many regards this is the most important statistical problem around.

- *Medical Diagnosis*. Patients with suspicion of heart attack arrive at UCSD medical center. We want to identify high risk patients (those likely to survive less than 30 days) based on values of 19 variables (blood pressure, age,...) measured upon arrival of patient. We are given a sample of patients for which both the measurements and the diagnosis are known.

- *Handwritten character recognition.* We want to automatically read zip-codes from mail envelopes. Subproblem: given a 16×16 greyscale image of a handwritten digit, identify the digit.

- *Dynamic signature verification.* People sign their names at credit card facilities such as supermarkets, and the signature is recorded on a pressure sensitive pen pad. We wish to classify the signature as genuine or a forgery.

- *Satellite image analysis.* We have multi-spectral images of the earth surface. We wish to automatically segment the images, i.e. assign each pixel to a number of classes (forest, grassland, water, road, ...). We are give a number of images for which the "ground truth' is known.

Let $P(X, G) = P(G|X)P(X)$ denote the joint distribution of X and G in the population. With knowledge of P, can we produce the best possible rule $d(X)$? We need to settle on what we mean by best. Let $L(j, k)$ be the cost or loss associated with misclassifying a class-j object as class k. A common way to evaluate a rule d is via the expected loss or risk:

$$\begin{aligned} R(d) &= E_{X,G}L(G, d(X)) \\ &= E_{G|X}d(G, d(X)) \\ &= E_X \sum_{j=1}^{J} P(G = j|X)L(j, d(X)) \end{aligned} \tag{1}$$

To minimize (1), it is sufficient to minimize the conditional risk $E_{G|X}d(G, d(X))$ at each value X:

$$d(X) = \text{argmin}_k \sum_{j=1}^{J} P(G = j|X)L(j, k); \tag{2}$$

this is the *Bayes optimal* rule.

In general the loss function will depend on the application, but often the 0/1 loss function is natural. It charges one unit for a misclassification, else zero. In this case the risk is the probability of a misclassifications in the population, and the Bayes rule is

$$d(X) = \text{argmax}_j P(G = j|X), \tag{3}$$

in other words assign to the class with the largest posterior probability.

Whatever loss function we use, optimal classification requires knowledge of the posterior density $P(G|X)$. Since $P(G|X) = P(X|G)P(G)/P(X)$, we equivalently need to know the class specific density functions $P_i(X) = P(X|G = i)$ and the prior class probabilities $\pi_i = P(G = i)$. In this case (for 0/1 loss) the decision rule is

$$d(X) = \text{argmax}_j P_j(X)\pi_j. \tag{4}$$

Many statistical pattern recognition procedures can be characterized as belonging to one of the two branches:

- those that model the class densities $P_i(X)$ separately, such as kernel methods and classical linear discriminant analysis, and
- those that model the posterior probabilities $P(G|X)$ directly, such as classification trees, linear and nonparametric logistic regression.

Although the development in this section follows the Bayes decision theory paradigm, the context here is different from the often more controversial Bayesian approach to modelling. In the latter case a prior distribution is used to characterize the uncertainty in model parameters ϕ for some family of probability distributions P_ϕ. Here the class variable G plays the role of ϕ. For a thorough treatment of the material in this section see McLachlan (1992), Fukunaga (1990) and Duda & Hart (1973).

2 Logistic Regression

Here we outline an approach to modelling $P(G|X)$ directly using nonparametric regression as a building block. Initially we focus on the case where $J = 2$, and then discuss the multiple class case in less detail.

The classical linear logistic regression model has the form

$$\begin{aligned} \text{logit}P(G=1|X) &\stackrel{\text{def}}{=} \log\frac{P(G=1|X)}{P(G=2|X)} \\ &= \beta_0 + \beta^T X \end{aligned} \tag{5}$$

(McCullagh & Nelder 1989). The log transformation guarantees that $P(i|X)$ lie in $[0, 1]$ and sum to 1, and allows us to model the *linear predictor* $\eta(X) = \beta_0 + \beta^T X$ without constraint. This looks like we can model the probabilities by doing ordinary regression on the logistic scale; we will see that this is almost the case.

An obvious way to generalize (5) is to replace the linear predictor $\beta_0 + \beta^T X$ by a nonparametric version $\eta(X)$, such as

- an arbitrary regression surface (for low dimensional X), estimated using a surface smoother;
- a more structured high dimensional regression surface estimated using procedures such as Friedman's MARS;
- an even more structured nonparametric model such as an additive model: $\eta(X) = \sum_k f_k(X_k)$, where the subscripts k refer to the coordinates of X.

The first part of this two-part series of papers focuses on fitting nonparametric regression models—in particular additive models. We now show how these algorithms can be used directly to fit the non-parametric logistic regression model.

2.1 Fitting Logistic Regression Models

Maximum likelihood is the most popular method for estimating the linear logistic model. For the present problem the log-likelihood has the form

$$l(y,\beta) = \sum_{i=1}^{n}\{y_i \log p_i + (1-y_i)\log(1-p_i)\} \tag{6}$$

where y_i is a 0/1 coded version of g_i, and $p_i = P(Y = 1|x_i)$. This uses the fact that $P(G|X)$ is Bernoulli, which has to be the case for a two class problem with independent trials.

The log-likelihood is concave, with score equation,

$$\frac{\partial l}{\partial \beta} = \sum_{i=1}^{n} x_i(y_i - p_i) = 0, \tag{7}$$

nonlinear in the parameters β, and consequently one has to find the solution iteratively.

The Newton-Raphson iterative method can be expressed in an appealing form. Suppose the current estimates are $\hat{\beta}$, yielding estimated probabilities p_i. We form the linearized response $z_i = \hat{\beta}^T x^i + (y_i - p_i)/\{p_i(1-p_i)\}$ and weights $w_i = p_i(1-p_i)$. A new $\hat{\beta}$ is obtained by weighted linear regression of z_i onto the x^i with weights w_i. This is repeated till $\hat{\beta}$ converges.

A motivation for this procedure is as follows. Suppose that instead of observing y_i, we observed a proportion r_i based on a number of counts. Then we could simply apply the logit transform to the r_i, provided $r_i \in (0,1)$, and use linear regression (perhaps with weights). However, in the extreme case of only one count per observation, or when the observed proportions are one or zero, the logit transform is not defined. The quantity z_i represents the first-order Taylor's series approximation to logit(y_i) about the current estimate p_i. If $\hat{\beta}$ and hence p_i are fixed, the variance of z_i is $1/\{p_i(1-p_i)\}$, and hence the weights w_i.

This iterative regression algorithm lends itself ideally to the additive model or other nonparametric regression generalizations. We define $z_i = \alpha + \sum_{j=1}^{p} f_j(x_{ij}) + (y_i - p_i)/\{p_i(1-p_i)\}$, where the f_j are the current estimates for the additive model components and $p_i = \exp\{\alpha + \sum f_j(x_{ij})\}/[1 + \exp\{\alpha + \sum f_j(x_{ij})\}]$. Weights w_i are defined as before. New functions α and f_j are computed by fitting a weighted additive model to z_i. Of course, this additive model fitting procedure is iterative as well, so there is potentially a lot of computing to be done. Fortunately, the functions from the previous nonlinear step are good starting values for the next step. This procedure is called the *local-scoring* algorithm; see Hastie & Tibshirani (1990) for further details. The new functions from each local-scoring step are monitored, and the iterations are stopped when their relative change is negligible.

2.2 Example: Kyphosis in Children

Figure 1 shows a simple example of this procedure in operation on a small dataset. Depicted here are two predicted variables, *Start* and *Age*, believed to be important

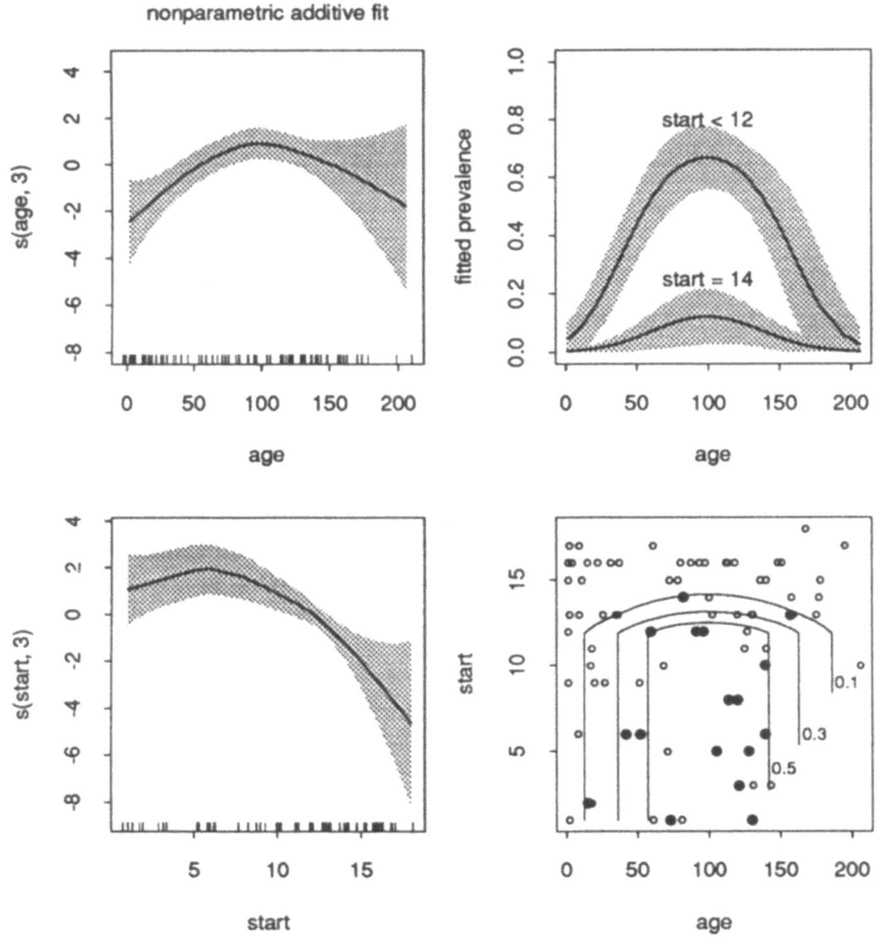

Fig. 1. The two functions on the left are those fitted for the additive logistic regression model for the *Kyphosis* data. The lower-right panel shows the data, with the class label indicated by a black dot. The upper-right panel depicts the fitted posterior probabilities as a function of the two predictors.

in predicting the success or failure of an operation to straighten the spine in young children. The bent spine condition is known as *Kyphosis*, and the black dots in the bottom right panel indicate the cases for which the operation was not successful. *Start* is the index of the vertebra at which the bending first begins, and *Age* is the age in months of the child at the operation. The two functions on the left are the estimated component functions of the additive logistic model

$$\text{logit}P(Kyphosis|Age, Start) = \beta_0 + f_{Age}(Age) + f_{Start}(Start) \tag{8}$$

Pointwise twice-standard-error shaded bands are included in the plots. The fitted posterior probabilities are indicated in the top-right plot, and shows that the risk of *Kyphosis* is much higher for lower values of *Start*. The contours in the lower right plot give an indication of the ability of this model to classify patients based on the two predictors.

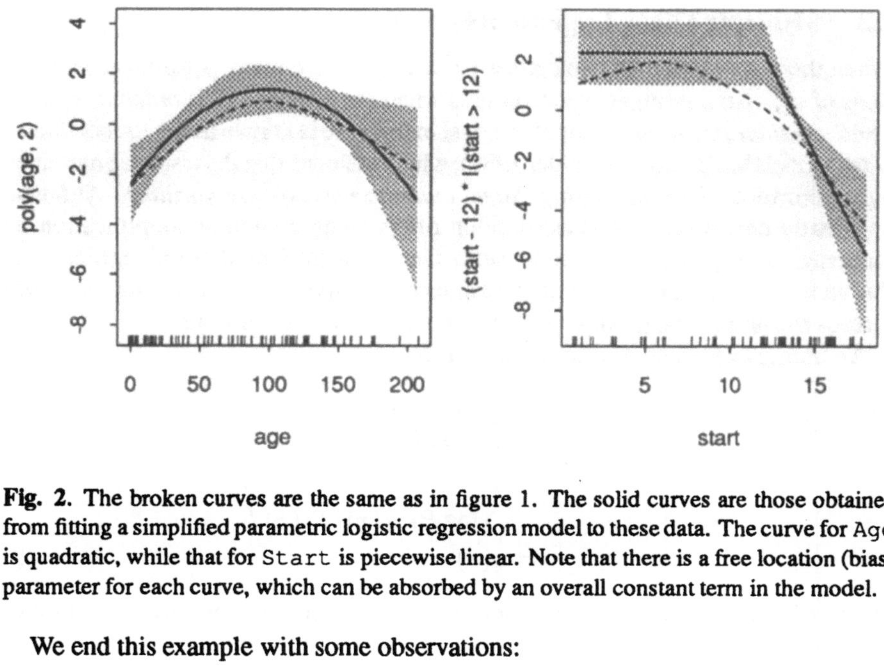

Fig. 2. The broken curves are the same as in figure 1. The solid curves are those obtained from fitting a simplified parametric logistic regression model to these data. The curve for `Age` is quadratic, while that for `Start` is piecewise linear. Note that there is a free location (bias) parameter for each curve, which can be absorbed by an overall constant term in the model.

We end this example with some observations:

- The sample size is small, and thus does not support a very rich model; the structure imposed by additivity can be helpful here.
- In cases such as this, the investigators are interested in the role of the predictors, and once again the additive structure is helpful.
- Although the lower right figure suggest that a threshold of about 0.3 on the posterior probabilities might produce a good decision boundary, these data were used in the fitting of the model, and hence we should suspect some bias.

- The horizontal label of the left lower plot is `s(start,3)`; this is the automatic label generated when this model is fitted and plotted in the S modelling environment. The "3" indicates that 3 *equivalent degrees of freedom* were used in producing this term—equivalent in complexity to a cubic polynomial.
- A typical strategy is to simplify the model even further after seeing the non-parametric fits. Figure 2 shows the parametric approximation that was our final fit to these data.

The fitted posterior probabilities can be used for classification as in (1). Often the goal is not classification; rather the model fitting is used to understand the relationship between the different predictors and the response, such as in medical risk-factor studies. In cases such as these, structure such as that imposed by an additive model, can be helpful. When classification is the goal and we have sufficient data, then the richer classes of nonparametric models are more attractive.

2.3 Multiple Class Logistic Regression

When there are more than two classes ($J > 2$) there are many possible generalizations of (5). An important special case is when the response G is *ordered*, such as *small, medium* and *large*. A popular model in this case is known as the *Proportional-Odds* model (McCullagh & Nelder 1989), which assumes that the response measures a discretization of an *underlying, latent quantitative response variable*. Although apparently complicated, this assumption offers some structural simplification by reducing the response to one dimension. One essentially models the regression of this underlying variable, based on the grouped response. Hastie & Tibshirani (1990) discuss the proportional-odds model and nonparametric extensions.

An unrestricted generalization has the form

$$\begin{aligned} \text{Logit}P(x) &= \begin{pmatrix} \log P_1(x)/P_J(x) \\ \log P_2(x)/P_J(x) \\ \vdots \\ \log P_{J-1}(x)/P_J(x) \end{pmatrix} \\ &= \eta(x) \end{aligned} \tag{9}$$

where η is a $J-1$ component vector of functions. Inversely, the class probabilities are given by

$$P_j(x) = \frac{\exp(\eta_j(x)}{\sum_{k=1}^{J}\exp(\eta_k(x))},$$

(where $\eta_J(x)$ is taken to be 1.) In the case of linear functions $\eta_j(x) = \beta_j^T x$, this is equivalent to a neural-network model with no hidden layer and probabilities formed via *Softmax*. More generally the functions $\eta_j(x)$ can be modelled nonparametrically; one could use nonparametric smooth functions, additive models, MARS type decompositions, or a neural network architecture. The authors are currently exploring additive and projection-pursuit models in this context.

The estimation proceeds in principle like in the two group logistic regression model. We use the multinomial log-likelihood:

$$l(y,\beta)=\sum_{i=1}^{n}\sum_{j=1}^{J} y_{ij}\log p_{ij} \tag{10}$$

where the elements y_{ij} of the $n \times J$ indicator response matrix Y code the responses g_i.

The simplicity stops here. Unlike in the two group case (with one regression function $\eta(x)$), the estimation of the components of $\eta_j(x)$ cannot be uncoupled. So in the linear case with p predictors of inputs in x, one ends up solving for a $(J-1)p$ vector of coefficients, with its associated square Hessian. This has tended to hold back modular generalizations to other nonparametric regression procedures, a step that was easy in the two group case.

3 Discriminant Analysis

One of the oldest statistical methods for classification is Fisher's linear discriminant function, which is based on modelling $P(X|G)$. Assume these class specific densities $P_j(X)$ are multivariate Gaussian with means μ_i and common covariance $\text{cov}_j(X)=\Sigma\,\forall j$. Taking logs, the rule (4) becomes

$$d(X)=\text{argmax}_j X^T\Sigma^{-1}\mu_j-\frac{1}{2}\mu_j^T\Sigma^{-1}\mu_j+\log\pi_j \tag{11}$$

Note that the decision boundaries between the different classes are linear in X. Inspection of (9) shows that this is true for the linear logistic regression model as well; however, the boundaries are estimated differently.

There is a simple way to state what is going on in (11), especially if the π_j are all the same. Using $d(X)$ amounts to assigning to that class j for which the *Mahalanobis distance* $(X-\mu_j)^T\Sigma^{-1}(X-\mu_j)$ is smallest. We first "sphere" the data via the linear transformation $Z\leftarrow\Sigma^{-\frac{1}{2}}X$, and then classify to the closest centroid in this space. Discriminant analysis can thus be viewed as a simple *prototype* method for classification.

In computing the closest centroid, we need only consider distances confined to the (at most) $J-1$ dimensional subspace spanned by them. This leads to the more useful version of Fisher's approach:

> *In the sphered space, find the $K<J-1$ dimensional subspace that best separates the centroids*

For small K we can produce plots of projected data that highlight the class separation — figure 3 gives some examples. The solution is characterized by the stationary points of eigenvalue problem:

$$\max_u u^T\Sigma_B u \text{ subject to } u^T\Sigma u=1 \tag{12}$$

where Σ_B is the between groups covariance matrix (covariance of the centroids themselves). The sequence of solutions u_k (orthogonal in the metric Σ) span the ordered sequence of subspaces for optimal separation.

How do we generalize this procedure via nonparametric regression? Breiman & Ihaka (1984) showed the way, followed by more recent developments by Hastie, Tibshirani & Buja (1992) and Ripley & Hjort (1994).

Consider the *optimal scoring* problem

$$\min_{\theta,\beta} \sum_{i=1}^{n} (\theta(g_i) - \beta^T x_i)^2 \tag{13}$$

with the normalization $\sum_i \theta(g_i)^2 = 1$. It can be shown that the optimal β is a scalar multiple of the optimal u in the discriminant problem (12). As in (12), there are a sequence of solutions, and they all corresponds in a similar way. Now an obvious generalization suggests itself—we replace the linear regression $\beta^T X$ in (13) by a nonparametric regression, such as MARS, an additive model, a neural-network model, etc.

Here follows a summary of the important aspects of this generalization.

1. For most versions of non-parametric regression, we can view the operation as 1) expanding the original predictors X into a carefully chosen set of basis functions, and 2) performing the usual discriminant analysis in this new space.

2. Often the dimension of the basis set is extremely high, and we compensate by using a *penalized* discriminant analysis. This is the case when penalization-based nonparametric regression procedures are used in the generalization.

3. These operations are equivalent in some cases (when penalization is not used) to applying the nonparametric regression procedures to the *dummy* response matrix, and the fitted values are then used as inputs to the discriminant analysis. This often results in a dramatic data reduction, and allows the regression procedure to be viewed as a *black box.*

4. One can show why in most cases this subsequent discriminant analysis gives improved classification results over using the regression fits directly via *soft-max.*

5. the resulting decision boundaries are linear in the expanded space, but typically nonlinear in the original space.

6. We can plot the data in the optimal subspaces as before (see figure 4), and often the choice of K can be treated as a regularizer—using $K < J - 1$ dimension for classification can lead to better prediction results (see table 1).

7. Using the gaussian densities, we can convert the distances in the expanded space back into posterior probability estimates, if these are required.

We end this section with an example taken from Hastie et al. (1992), who describe this approach to classification in more detail.

3.1 Example: Speech Recognition

This speech example is a popular benchmark for neural network algorithms, and consists of training and test data with 10 predictors and 11 classes. We obtained the data from the collection maintained by Scott Fahlman at Carnegie Mellon University. The data were contributed by Anthony Robinson (see Robinson, 1989). The 11 classes are different vowel sounds. Each word was uttered six times by each of fifteen speakers. Four male and four female speakers were used to train the networks, and the other four male and three female speakers were used for testing the performance.

Table 1. *vowel recognition data*

	Technique	Error rates	
		Training	Test
(1)	LDA	0.32	0.56
	Softmax	0.48	0.67
(2)	QDA	0.01	0.53
(3)	CART	0.05	0.56
(4)	CART (linear combination splits)	0.05	0.54
(5)	Single-layer Perceptron		0.67
(6)	Multi-layer Perceptron (88 hidden units)		0.49
(7)	Gaussian Node Network (528 hidden units)		0.45
(8)	Nearest Neighbor		0.44
(9)	FDA/BRUTO	0.06	0.44
	Best reduced dimension (=3)	0.12	0.44
	Softmax	0.11	0.50
(10)	FDA/MARS (degree = 1)	0.09	0.45
	Best reduced dimension (=2)	0.18	0.42
	Softmax	0.14	0.48
(11)	FDA/MARS (degree = 2)	0.02	0.42
	Best reduced dimension (=6)	0.13	0.39
	Softmax	0.10	0.50

The ten-dimensional feature vector represents a (complicated) digital transformation of the analog recorded speech signal for each spoken vowel.

The results of several classification procedures are shown in table 1. Lines (5)–(8) were taken from Robinson (1989); the first 3 performed the best among the neural network classifiers reported by Robinson. Lines (9)–(11) show the results of various FDA fits, which tend to dominate the performance of the procedures earlier in the table. The BRUTO and MARS postscripts to the FDA models indicate what regression method was used; BRUTO refers to an adaptive additive modelling procedure based on splines.

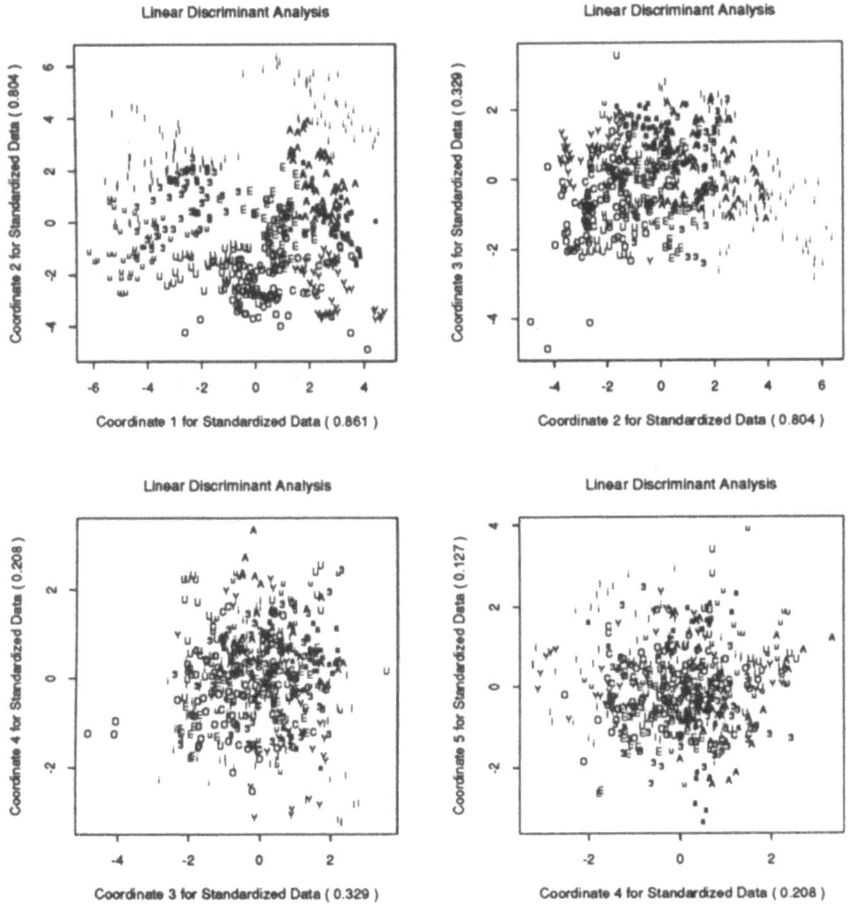

Fig. 3. *Some selected 2-dimensional projections of the LDA (Linear Discriminant Analysis) subspace computed for the vowel data; the eigenvalues for each coordinate are in parentheses, and indicate the strength of that variable in separating the groups. These plots show visually that most of the discrimination lies in the first few discriminant variables.*

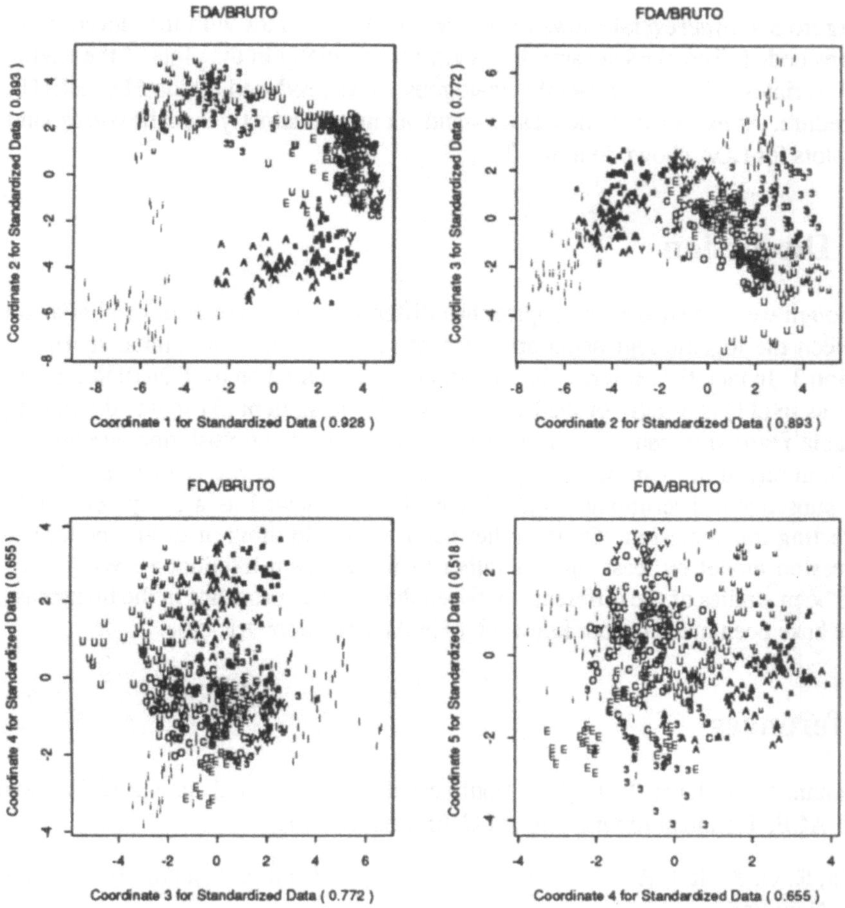

Fig. 4. *Some selected 2-dimensional projections of the discriminant variates derived from the FDA model fit to the vowel data; the eigenvalues for each coordinate are in parentheses, and indicate the strength of that variable.*

Figure 3 shows several views of the first 5 LDA variates with the eleven vowel classes coded. The class separation is evident, especially in the plots of the leading LDA variates. Figure 4 shows the analogous views produced by the FDA/BRUTO procedure. As expected, some classes stand out more distinctly than the corresponding plots for LDA shown in figure 3.

4 Discussion

Although we framed the two approaches differently, there are a lot of similarities between the logistic regression approach of section 2 and the optimal scoring of section 3. In fact, the posterior distribution $P(G|X)$ based on the Gaussian assumptions as in (11) is exactly of the linear logistic form. In item (3) above, the dummy variable regression can be seen as a naive estimate of the posterior probabilities (without regard to them being in $[0, 1]$), and using the squared error loss criterion. The subsequent discriminant analysis can then be viewed as a postprocessor for correcting this omission. On the other hand, we could think of fitting the logistic regression model by least squares rather than maximum-likelihood. While there have been studies of the difference between these two approaches in the linear case, none have been made (to our knowledge) in the nonparametric case.

References

Breiman, L. & Ihaka, R. (1984), Nonlinear discriminant analysis via scaling and ACE, Technical report, Univ. of California, Berkeley.

Duda, R. O. & Hart, P. E. (1973), *Pattern classification and scene analysis*, Wiley, New York.

Fukunaga, K. (1990), *Introduction to statistical pattern recognition*, Academic Press, Boston.

Hastie, T. & Tibshirani, R. (1990), *Generalized Additive Models*, Chapman and Hall.

Hastie, T., Tibshirani, R. & Buja, A. (1992), Flexible discriminant analysis, submitted.

McCullagh, P. & Nelder, J. A.. (1989), *Generalized Linear Models, Second Edition*, Chapman and Hall.

McLachlan, G. J. (1992), *Discriminant Analysis and Statistical Pattern Recognition*, Wiley, New York.

Ripley, B. D. & Hjort, N. (1994), Pattern recognition and neural networks—a statistical approach, in preparation—Cambridge University Press.

Robinson, A. (1989), Dynamic error propagation networks, Technical report, PhD. thesis, Elect. Eng., Cambridge University.

Neural Networks, Bayesian *a posteriori* Probabilities, and Pattern Classification*

Richard P. Lippmann

Room B-349, Lincoln Laboratory MIT, Lexington, MA 02173-9108 USA

Abstract. Researchers in the fields of neural networks, statistics, machine learning, and artificial intelligence have followed three basic approaches to developing new pattern classifiers. Probability Density Function (PDF) classifiers include Gaussian and Gaussian Mixture classifiers which estimate distributions or densities of input features separately for each class. Posterior probability classifiers include multilayer perceptron neural networks with sigmoid nonlinearities and radial basis function networks. These classifiers estimate minimum-error Bayesian *a posteriori* probabilities (hereafter referred to as posterior probabilities) simultaneously for all classes. Boundary forming classifiers include hard-limiting single-layer perceptrons, hypersphere classifiers, and nearest neighbor classifiers. These classifiers have binary indicator outputs which form decision regions that specify the class of any input pattern. Posterior probability and boundary-forming classifiers are trained using discriminant training. All training data is used simultaneously to estimate Bayesian posterior probabilities or minimize overall classification error rates. PDF classifiers are trained using maximum likelihood approaches which individually model class distributions without regard to overall classification performance. Analytic results are presented which demonstrate that many neural network classifiers can accurately estimate posterior probabilities and that these neural network classifiers can sometimes provide lower error rates than PDF classifiers using the same number of trainable parameters. Experiments also demonstrate how interpretation of network outputs as posterior probabilities makes it possible to estimate the confidence of a classification decision, compensate for differences in class prior probabilities between test and training data, and combine outputs of multiple classifiers over time for speech recognition.

Keywords. Neural Networks, Pattern Classification, Posterior Probabilities, Density Estimation, Prior Probabilities, Speech Recognition

---

*This work was sponsored by the Advanced Research Projects Agency. The views expressed are those of the authors and do not reflect the official policy or position of the U.S. Government

1. Introduction

The pace at which pattern classification algorithms have been successfully applied to new problems has increased dramatically over the past few years. Much of this recent activity has been motivated by developments in the field of artificial neural networks. Researchers in this field are enthusiastically attempting to match human performance in many applications. Their unique multi-disciplinary approach has led to new theoretical analyses and highly parallel algorithms with many simple processing elements which attempt to mimic the types of processing performed by biological nervous systems. Overviews of these algorithms are available in [5, 7]. They have been shown to be effective on real-world problems and are relatively simple to implement and apply.

One important characteristic of many neural network classifiers is that network outputs provide estimates of those posterior probabilities required in a minimum error Bayesian classifier [12]. When posterior probabilities are estimated accurately, classification error rate is minimized, outputs sum to one, and outputs can be treated as probabilities. Interpretation of network outputs as posterior probabilities makes it possible to estimate the confidence of a classification decision, compensate for differences in pattern class probabilities between test and training data, combine outputs of multiple classifiers over time for speech recognition, and implement simple rules for pattern rejection.

A second important characteristic of neural network classifiers is that they use discriminant training procedures. No underlying distributional form is assumed for class densities and the goal of training is either to directly estimate posterior probabilities or to directly minimize the overall error rate by forming decision regions. Discriminant training has the advantage of making weaker assumptions than most PDF approaches and of using cost functions that are directly related to the final classification error rate. It often permits the use of a smaller classifier with fewer parameters than are required by more conventional PDF approaches.

2. Three Approaches to Pattern Classification

The purpose of a pattern classifier is to assign every input pattern to one of a small number of discrete classes or groups. Figure 1 shows a block diagram of a simple pattern classification system. Inputs from sensors or processed information from computer data bases are fed into a preprocessor which extracts measurements or *features*. Features are tailored individually for each application. They simplify the classification task by eliminating irrelevant information and focusing only on those properties of the raw inputs which distinguish between classes. Input feature measurements $x_1, x_2, \ldots, x_D$ form a feature vector X with D elements in each vector. A feature vector or patterns is fed into a classifier which assigns the input to one of M prespecified classes denoted C_i using M outputs y_i.

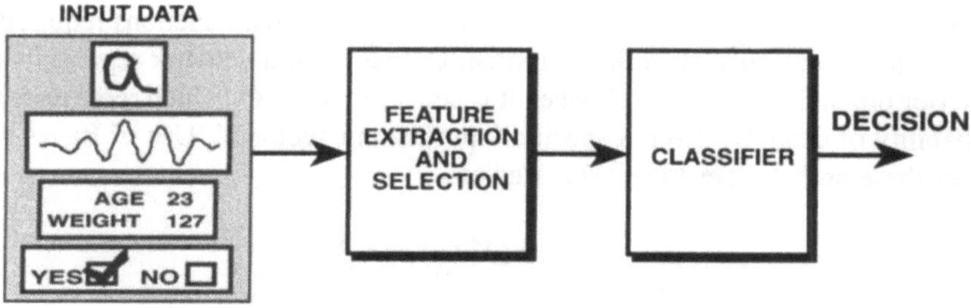

FIGURE 1. A simple pattern classification system with image, waveform, categorical, and binary inputs.

The input-to-output functions created by classifiers are called *discriminant functions*. When a classifier has continuous outputs, the decision rule is to select the class corresponding to the discriminant function or output with the highest value. All classifiers separate the space spanned by the input variables into *decision regions*. These correspond to regions in the input feature space where the classification decision remains constant as the input features change.

Three major approaches to developing pattern classifiers are to use *PDF*, *posterior probability*, or *boundary forming* strategies. These approaches differ in the statistical quantity their outputs model and in the procedures used for training as shown in Figure 2. PDF classifiers estimate class likelihoods, posterior probability classifiers estimate posterior probabilities, and boundary forming classifiers form decision regions. Figure 2 illustrates the shape of these functions for a simple problem with one input feature and two classes denoted A and B with Gaussian density functions. Likelihood functions formed by PDF classifiers on the left are Gaussian shaped. These functions represent the distributions of the input feature for the two classes. Posterior probabilities formed by many neural network classifiers have sigmoidal shapes. These functions vary from 0 to 1.0, sum to 1.0, and represent the probability of each class given a specific input feature vector. Binary indicator outputs of boundary forming classifiers separate the input into separate regions for classes A and B.

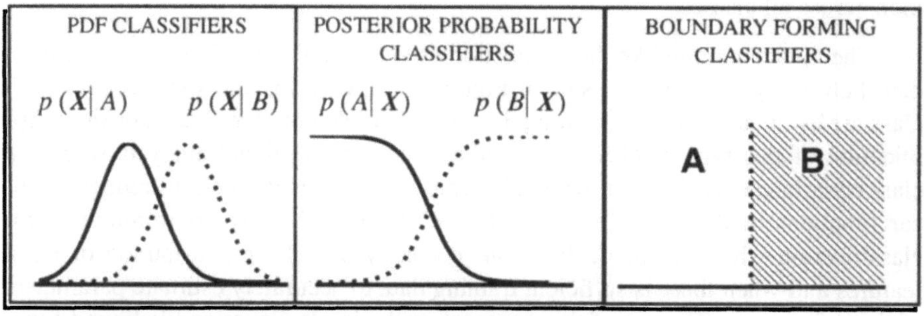

FIGURE 2. Discriminant functions formed by PDF, posterior probability, and boundary forming classifiers for a two-class problem with one input feature.

Bayesian *a posteriori* or posterior probabilities are those functions required to create a minimum-error Bayesian classifier. Output y_i of a network represents the posterior probability for class C_i when it is equal to $p(C_i|X)$ which represents the probability of class C_i given a specific input feature vector X. Use of Bayes rule allows these probabilities to be expressed as

$$p(C_i|X) = \frac{p(X|C_i)\,p(C_i)}{p(X)}. \tag{1}$$

In this equation, $p(X|C_i)$ is the likelihood or conditional probability of producing the input if the class is C_i, $p(C_i)$ is the *a priori* or prior class probability of class C_i, and $p(X)$ is the unconditional probability of the input. The prior class probability is the probability that a random selection of a new input pattern will come from a given class. These probabilities are normally obtained by measuring the relative frequency of occurrence of patterns from different classes. A classifier provides minimum classification error when the posterior probability is computed for each class and the classification decision is to respond with the class that produces the highest posterior probability.

Conventional PDF classifiers do not directly estimate posterior probability functions for each class. Instead, they estimate class likelihood functions and prior probabilities as shown in Figure 3. This Figure again assumes there are two classes denoted A and B. Training data for each class is plotted on the left in scatter diagrams which assume there are two input features. Training data for class A is used to estimate parameters of a prespecified likelihood function for class A. This trained likelihood function and the class prior probability for A is then used to form a discriminant function for class A equal to the numerator on the right side of Equation 1. The same procedure is followed separately for class B. Classification is performed by presenting a new pattern, computing the discriminant functions using the trained parameters, and selecting the class corresponding to the largest discriminant function. This comparison does not require the unconditional probability of the input (the denominator of the right side of Equation 1) because this term is common across all classes.

The most common likelihood function used for PDF classifiers is the Gaussian distribution shown in the left side of Figure 2 where means and variances for each class are estimated from the training data using simple non-iterative algorithms.Application of this type of classifier is called linear discriminant analysis when the class covariance matrices are identical because discriminant functions reduce to linear functions of the input features. This PDF approach provides minimum-error classification when likelihood functions correctly model the distribution of input features and when there is sufficient training data to accurately estimate parameters of these functions. The use of this approach with simple Gaussian likelihood functions provides good performance on many simple problems where input features do

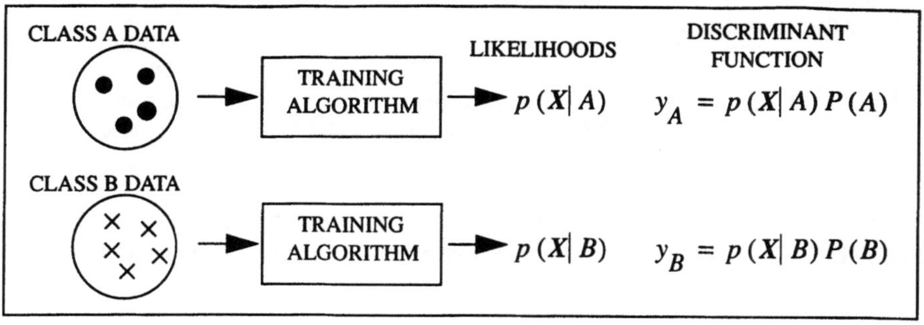

FIGURE 3. Training a PDF classifier using data for two classes denoted A and B.

have Gaussian distributions. Other approaches to classification can provide better performance, however, when training data is limited or when real-world feature distributions are not accurately modeled by Gaussian distributions.

Posterior probability classifiers include many neural network classifiers, polynomial classifiers, and many statistical classifiers which create nonlinear discriminant functions. These classifiers do not estimate posterior probabilities indirectly as in PDF classifiers. Instead, when the desired outputs are *1 of M* and a squared error or other cost function is used, posterior probabilities are estimated directly as shown in Figure 4. Training data for all classes is used simultaneously to produce output discriminant functions which approximate posterior probabilities. Neural network posterior probability classifiers are typically trained using a form of gradient descent called back-propagation which adjusts network parameters to minimize the squared-error between desired outputs of zero and one and actual network outputs [7]. After training is complete, classification is performed by presenting a new input and selecting the class corresponding to the highest output. This approach makes assumptions concerning the form of posterior probability functions. For example, a sigmoid network with linear input nodes feeding directly to sigmoid output nodes assumes a sigmoid posterior probability function. This type of function can be generated from Gaussian and other unimodal likelihood functions and leads to a type of analysis that is similar to logistic regression. When the functional form used by a

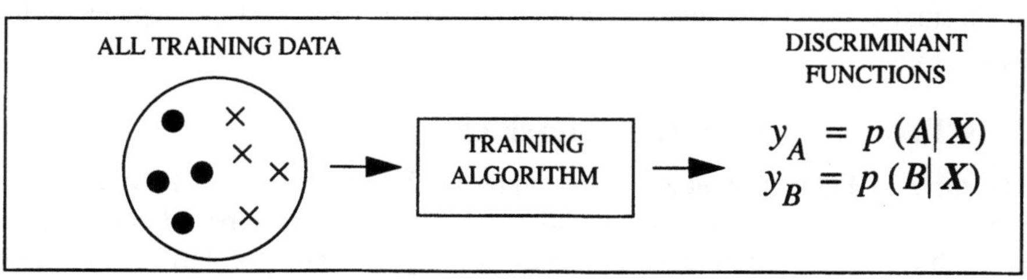

FIGURE 4. Training a posterior probability classifier using data for two classes denoted A and B.

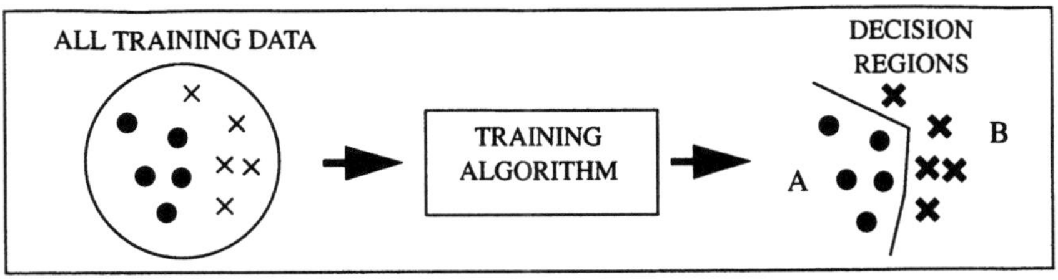

FIGURE 5. Training a boundary forming classifier using data for two classes denoted A and B.

neural network to estimate posterior probabilities is wrong, the training algorithm approximates the posterior probability function as closely as possible using the same cost function (e.g. squared error) used to train the network [12].

Boundary forming classifiers provide binary outputs which specify the class label to apply to each input as shown in Figure 5. Training involves examining all training data simultaneously and using a training algorithm which moves decision region boundaries in an attempt to minimize the number of classification errors. Boundary forming classifiers can form decision region boundaries using hard limiting nonlinearities as in the original single-layer perceptron [14] and in CART decision trees [1], using hyperspheres as in RCE networks [11], or using distances to specially selected exemplar training patterns as in nearest neighbor and Learning Vector Quantizer (LVQ) classifiers [6]. Although many boundary-forming classifiers can provide estimates of posterior probabilities, these estimates are much less accurate and variable than those formed by PDF or posterior probability classifiers. A new approach to training boundary forming classifiers called differential or classification figure of merit (CFM) training was recently developed by Hampshire [3, 4]. This approach can be used with many types of neural networks that are normally trained using back-propagation. Instead of minimizing the squared error across all outputs, differential training adjusts network parameters until the difference between the correct network output for each training pattern and the next highest output is positive for all training patterns. It stops training when no errors occur on the training data and can sometimes provide low error rates with networks that are much smaller than those required using more conventional back-propagation training.

3. A Taxonomy of Pattern Classifiers

The table in Figure 6 contains a taxonomy of the most common PDF, posterior probability, and boundary forming classifiers. The first three types of classifiers in this table produce continuous probabilistic outputs while the last two produce binary indicator outputs. The first row in Figure 6 represents conventional PDF classifiers which model distributions of pattern classes separately using assumed distributional forms. The bottom four rows in Figure 6 include both posterior probability and boundary forming classifiers created from the fields of neural networks,

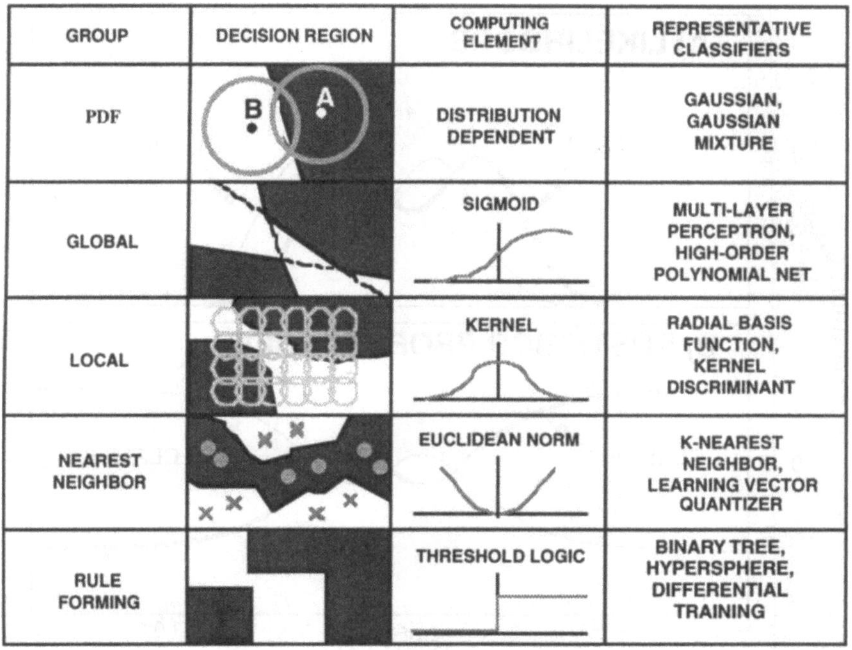

FIGURE 6. A pattern classification taxonomy.

statistics, and machine learning. *Global* posterior probability classifiers form output discriminant functions from internal computing elements or nodes that use sigmoid or polynomial functions which have "high" nonzero outputs over a large region of the input space. These classifiers include multilayer perceptron (MLP) networks trained with back-propagation, Boltzmann machines, and high-order polynomial networks. *Local* posterior probability classifiers form output discriminant functions from internal computing elements that use Gaussian or other functions which have "high" nonzero outputs over only a localized region of the input space. They include radial basis function (RBF) networks and kernel discriminant classifiers. Local and global posterior probability classifiers make no strong assumptions concerning underlying distributions. They can form complex decision regions with only one or two hidden layers of computing elements and are typically trained to minimize the mean-squared error between desired and actual discriminant function outputs.

The bottom two rows of Figure 6 contain boundary forming classifiers. *Nearest neighbor* classifiers perform classification based on the distance between a new unknown input and previously stored exemplars. Conventional k-nearest neighbor classifiers and LVQ neural network classifiers are examples. These types of classifiers train extremely rapidly but can require large amounts of computation time on a serial processor for classification and also large amounts of memory. *Rule forming* classifiers partition the input space into labeled regions using threshold-logic nodes

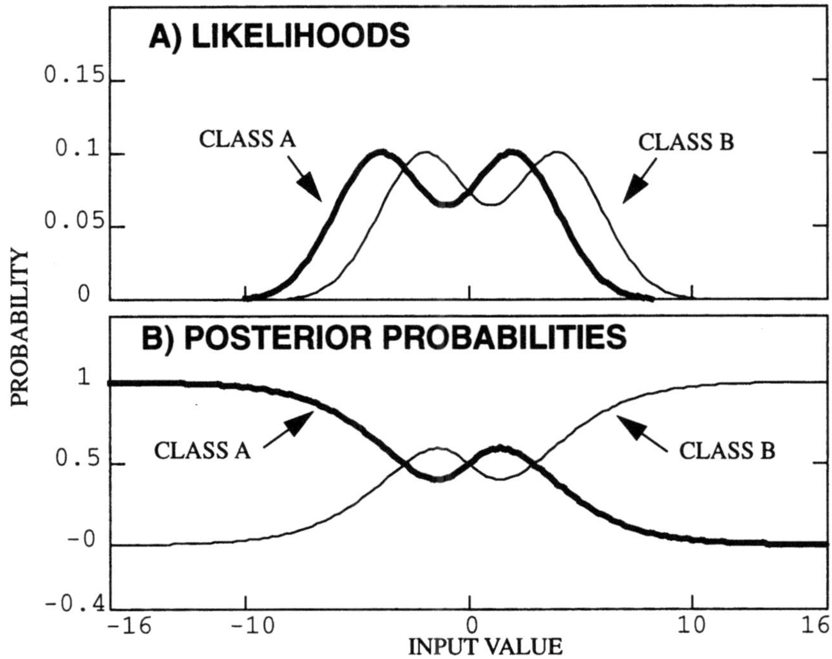

FIGURE 7. (A) Likelihoods and (B) Posterior probabilities for a two-class problem with one input feature.

or rules. Inputs are classified using labels assigned to the different decision regions. These classifiers have binary outputs and include binary decision trees such as CART, the hypersphere classifier, perceptrons with hard-limiting nonlinearities trained using the perceptron convergence procedure, sigmoidal or radial basis function networks trained using differential training, and many machine learning approaches that result in a small set of classification rules.

4. Accuracy of Neural Network Posterior Probability Estimation

Classifiers with outputs that accurately estimate posterior probabilities are much more useful and flexible than classifiers with binary indicator outputs. Many papers have proven that neural networks which use squared-error, cross-entropy, or maximum-likelihood cost functions and desired outputs of zero and one estimate posterior probabilities if the training algorithm is successful in minimizing these cost functions. These results are summarized in [12]. Proofs, however, do not indicate how accurately posterior probabilities are estimated with finite training data and non-optimal back-propagation training. Network outputs provide good posterior probability estimates only if sufficient training data is available, if the network is complex enough, and if classes are sampled with the correct prior class probabilities in the training data.

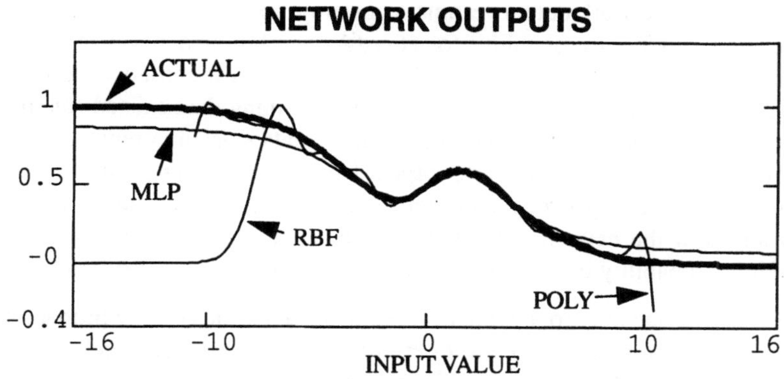

FIGURE 8. Actual posterior probability (thick curve) and outputs of multilayer perceptron (MLP), radial basis function (RBF), and high-order polynomial (POLY) networks.

Experiments performed to illustrate the accuracy with which neural networks can estimate posterior probabilities are described in [12]. One set of experiments used data generated for a two-class problem with one input feature whose distribution for the two classes was bimodal as shown in the top of Figure 7. The posterior probabilities calculated from these likelihoods are shown in the bottom of Figure 7. Note that for each input value, the posterior probabilities sum to one. Also, since prior class probabilities are equal, for each input value the posterior probability is largest for that class for which the corresponding likelihood is largest, and smallest for that class for which the corresponding likelihood is smallest.

Data generated according to these prespecified and known posterior probabilities were used with MLP networks trained with back-propagation, RBF networks trained with a matrix pseudoinverse technique, and high order polynomial networks (POLY) trained using the group method of data handling as described in [9]. All experiments used one continuous-valued input. Actual posterior probabilities were used to generate training and test data. For the MLP network, various topologies, with both one and two hidden layers, were tested. Of the topologies tested, one with a single hidden layer of twenty-four nodes offered the best training-time/estimation-accuracy trade-off. Results shown were obtained with this topology, a step size of 0.01, and momentum of 0.6. The RBF network contained one hidden layer with Gaussian basis function nodes. Gaussian means and variances were obtained using a clustering technique based on the Estimate-Maximize (EM) algorithm as in [9]. Weights between basis function and output nodes were determined using a matrix pseudoinverse approach. Twenty-four hidden nodes were used to facilitate comparison with the MLP network.

Figure 8 depicts the actual posterior probabilities for class A and the corresponding network outputs for the two-class problem. Four thousand training samples were used for each class. For the MLP network, each training sample was used only once for training because of the good convergence that resulted without repeating samples. Network outputs estimate posterior probabilities best in regions where the input has high probability for at least one class and worst in regions where the input has low probability for all classes. This is a consequence of the squared-error cost function used for training. Much training data existed (on average) in regions of high probability and little training data existed in regions of low probability. Deviations of the network outputs from the posterior probabilities in regions of high probability strongly impact the squared-error cost function. Similarly, deviations of the network outputs from the actual posterior probabilities in regions of low probability only weakly influence the squared-error cost function.

MLP network outputs provide the best estimates in regions of low probability. The polynomial network outputs behaves erratically in these regions, and the RBF network outputs quickly approach zero independent of the actual posterior probabilities. RBF network outputs approach zero because hidden node centers are in or near regions of high probability, and hidden node outputs approach zero for input samples far from node centers.

Network outputs should sum to one for each input value if outputs accurately estimate posterior probabilities. For the MLP network, the value of each output necessarily remains between zero and one because sigmoid functions are incorporated in output nodes. However, the criterion used for training did not require the outputs to sum to one. In contrast, there were no constraints on the outputs of the RBF and high-order polynomial networks. Nevertheless, as shown in Figure 9, the summed outputs of the MLP network are always close to one and the summed outputs of the RBF and high-order polynomial networks are close to one in regions where the input has high probability for at least one class. The accuracy of posterior probability estimation in this artificial problem falls off if networks don't have sufficient numbers of free parameters (hidden nodes and weights) to model the probabilities accurately and if there is insufficient training data as shown in [12].

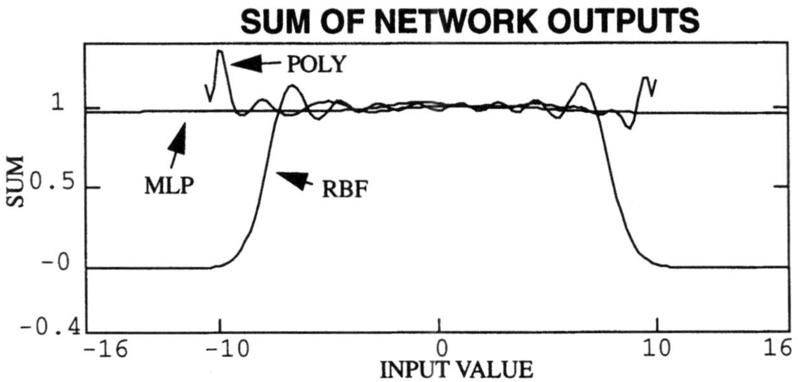

FIGURE 9. Summed outputs of multilayer perceptron (MLP), radial basis function (RBF), and high-order polynomial (POLY) networks.

5. Using Posterior Probabilities for Speech Recognition

Many researchers are using neural networks to estimate local per-frame probabilities required in hidden Markov model (HMM) speech recognizers [8, 15, 17]. These probabilities were previously estimated using non-discriminant training with Gaussian and Gaussian mixture PDF models. The assumption that network outputs are posterior probabilities allows networks to be tightly integrated with HMM and other statistical approaches. Figure 10 shows the hybrid neural-network/HMM speech recognizer described in [15, 16] which combines RBF networks and HMMs for isolated-word speech recognition. RBF networks in this system produce posterior probabilities which represent the probability of a specific sub-word acoustic speech unit given input features from a 10 msec input speech frame. These network outputs are normalized to be scaled likelihoods by dividing by class prior probabilities. Scaled likelihoods are fed to Viterbi decoders which perform nonlinear time alignment to compensate for varying talking rates and differences in word pronunciation. Viterbi decoders align input frames with labels of sub-word speech units and specify desired class labels for all frames. One Viterbi decoder for each word produces an accumulated output log likelihood score for every word at the end of each input utterance by assuming probabilities across frames are independent. This hybrid system was tested on a difficult talker-independent E-set recognition task where the goal is to recognize those spoken letters of the alphabet that contain the vowel "E". This system provided error rates that were lower than those provided by a state-of-the-art high-performance Gaussian tied-mixture recognizer with an equal number of trainable parameters [15, 16].

The good performance provided by this and other hybrid recognizers suggests that network outputs do closely approximate posterior probabilities. The accuracy of posterior probability estimation for this system was tested using three approaches. One necessary condition for network outputs to be posterior probabili-

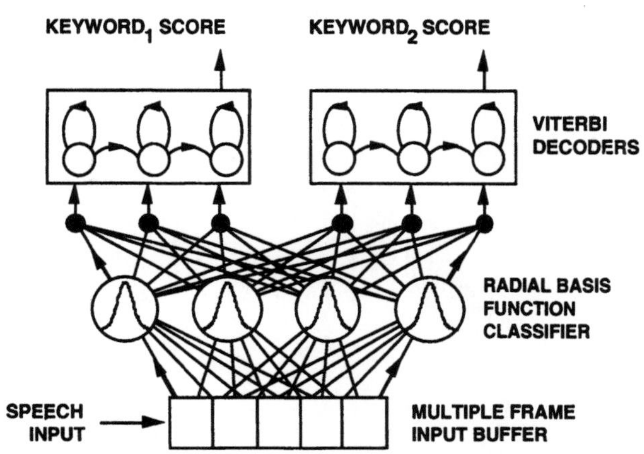

FIGURE 10. A hybrid isolated-word recognizer using radial basis function networks to generate posterior probabilities for a statistical Viterbi decoder.

ties is that they sum to 1.0 across all classes. This was tested by computing the RMS error between the sum of the RBF outputs and unity over all frames of the test data. The RMS error was low (less than 0.0001). This was true even though RBF outputs are not restricted to lie between zero and one. A second condition for network outputs to be posterior probabilities is that the average output of RBF networks should equal the prior probability of the class associated with that output. Average outputs were computed and found to equal prior probabilities closely. The RMS error was again low averaged over all frames (less than 0.00001).

A more direct third approach was used to measure the accuracy of posterior probability estimation as a function of the level of network outputs. If network outputs represent posterior probabilities, then a specific network output value (between 0.0 and 1.0) should reflect the relative frequency of occurrence of correct classifications of frames which produce that output value. If posterior probability estimation is exact, then the relative frequency of occurrence of correct classifications should exactly match the network output value. Because there is only a finite amount of data, outputs were partitioned into 100 equal size bins between 0.0 and 1.0. RBF outputs selected bins whose counts were incremented on every frame. In addition, the single correct-class bin count for the one bin which corresponded to the class of the input pattern was incremented on every frame. The ratio of the correct-class count to the total count for each bin was then computed and compared to the value of the bin center. For example, data indicated that for the 61,466 frames of training tokens, outputs of the RBF net in the range 0.095-0.105 occurred 29,698 times and were correct classifications 3,067 times. The relative frequency of correct labeling in this bin was thus 0.103 which is close to 0.10, the bin center. A plot of the relative frequencies of correct labeling for each bin versus bin centers gives a measure of the accuracy of posterior probability estimation by the RBF neural network.

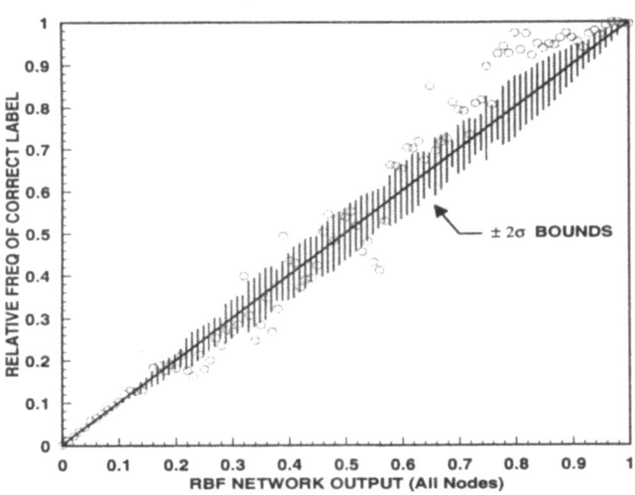

FIGURE 11. Comparison of RBF network outputs to posterior probabilities.

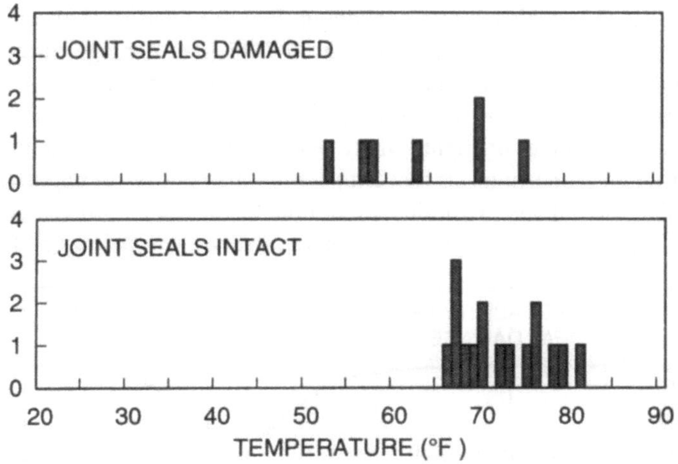

FIGURE 12. Histograms of the number of Space Shuttle flights where seals in the rocket booster field joints were damaged (top) or remained undamaged and intact (bottom).

Measured relative frequencies of correct labeling for the RBF net and 2σ bounds for the binomial standard deviation of each relative frequency are shown in Figure 11. Network outputs below 0.0 and above 1.0 are fixed at 0.0 and 1.0, respectively. Relative frequencies tend to be clustered around the diagonal and many are within the 2σ bounds. The lack of systematic deviation of relative frequencies from the diagonal and the good speech recognition performance provided by these RBF networks suggest that posterior probabilities are closely estimated. Goodness-of-fit measurements using the χ^2 test, however, indicate that the fits fail at significance levels below 0.01. This suggests that improvements in training or in structuring the network architecture could increase the accuracy of posterior probability estimation.

6. Using Posterior Probabilities for Fault Prediction

Probability estimates produced by network outputs can be used directly for fault prediction and prevention. A postmortem analysis of data from the U.S.A. NASA Space Shuttle program after the explosion of the Space Shuttle Challenger on 29 January 1986 demonstrates the usefulness of such probability estimates. In this example, the one input feature is the temperature of the field joints on the Space Shuttle rocket booster at launch, one class corresponds to damage occurring to one or more seals in these joints, and the second class corresponds to joints remaining intact after launch. A detailed analysis of all aspects of the Space Shuttle by a presidential commission [13] indicated that failure of the O-rings used to seal joints between separate sections of the solid-fuel rocket boosters led to the Challenger explosion. Although O-ring seals had been damaged on previous flights, the importance of this information was not realized until after the accident.

Figure 12 shows histograms containing data provided in [13] which demonstrate the effect of temperature at launch on field joint damage during all space shuttle flights up to the Challenger flight. The upper histogram shows the number of flights where O-ring seals on the field joints were damaged and the lower histogram shows the number of flights where seals remained intact. Examination of the upper histogram alone suggests that temperature may not be an important factor in causing joint seal damage. Examination of both histograms, however, demonstrates that joints were always damaged when the temperature was below 65 °F.

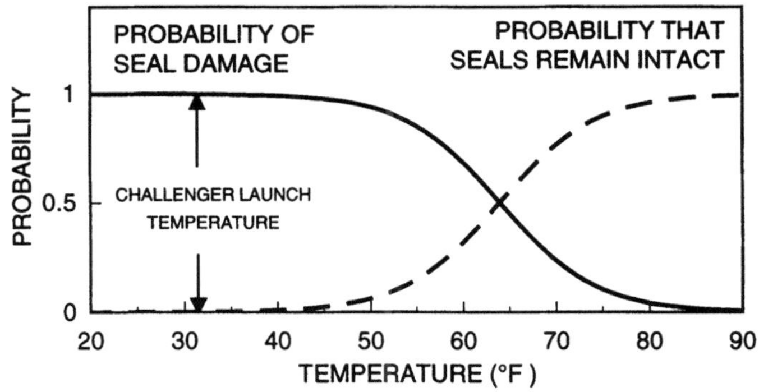

FIGURE 13. Probability of damage as a function of temperature as estimated by a neural network classifier.

A simple neural network classifier trained on this data classifies input patterns as predicting damage when the input temperature is below 65 °F and as predicting no damage otherwise. This classifier produces the output shown in Figure 13 which estimates the probability of damage given the launch temperature. This output indicates that the probability of joint damage increases as the temperature decreases and approaches certainty as the temperature drops below 65 °F. Although the network is extrapolating into a region where there is no training data, this type of analysis would have indicated that low launch temperatures are potentially dangerous. It might have prevented the fatal launch of the Challenger at the lowest launch temperature ever recorded of 32 °F if it had lead to an improved understanding of the physical mechanism that relates temperature to joint failure. This type of analysis can be applied to many other situations where a large, complex, process is monitored to detect dangerous or unusual situations or faults which may lead to undesirable results. The availability of posterior probabilities makes this approach much more acceptable in fault prevention applications, in medical decision making, and in other applications when human experts use networks to make complex decisions.

7. Scaling Posterior Probabilities by Class Priors

The prior probability of a class is the expected probability of obtaining a pattern from that class when patterns are presented randomly to a network. Prior probabilities can differ dramatically across classes for many applications such as medical diagnosis problems when only a small percentage of the population has a particular disease or for satellite surveys when different numbers of pixels in a satellite image represent water, land, trees, and other types of terrain. Prior probabilities can also differ dramatically between training and testing data. For example, in medical diagnosis, training data may sample diseased and normal patients evenly because it is expensive to administer medical tests on normal patients. In satellite surveys, the percentage of pixels representing water, land, and trees differs dramatically as the satellite moves across the earth's surface. It is relatively simple to compensate for different training and testing prior probabilities for neural networks that estimate posterior probabilities.

Networks with outputs that estimate posterior probabilities don't explicitly estimate the three terms on the right of Equation 1 separately. The output $y_i(X)$ is implicitly the corresponding prior class probability $p(C_i)$ times the class likelihood $p(X|C_i)$ divided by the unconditional input probability $p(X)$. It is possible to vary prior class probabilities during classification without retraining, since these probabilities occur only as multiplicative terms in producing the network outputs. As a result, class probabilities can be adjusted during use of a classifier to adjust class probabilities to those that occur in the real world. Correct class probabilities can be used during classification by first dividing network outputs by training-data prior probabilities and then multiplying by the test-data prior class probabilities. Training-data class probabilities can be estimated as the frequency of occurrence of patterns from different classes in the training data. Test-data class probabilities can be obtained from an independent set of training data that only needs to contain class labels and not input patterns. Such data is often readily available. For example, word frequency counts useful for spoken word recognition can be obtained from computer-based text data bases and the frequency of occurrence of various diseases for medical diagnosis can be obtained from health statistics.

Small differences between training and testing prior class probabilities normally increase overall error rates little. Large differences, however, can seriously degrade classification performance. These large differences can occur in satellite survey and medical diagnosis applications as noted above. The first two conditions in Figure 14 labeled "TRAIN 10:1" and "TRAIN 1:1" illustrate the increase in error rate that occurs when there is a large mismatch between training and testing prior probabilities. The last two conditions labeled "SAMPLE" and "SCALE BY PRIORS" demonstrates that this increase in error rate can be eliminated using two approaches. Training data can be sampled randomly using the correct test prior probabilities for any classifier. Alternatively, the continuous outputs of classifiers that estimate likelihoods or posterior probabilities can be multiplied by scale factors to apply the correct prior probabilities during testing. Results in Figure 14 were produced using a two-class two-input-feature problem where input feature vectors for both classes had multivariate Gaussian distributions with diagonal covariance

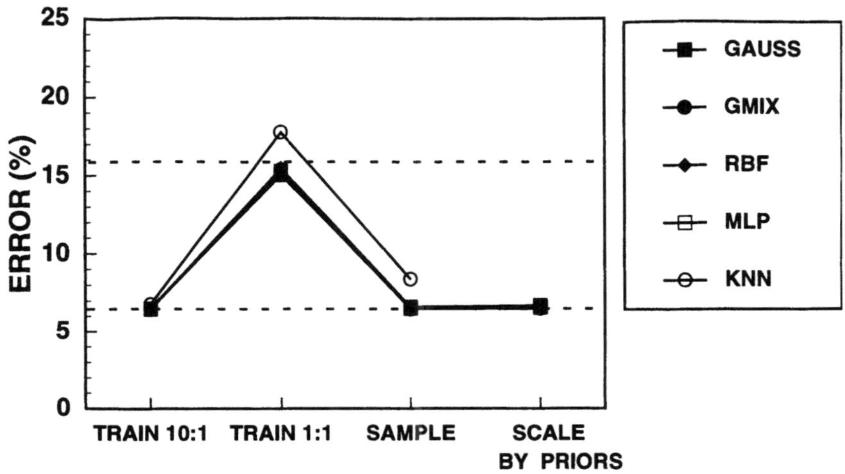

FIGURE 14. Testing error rates on a 2-class Gaussian problem for Gaussian, Gaussian Mixture, Radial Basis Function, Multi-Layer Perceptron, and K Nearest Neighbor Classifiers when training and testing class prior probabilities are correct, mismatch, and are corrected by sampling training data or scaling network outputs.

matrices and all variances were 1.0. The separation of the means for the two classes denoted as class A and B was 2.0. All classifiers were tested using a 10:1 sampled database containing 2000 patterns from class A and 200 patterns from class B.

In the first condition of Figure 14 labeled "TRAIN 10:1," classifiers were trained using a 10:1 sampled training data base where the relative frequency of occurrence of class A and B patterns had a 10 to 1 ratio. The theoretical minimum-error rate for this condition where training and testing priors are matched is 6.5% as shown by the dotted line. Error rates for Gaussian, Gaussian Mixture, Radial Basis Function, Multi-Layer Perceptron and K Nearest Neighbor classifiers are all near this theoretical value. Error rates increase dramatically, however, for the "TRAIN 1:1" mismatch condition when classifiers are trained assuming classes have equal prior probabilities using evenly sampled 1:1 training data but tested using data with a 10 to 1 inequality in prior probabilities. Error rates of all classifiers are near the theoretical error rate of 15.9% shown by the dotted line that results from this mismatch in prior probabilities.

The difference between class probabilities during training and testing can be corrected by randomly sampling the 1:1 training data non uniformly to produce the testing prior class probabilities or by scaling the outputs of classifiers with continuous outputs. Scaling consists of multiplying network outputs of MLP and RBF classifiers by the ratio of testing to training prior probabilities and multiplying likelihoods produced by Gaussian and Gaussian mixture classifiers by the testing prior probabilities. Random sampling can be applied successfully to all classifiers including boundary-forming classifiers while scaling by priors can only be applied

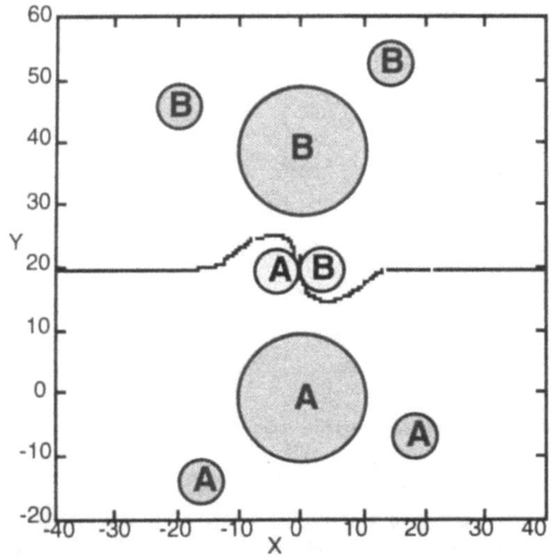

FIGURE 15. Distributions of patterns for two classes for the "Four-Cluster" artificial data base.

to classifiers with continuous outputs. As can be seen in Figure 14, under the conditions "SAMPLE" and "SCALE BY PRIORS," both approaches are successful in bringing classification error rates back down to values near the theoretical minimum error rate achieved when training and testing class priors are similar. These results again demonstrate that multilayer perceptron and RBF classifiers provide outputs which estimate posterior probabilities. They also demonstrate the added flexibility provided when classifiers estimate probabilities.

8. Posterior Probabilities can be Less Complex than Likelihoods

Many studies have demonstrated that neural network MLP and RBF classifiers used in hybrid speech recognizers can provide error rates near those of more complex Gaussian mixture classifiers but with many fewer trainable parameters [8, 15]. These results suggest that classifiers trained using neural network cost functions may require fewer trainable parameters than conventional PDF classifiers. This can occur when class distributions are complex, but posterior probability functions are simple because distributions overlap only in a small part of the input space. In such situations, a neural network classifier models relatively simple posterior probability functions which are either "high" and near 1.0 or "low" and near 0.0 over most of the input space. Alternatively, likelihood functions modeled by PDF classifiers may vary in a complex manner over large regions of the input space. The two-class "Four-Cluster" artificial data base shown in Figure 15 is an example of a classification problem where class likelihood functions are complex but the posterior functions are relatively simple.

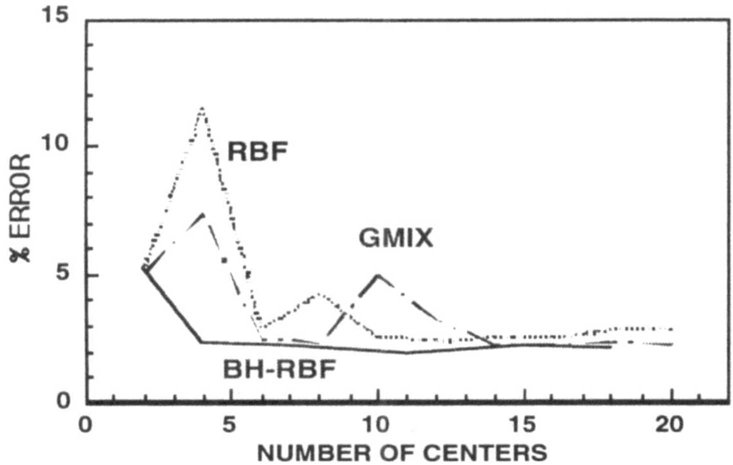

FIGURE 16. Testing error rates for radial basis function (RBF), Gaussian Mixture (GMIX), and boundary-hunting radial basis function (BH-RBF) classifiers on the Four-Cluster data.

There are two classes in the four-cluster problem. Each class consist of one large Gaussian cluster with 700 random patterns and three smaller clusters with 100 patterns each. Figure 15 shows the distribution of the data and the ideal decision boundary if the actual centers and variances are used to train a Bayesian minimum error classifier. These data were used to train a neural network boundary-hunting radial basis function (BH-RBF) classifier described in [2], a more conventional neural network RBF classifier, and a Gaussian mixture classifier. All classifiers were trained using from 1 to 10 centers or Gaussian functions per class. Classifiers were trained using 2000 training patterns and tested using a separate set of 2000 test patterns. All classifiers compute discriminant functions using sums of Gaussian functions and thus can be simply compared by counting the number of centers used. The only difference between the classifiers is the method used to train parameters. The BH-RBF classifier uses discriminant training to position Gaussian hidden nodes and train weights, the conventional RBF classifier uses discriminant training only to train weights and positions hidden nodes using k-means clustering, and the Gaussian mixture classifier is trained using the non-discriminant EM algorithm. The theoretically optimal Bayesian classifier for this database provides the error rate of 1.9% on the test set. This optimal Bayesian classifier is obtained using the actual centers, variances, and prior class probabilities used to generate the data in a Gaussian mixture classifier. In a real classification task, these center parameters are not known and have to be estimated from training data.

Figure 16 shows the testing error rate of the three different classifiers. The BH-RBF classifier provides the best performance with the fewest parameters. It provides a 2.3% error rate with only 4 centers and the error rate gradually decreases to 2.1% with 15 centers. The BH-RBF classifier performs well with few centers because it allocates these centers near the boundary between the two classes in an attempt to model posterior probabilities only were they vary substantially. On the other hand, the performance of the RBF classifier and the Gaussian mixture classifier is worse with few centers because these classifiers allocate centers in interior regions that have many patterns. The non-discriminant training algorithms used to position Gaussian means for these classifiers do not distinguish between patterns that are easily confusable between classes (i.e. near the class boundary) and patterns that clearly belong in a given class. Instead, they place Gaussian functions in regions where class probability density functions are high. Only after the number of centers increases above 14, and there are many parameters in all classifiers, do error rates converge. These results on a simple artificial problem demonstrate the reduction in classifier parameters than can be obtained by modeling posterior probabilities. They suggest that neural network classifiers may require fewer parameters than PDF classifiers when class densities are complex, and the overlap between class densities is small.

9. Differential Training for Reduced Network Complexity

Posterior probabilities or class likelihoods are not required in some classification applications. For example, a decoder in a modem that determines whether an input waveform corresponds to a binary 1 or 0 outputs a single binary bit. High-level error correction compensates for errors made at the bit level. A relatively new approach to training neural network classifiers called differential training can be used in these applications to design a small network that provides good performance [3, 4]. Differential training maximizes a function of the difference between the correct network output and the next highest output as shown in Figure 17. The

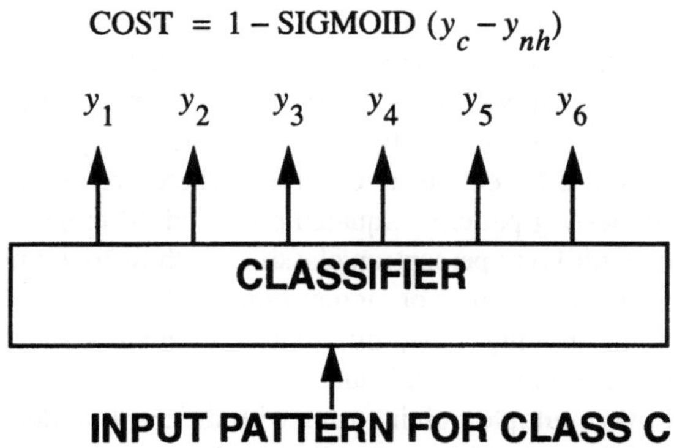

FIGURE 17. The cost function for differential training is a sigmoid function of the difference between the correct classifier output (y_c) and the next highest classifier output (y_{nh}).

cost function used in this approach is an approximation to the number of errors in the training set and attempts to minimize these misclassification errors as in the original perceptron convergence procedure. Differential training bridges the gap between these older classifiers and conventional back-propagation classifiers by allowing sigmoid, radial basis function, and high-order networks to be trained to minimize the number of misclassifications on the training set. Two experiments were performed to demonstrate the reduction in classifier complexity that can be provided with differential training. Other experiments performed by John Hampshire who originally developed this approach are described in [3, 4].

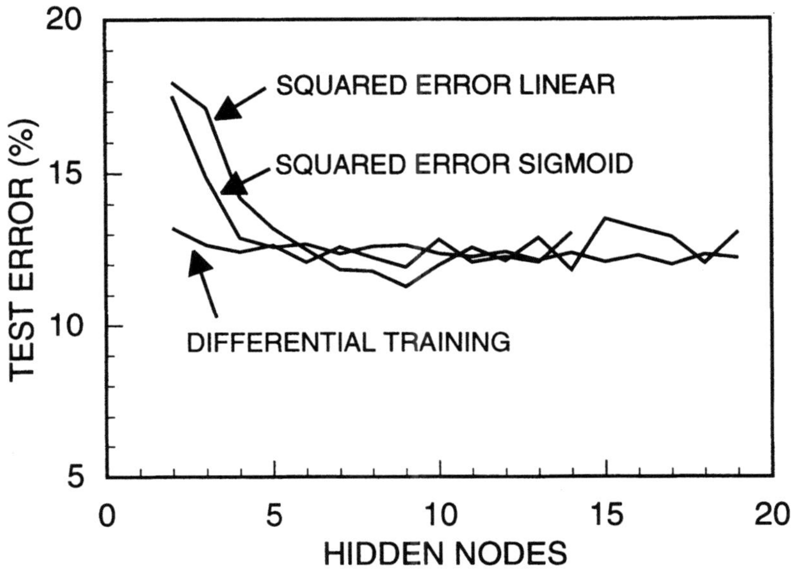

FIGURE 18. Test set error on the seismic data base.

One set of experiments was performed using a seismic data base generated with 14 continuous and binary input features derived from seismic waveform signals. These features are used to classify a waveform as belonging to one of seven classes which represent different seismic phases. There are 1000 training, 1000 evaluation, and 1000 testing patterns. Squared error and differential cost functions were used to train a multilayer perceptron classifier with different numbers of hidden sigmoid nodes and with linear or sigmoid output nodes. Training parameters (stepsize, momentum, training time, differential training gain) were carefully selected using cross-validation with this and a vowel data base data base and error rates are averaged over multiple training runs with different random initial weight settings. Results are shown in Figure 18. All classifiers provide similar error rates when there are many hidden nodes. Differential training with only two or three hidden nodes provided an error rate as low as that provided by back propagation classifiers with five or more hidden nodes.

A second set of experiments was performed using the original Peterson and Barney vowel classification data [10] with four inputs (first, second, and third formant frequencies and pitch), 10 classes, 896 test patterns, 300 evaluation patterns, and 300 test patterns. Similar error rates of 12.7% were provided by a Gaussian classifier and a back-propagation classifier using a squared error cost function with 25 hidden nodes. Differential training, however, was capable of training a single-layer back-propagation classifier with no hidden nodes to provide the same error rate. These two results demonstrate that differential training can reduce the size of a network required for good performance when output probabilities are not necessary.

10. SUMMARY

Classifiers have been developed using PDF, posterior probability, and boundary forming approaches to pattern classification. Many neural network classifiers approximate Bayesian a posteriori (posterior) probabilities while boundary forming classifiers minimize the overall classification error rate. PDF classifiers are trained using maximum likelihood approaches which individually model class distributions. The understanding that neural networks produce posterior probabilities greatly increases the flexibility and utility of neural network classifiers. As demonstrated in experiments, posterior probabilities from neural networks make is possible to provide a confidence measure for each classification decision, to compensate for differences in prior class probabilities between test and training data, and to combine outputs of multiple classifiers for higher-level decision making and across time. In addition posterior probabilities make it possible to use alternative risk functions different from minimum-error risk and to implement simple rules for pattern rejection. Analytic results for artificial and real-world speech problems demonstrate that neural network classifiers can provide lower error rates than PDF classifiers using the same number of trainable parameters when posterior probability functions are less complex than class likelihoods and thus simpler to model. Finally, experiments demonstrate that when posterior probabilities are not required, an approach to training called differential training can reduce network complexity while maintaining low error rates.

ACKNOWLEDGMENTS

Many experiments described in this paper were performed using LNknet software which was developed cooperatively with Linda Kukolich and Dave Nation. Many other people contributed to the experiments and systems described in this paper including Eric Chang, Charles Jankowski, Yuchun Lee, Rick Rose, and Elliot Singer.

REFERENCES

1. L. Breiman, J. H. Friedman, et al., *Classification and Regression Trees*. Belmont, CA: Wadsworth International Group (1984).
2. Eric I. Chang and Richard P. Lippmann, "A Boundary Hunting Radial Basis Function Classifier Which Allocates Centers Constructively," in *Neural Information Processing Systems 5*, Morgan Kaufmann: 139-146, 1993.

3. John B. Hampshire, *A Differential Theory of Learning for Efficient Statistical Pattern Recognition*, Carnegie Mellon University, Ph.D., 1993.
4. John B. Hampshire and Alexander H. Waibel, "A Novel Objective Function for Improved Phoneme Recognition Using Time-Delay Neural Networks," in *IEEE Transactions on Neural Networks*, 216-228, 1990.
5. Don R. Hush and Bill G. Horne, "Progress in Supervised Neural Networks," *IEEE Signal Processing Magazine*, 10(1), 8-39, 1993.
6. T. Kohonen, "An Introduction to Neural Computing," *Neural Networks*, 1, 3-16, 1988.
7. Richard P. Lippmann, "An Introduction to Computing with Neural Nets," *IEEE Signal Processing Magazine*, 4(2), 4-22, 1987.
8. Nelson Morgan and Herve Bourlard. "Continuous Speech Recognition Using Multilayer Perceptrons with Hidden Markov Models," in *International Conference on Acoustics Speech and Signal Processing*. 1990.
9. Kenney Ng, *A Comparative Study of the Practical Characteristics of Neural Network and Conventional Pattern Classifiers*, MIT, Master's Thesis, 1990.
10. Gorden E. Peterson and Harold L. Barney, "Control Methods Used in a Study of Vowels," *The Journal of the Acoustical Society of America*, 24(2), 175-84, 1952.
11. D. L. Reilly, L. N. Cooper, and C. Elbaum, "A neural model for category learning," *Biological Cybernetics*, 45, 35-41, 1982.
12. Mike D. Richard and Richard P. Lippmann, "Neural Network Classifiers Estimate Bayesian a Posteriori Probabilities," *Neural Computation*, 3, 461-483, 1992.
13. W. Rogers, N. Armstrong, et al., *Report of the Presidential Commission on the Space Shuttle Challenger Accident*. Washington D.C.: U.S. Government (1986).
14. Frank Rosenblatt, *Principles of Neurodynamics: Perceptrons and the Theory of Brain Mechanisms*. Spartan Books (1962).
15. Elliot Singer and Richard P. Lippmann, "Improved Hidden Markov Model Speech Recognition Using Radial Basis Function Networks," in *Neural Information Processing Systems 4*, J. Moody, S. Hanson, and R. Lippmann, (Eds.), Morgan Kaufmann: San Mateo, California, 1992.
16. Elliot Singer and Richard P. Lippmann. "A Speech Recognizer Using Radial Basis Function Neural Networks in an HMM Framework," in *Proceedings International Conference on Acoustics Speech and Signal Processing*. San Francisco: IEEE, 1992.
17. Torsten Zeppenfeld and Alex Waibel. "A Hybrid Neural Network, Dynamic Programming Word Spotter," in *Proceedings International Conference on Acoustics Speech and Signal Processing*. San Francisco: IEEE, 1992.

Flexible Non-linear Approaches to Classification

B. D. Ripley

Professor of Applied Statistics, University of Oxford
1 South Parks Road, Oxford OX1 3TG, UK. ripley@stats.ox.ac.uk

Abstract. Neural networks are one of a class of classifiers which construct a non-linear function from inputs to targets. There are a series of questions common to all members of the class, including how best to use the outputs to classify, how to fit the class of functions and also how to choose between classes. These questions are explored via some theory and three real examples. We also discuss the analysis of comparative experiments.

1 Statistical pattern recognition

The most widely accepted paradigm in classification is that of statistical decision theory (Berger, 1985; McLachlan, 1992; Ripley & Hjort, 1994) also known as statistical pattern recognition (Fukunaga, 1990). We suppose that there is a feature space $\mathcal{X}$ of potential observations, and to each we should assign a label, either that of one of K classes or 'doubt' $\mathcal{D}$ or 'outlier' $\mathcal{O}$. 'Doubt' is used when more than one class seems plausible and 'outlier' when no class is plausible. (Doubt options are particularly useful when there is a second line of classification, for example to make a more expensive test or to consult a human expert.) Let $\mathcal{Y} = \{1, \ldots, K, \mathcal{D}, \mathcal{O}\}$ be the space of possible decisions; a *classifier* is then a map from $\mathcal{X}$ to $\mathcal{Y}$.

This paradigm assumes cases $(\mathbf{X}, Y)$ are drawn independently from a probability distribution; we call the random variable $\mathbf{X}$ the *pattern* and Y the true decision (which usually does not take the value $\mathcal{D}$). The *training set* $\mathcal{T}$ is a set of n classified cases. Future cases will present a pattern $\mathbf{X}$ for the classifier to compute a decision.

The probability distribution of pairs $(\mathbf{X}, Y)$ can be specified in a number of ways. The *sampling paradigm* (in the terminology of Dawid, 1976) gives a prior distribution π_k over classes and the class-conditional densities $p_k(\mathbf{x})$. The *diagnostic paradigm* gives the posterior densities $p(k \,|\, \mathbf{x})$ and the marginal density $p(\mathbf{x})$ of $\mathbf{X}$. These specify the same information, for the joint density is $\pi_k p_k(\mathbf{x}) = p(k \,|\, \mathbf{x}) p(\mathbf{x})$.

Statistical decision theory assigns costs to decisions. We assume that correct decisions have no cost, incorrect ones unit cost and 'doubt' costs

$0 < d \le 1$. Then the rule with minimum expected cost, the *Bayes rule*, is specified by

$$y(\mathbf{x}) = \begin{cases} k & \text{if } p(k \mid \mathbf{x}) = \max_j p(j \mid \mathbf{x}) > 1 - d \\ \mathcal{D} & \text{if } \max_j p(j \mid \mathbf{x}) \le 1 - d \end{cases}$$

Note that the Bayes rule does not depend (directly) on $p(\mathbf{x})$. The expected loss under the Bayes rule, the *Bayes risk* represents the best achievable performance in the problem. (We can include different costs for incorrect decisions by replacing $p(k \mid \mathbf{x})$ by $1 - \sum_{k \ne j} C_{jk} p(j \mid \mathbf{x})$, where C_{kj} is the cost of confusing class k with j.) The posterior probabilities $p(k \mid \mathbf{x})$ are central.

It is less clear-cut how to treat outliers in the decision-theory framework. The purist approach would be to consider outliers to form another class, but then it is necessary to specify the class-conditional density $p_{\mathcal{O}}(\mathbf{x})$ of outliers. A less rigorous approach is to class as outliers those patterns $\mathbf{x}$ for which $p(\mathbf{x})$ is small. This needs the overall density $p(\mathbf{x})$ to be estimated, for example by a kernel density estimator. (Smyth, 1993, takes this approach.)

Most classifiers can be seen as approximations to the Bayes rule. Let $f_k(\mathbf{x}) = p(k \mid \mathbf{x}) = E(I(Y = k) \mid \mathbf{X} = \mathbf{x})$ and $\mathbf{f}(\mathbf{x}) = (f_k(\mathbf{x}))$. The Bayes rule chooses a maximizer of $f_k(\mathbf{x})$ over k. So if we can estimate $\mathbf{f}(\mathbf{x})$ or any monotonic function of it such as $g_k(\mathbf{x}) = -\log f_k(\mathbf{x})$, we can find an approximation to the Bayes rule. Define *target* $\mathbf{t}_k$ to be the kth unit vector. Since

$$\|\mathbf{f}(\mathbf{x}) - \mathbf{t}_k\|^2 = -2 f_k(\mathbf{x}) + 1 + \|\mathbf{f}(\mathbf{x})\|^2$$

the Bayes' rule amounts to finding the nearest target to $\mathbf{f}(\mathbf{x})$. (Note that unlike common practice for neural networks, doubt is not expressed by the distance from a target.)

The difficulties emerge when (as is usual) the distributions are unknown but have to be estimated from the training set $\mathcal{T}$. Suppose that we have a family of distributions parametrized by θ. The commonest approach is the *plug-in* approach, to compute the Bayes rule based on $p(k \mid \mathbf{x}; \hat{\theta})$, where $\hat{\theta}$ is an estimate of θ. This is not strictly correct as the uncertainty in $\hat{\theta}$ is not taken into account. The *predictive* approach uses

$$\begin{aligned} P(Y = k \mid \mathbf{X} = \mathbf{x}, \mathcal{T}) &= \int p(k \mid \mathbf{x}; \theta) p(\theta \mid \mathcal{T})\, d\theta \\ &\propto \int p(k \mid \mathbf{x}; \theta \prod_{p=1}^{n} p(\mathbf{x}^p, y^p; \theta))\ p(\theta)\, d\theta \\ &\propto \int p(k \mid \mathbf{x}; \theta) \prod_{p=1}^{n} p(y^p \mid \mathbf{x}^p; \theta) p(\mathbf{x}^p; \theta)\ p(\theta)\, d\theta \quad (1) \end{aligned}$$

and this needs a prior distribution over θ. This full Bayesian approach has been tried for regression neural networks (e.g. Neal, 1993, who uses a Monte Carlo method.). MacKay (1992a,b,c) uses a series of approximations to this approach to make it more computationally tractable. Note that 'model choice' such as choosing the number of hidden units or the network topology is contained in θ; in principle we do not select models but take a weighted average over all models. (In practice we average over a few good models.)

In the diagnostic paradigm it is usual to work conditionally on $\mathbf{X}$. As we have seen, the Bayes rule does not depend on the marginal distribution of $\mathbf{X}$, but the likelihood of θ given $\mathcal{T}$ will unless $p(\mathbf{x};\theta)$ does not depend on θ, and so there is usually a loss of information (in the technical sense), balanced by having to specify less of the model. One loss which may be considerable is the inability to estimate $p(\mathbf{x};\theta)$ from unclassified samples. (In some fields examples are readily available but producing accurate classifications is slow, expensive or both.) We have already noted that $p(\mathbf{x})$ may be needed to detect outliers.

There are pure nonparametric approaches based on the sampling paradigm estimating the class-conditional densities, including kernel discrimination (Hand, 1982; Coomans & Broeckaert, 1986, also known as ***probabilistic neural networks***, Specht, 1990; Wasserman, 1993) and using mixture distributions (Titterington *et al.*, 1985). The latter is closely related to, but differs from, the use of Gaussian radial basis functions.

Since the Bayes risk represents the best possible performance, it is worth making some effort to estimate it. The theory of k-nearest neighbour rules provides asymptotic bounds which with careful choice of metric can give a useful idea of the Bayes risk (Fukunaga, 1990, §7.4).

Discrimination

In some problems the primary aim of producing a classifier is not to predict future observations but to encapsulate the essential differences between the groups. In the statistical literature this is sometimes known as ***discrimination*** against ***allocation*** or ***classification***, but the concepts and ideas are often jumbled.

It seems not to be widely known that Fisher's original purpose in studying the (in)famous Iris data in his 1936 paper was discrimination rather than classification. His genetical hypothesis was that *Iris versicolor* had been formed as a 2:1 mixture of *I. virginica* and *I. setosa*. He used the 'Fisher linear discriminant' to find the best linear combination of measurements separating the two putative parents, and then test whether *I. versicolor* lay 2:1 between them on that combination. (It did.)

2 Flexible function fitting

Several families of functions $\mathbf{f}(\ ;\theta)\colon \mathcal{X} \to \mathbf{R}^{\mathrm{d}}$ are known to be universal approximators over compact sets, including single-hidden-layer neural networks (e.g. Cybenko, 1989; Jones, 1990), projection-pursuit regression (Friedman

& Stuetzle, 1981; Diaconis & Shahshahani, 1984) and sub-classes of radial basis functions (Girosi & Poggio, 1990; Park & Sandberg, 1991, 1993). There are other recent approaches such as MARS (Friedman, 1991) and the Π and hinging hyperplane methods (Breiman, 1991, 1993). Splines (Wahba, 1990) also have a place although they are much less convenient in more than one dimension. The close conceptual relationship between projection-pursuit regression and neural networks is discussed by Hwang *et al.* (1992, 1993) and Ripley (1993a, 1994b).

There are several papers (e.g. Gish, 1990; Hampshire & Pearlmutter, 1990; Miller *et al.*, 1993; Richard & Lippmann, 1991; Ruck *et al.*, 1990) which consider large samples and show that provided the parametric family is such that $f(\mathbf{x};\theta)$ can approximate the true $f(\mathbf{x})$, the classifier will approximate the Bayes rule. Of course, in large samples we expect the distribution of $p(\theta \mid \mathcal{T})$ to concentrate near a single point, and subject to continuity conditions the plug-in and predictive approaches become equivalent.

For finite samples there are trade-offs between the flexibility of $\mathbf{f}(\mathbf{x};\theta)$ and the spread of $p(\theta \mid \mathcal{T})$ (e.g. Geman *et al.*, 1992). We will need to impose limits on the degree of flexibility of the function, such as restrictions on the number of parameters (for example by restricting the number of hidden units or the number of radial bases) or to penalize rough functions. For the latter we can impose regularization penalties (Bishop, 1991, 1993; Poggio & Girosi, 1990) or use a prior over θ (Buntine & Weigend, 1991; MacKay, 1992a,b). An example is weight decay for neural networks which I see as important enough to use routinely (Ripley, 1993a,b). Regularization penalties themselves usually have one or more free parameters, which can be seen as parameters in a prior and themselves gives a (hyper)prior.

We can learn a lot from the case of *linear functions*. There the diagnostic paradigm uses linear models for $g_k(\mathbf{x}) = \log p(k \mid \mathbf{x})$ which in the case of two classes reduces to logistic regression. For classes 0 and 1 the deviance (the difference between twice log likelihood and its maximum) is

$$D(\theta;\mathcal{T}) = 2\sum_{p=1}^{n}\left[y^p \log\frac{y^p}{p(1\mid\mathbf{x}^p)} + (1-y^p)\log\frac{\{1-y^p\}}{\{1-p(1\mid\mathbf{x}^p)\}}\right]$$

This form has frequently been suggested in the neural network literature (Solla *et al.*, 1988; Hinton, 1989; Bridle, 1990; Spackman, 1992; van Ooyen & Nienhuis, 1992) from both likelihood and entropy principles. Surprisingly, it is common there to use a logistic model for *each* class, which does not ensure that the probabilities sum to one. The log-linear approach gives rise to what Bridle (1989, 1990) terms *softmax* and expressed equivalently as

$$p(k \mid \mathbf{x}) = \frac{\exp g_k(\mathbf{x};\hat\theta)}{\sum_j \exp g_j(\mathbf{x};\hat\theta)} \qquad (2)$$

and in any case the classifier chooses the class maximizing $g_k(\mathbf{x};\hat\theta)$.

The sampling-paradigm model of normal distributions for the classes with different means but a common variance matrix gives rise to a log-linear model. However, the parameters are estimated from the joint distribution $p(\mathbf{x}, y)$ whereas logistic regression uses the conditional distribution $p(y \mid \mathbf{x})$. Efron (1975) showed that the information loss in ignoring the marginal distribution of $\mathbf{X}$ is appreciable asymptotically. (Later work is discussed by McLachlan, 1992, §8.5.) Remarkably, for this model the plug-in estimate from the sampling paradigm can be found by linear regression. For two classes it has been known since Fisher (1936) that regression of the indicator of class 1 on $\mathbf{X}$ gives a linear rule which can be thresholded to give the plug-in sampling-paradigm classifier. (The threshold is not in general 1/2 but very close to it: Ripley, 1993b; Ripley & Hjort, 1994.)

For more than two classes Breiman & Ihaka (1984) developed this approach, and their work has been extended by Hastie, Tibshirani (see their papers in this volume) and by myself. This shows that the predicted values of linear regression of the class indicators for the K classes on $\mathbf{x}$ can be used to reduce the space $\mathcal{X}$ to the space $\mathcal{X}^*$ of at most $K - 1$ dimensions, and within $\mathcal{X}^*$ classification can be done either via a Mahalanobis distance to the class means or via another distance to the targets $\mathbf{t}_k$. (In each case there are constants to be subtracted for each class before minimizing.) Thus an inappropriate linear model for $f(\mathbf{x})$ is compensated for by using a different classification procedure to give exactly the sampling-paradigm estimate of the log-linear model. (Unfortunately this is often not done in the pattern recognition literature where Euclidean distance from the fitted values to the targets is used.)

This suggests two useful procedures to employ flexible families $f(\mathbf{x}; \theta)$:

1. Model the log-probabilities and classify by the class with the largest coordinate. Fit the model using softmax and maximizing the conditional likelihood
$$\ell(\theta; \mathcal{T}) = \prod_p p(y^p \mid \mathbf{x}^p)$$
possibly 'penalized' by a regularizing term such as the log prior probability.

2. Model $E(I(Y = k) \mid \mathbf{X} = \mathbf{x})$, fit by (possibly penalized) least-squares but classify by a distance in the space of predicted values. We can think of this as choosing a transformation of the space $\mathcal{X}$ to a space in which we use linear methods. (It allows the direct use of regression methods and software.)

Note that the distance in the second procedure is *not* the Euclidean distance to the targets and does not correspond to choosing the largest component, which is the common practice in the neural networks literature. The linear case suggests that the second of these procedures may be preferable (but see below).

The predictive approach

In the predictive approach we compute

$$p(k \mid \mathbf{x};\theta) = \frac{\exp g_k(\mathbf{x};\theta)}{\sum_j \exp g_j(\mathbf{x};\theta)}$$

and then average over the posterior distribution of θ given the training set $\mathcal{T}$. For a neural network the result is not expressible in closed form, but if $E(\theta;\mathcal{T})$ denotes the sum of the log-likelihood and the log-prior (the regularizing term), and H is its Hessian at a local minimum, then locally the posterior density is proportional to

$$\exp -E(\theta) \approx \exp - \left[E(\hat{\theta}) + (\theta-\hat{\theta})^T H(\theta-\hat{\theta})/2\right]$$

and integration over this peak suggests weighting the local minimum proportionally to

$$|H|^{-1/2} \exp -E(\hat{\theta}) \tag{3}$$

So one approximation is to find as many local minima as possible, and weight the $p(k \mid \mathbf{x};\hat{\theta})$ proportional to (3). We may also want to consider the variation of $p(k \mid \mathbf{x};\theta)$ across a peak. A simple idea is to note that approximately we have

$$\theta \sim N(\hat{\theta}, H^{-1}),$$

so we can sample from this distribution and average the predicted $p(k \mid \mathbf{x};\theta)$. It makes sense to sample proportionally to the weight given to the peak, the approach taken in our examples.

2.1 Fitting neural networks *via* softmax

Since using softmax with neural networks is not in most texts, we give the details here to show that it is only slightly more complicated than the usual approach of fitting separate logistic regressions for each class versus the rest. We will consider a feed-forward neural network with *linear* output units providing a output y_k for each class.

The measure of fit is

$$E = \sum_k t_k \log \frac{t_k}{p(k \mid \mathbf{x})}$$

summed as usual over patterns. The targets t_k will usually be one for the correct class, and zero for the others, and the probabilities are given by (2) computed from (y_k).

To use back-propagation, or any other optimization method that uses derivatives, we need to find $\delta_k = \partial E/\partial y_k$, where y_k denotes $g_k(\mathbf{x};\theta)$. It follows immediately that

$$\delta_k = \left(\sum_j t_j\right) p_k - t_k, \qquad p_k = \frac{\exp y_k}{\sum_j \exp y_j} \tag{4}$$

This is the initial step needed for back-propagation. Note that the outputs (y_k) can be shifted by a constant without altering the fitted probabilities. The most efficient way to avoid this over-parameterization is to drop one class (say class one) and set its output to zero, but include it in the sums in (4). This will, however, cause difficulties with the use of a weight-decay penalty.

3 Robustness

A strong warning is needed that the theory only applies if the models and data are correct. Even one incorrect classification in the training set can cause havoc in fitting $\mathbf{f}(;\theta)$. I strongly advocate the use of robust methods of fitting (e.g. Staudte & Sheather, 1990). Some ideas for models for misclassification are given by Copas (1988) and its discussion. In particular, procedure 2 above is only reasonable if the distributions in the space $\mathcal{X}^*$ are approximately normal with the same covariance matrix, and a robust estimate of the covariance matrix (e.g. Rousseeuw & van Zomeren, 1990) is needed to avoid a single bad fit grossly distorting the process.

Another area where robustness is needed is in choosing the complexity of the model; it is easy to choose complex models to fit cases which are actually wrongly classified. (This applies also to the predictive approach, which will give too much posterior weight to complex models unless misclassification is modelled.)

4 Tree-structured classifiers

Another approach which can also approximate $\mathbf{f}(\mathbf{x})$ and the Bayes classifier arbitrarily well in large samples is to design a partition $\mathcal{P}$ of $\mathcal{X}$, and to approximate the posterior probabilities (and hence the Bayes rule) within each cell of the partition by the frequencies of the classes of the training case which fall within that cell. Because general partitions are hard to work with, most procedures in this category use *decision trees* to specify the partition. These successively divide the space $\mathcal{X}$ and the training set on the levels of an attribute. The best-known approach within statistics is that of Breiman *et al.* (1984); there are also strands within the machine learning community (Dietterich, 1990; Quinlan, 1986, 1990, 1993) and in engineering (Chou *et al.* 1989; Chou, 1991; Gelfand & Delp, 1991; Safavian & Landgrebe, 1991).

These approaches differ principally in how they choose the model complexity, the size of the tree. Breiman *et al.* (1984) and Chou *et al.* (1989) use cost-complexity pruning, which is a backwards selection process with a penalty analogous to Mallow's C_p in regression (which penalizes the residual sum of squares by a constant times the number of parameters). Others (Crawford, 1989; Gelfand & Delp, 1991) prune with respect to an 'honest' measure of error rate. Buntine (1992) allows restricted n-ply lookahead and follows an approximation to the full Bayesian approach by averaging posterior distributions over many plausible trees.

One difficulty with tree methods is to allow a sufficiently large class of attributes on which to split; approximating partitions by splits along the axes may need very many cells. Allowing linear combinations of variables goes back at least to Henrichon & Fu (1969), and is part of the CART methodology of Breiman *et al.* (1984). Later authors have taken this up, sometimes under the name of *perceptron trees,* and non-linear functions are now proposed, for example small neural networks by Strömberg *et al.* (1991) and Guo & Gelfand (1992). These ideas replace a combinatorial choice over features and split-points by a continuous optimization over parameters of a (linear or non-linear) function.

Tree-classifiers have also been related to neural nets by Brent (1991) and Sethi (1990, 1991). They had essentially the same idea. Suppose we have binary tree with t splits and so $t+1$ leaves. The splits compute and threshold t functions of $\mathbf{x}$. Think of a network in which the first hidden layer of t nodes computes the split functions, and the second hidden layer has a node for each of the $t+1$ paths to a leaf which ANDs the (possibly inverted) outputs of the nodes on the path. The output layer then ORs leaves with the same class. Sethi proposes replacing the threshold nodes by logistic ones and re-training the network.

5 Examples

We include 3 small examples chosen to reflect some of the difficulties of relating our theoretical considerations to practice. A fixed weight-decay parameter chosen from past experience was used for each neural-network method.

5.1 *Leptograpsus* Crabs

Campbell & Mahon (1974) studied rock crabs of the genus *Leptograpsus.* One species had been split into two new species, previously grouped by colour form, orange and blue. Data are available on 50 specimens of each sex of each species. Each specimen has measurements on the width of the frontal lip, the rear width, length along the midline and the maximum width of the carapace and the body depth.

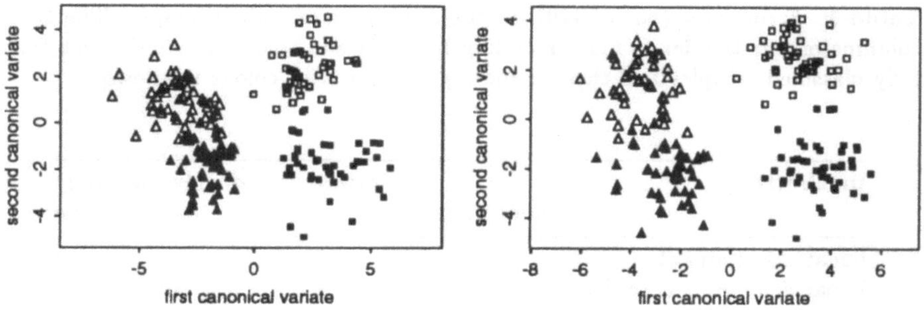

Fig. 1. Canonical variate plots for the *Leptograpsus* crab data. Left on original variables and right on $\log_{10}$ scale. The blue species is shown by triangles, the orange species by squares, and the symbols for females are filled.

The data are plotted on the first two canonical variates in figure 1. (The canonical variates are the variables produced by a linear discrimnant analysis, and successively best separate the group means.) As the measurements are scales, we also considered taking logarithms, and as the figure shows this does increase slightly the separation between the groups. As there are four groups, the canonical variates span three dimensions, and on log scale the ratios of between- to within-group standard deviations are 25.5, 16.9 and 2.9 on the three variates. Thus the first two show 99.1% of the variation between the groups. Clearly the first canonical variate expresses the difference between the species, the second that between the sexes. This is almost a textbook example of multivariate normal populations with equal covariances. Applying that model and classifying 5,000 simulated examples estimated the Bayes risk at 1.5%, with errors between species having rate less than 0.1%. The k-nearest neighbour method estimated a lower bound for the Bayes risk as 1.4%.

The 200 examples were divided as 20 of each class for a training set and the remaining 120 as a test set. To make this a less standard problem, we also considered ignoring the colour forms and classifying on sex. Table 1 gives the number of errors (out of 120). (The statistical significance of these results is discussed in section 6.) In this example a classification tree is hopeless unless allowed to take linear combinations of measurements. All the neural networks considered had skip-layer connections and had two units in the hidden layer. Maximum-likelihood fitting was used with softmax or logistic output units (there being no difference for two classes); we also tried a regression neural network and classification by the nearest target and after post-processing by linear discriminant analysis.

BRUTO (Hastie & Tibshirani, 1990) is a specific method of fitting a smooth additive model, which is able to choose any smooth transformation for each variable, hence a logarithm. However, it does not know to choose the same transformation for each variable, and here differs negligibly from linear dis-

Table 1. Error rates (out of 120) for the *Leptograpsus* crabs example. The three columns of results refer to first predicting both sex and colour, predicting sex from fully classified samples and then predicting just sex with colour unknown.

methods	4-way	sex only	sex only
colour given	yes	yes	no
linear discriminant	8	8	8
linear discriminant on log variables	4	4	4
quadratic discriminant	11	9	8
quadratic discriminant on log variables	9	7	7
neural network	6	5	2
linear, nearest target	12	12	8
post-processed by LDA	19	15	–
softmax on log variables	3	3	3
predictive	6	5	3
PP regression (4 ridge functions)	10	3	6
BRUTO	8	8	7
MARS (degree = 1)	10	8	4
MARS (degree = 2)	12	10	7
MARS (degree = 5)	19	15	7

crimination. In all the examples the PP regression, BRUTO and MARS methods used regression programs and option 2. above.

Note that despite the expectation from theory, we do better to classify the results of a neural network regression by Euclidean distance than via post-processing. To see why, consider a fit which occurred three of the five times when fitting the four-way classification, which had 12 errors using Euclidean distance and 23 errors via post-processing. The increase in errors comes from classifying one third of the blue males as orange females, a very rare confusion in other methods. Figure 2 shows why; the within-groups covariance matrices are far from equal. The sample size is too small for the robust version of the method to be able to help much; it still has 20 errors.

5.2 Forensic glass

This set of data was collected by B. German on 214 fragments of glass, and appears in Murphy & Aha (1992). Each has a measured refractive index and chemical composition (weight percent of oxides of Na, Mg, Al, Si, K, Ca, Ba and Fe). The fragments were originally classed as seven types, but some are infrequent or absent, and I re-grouped them as window float glass (70), window non-float glass (76), vehicle window glass (17) and other (22), omitting headlamp glass which seemed rather distinct in some preliminary

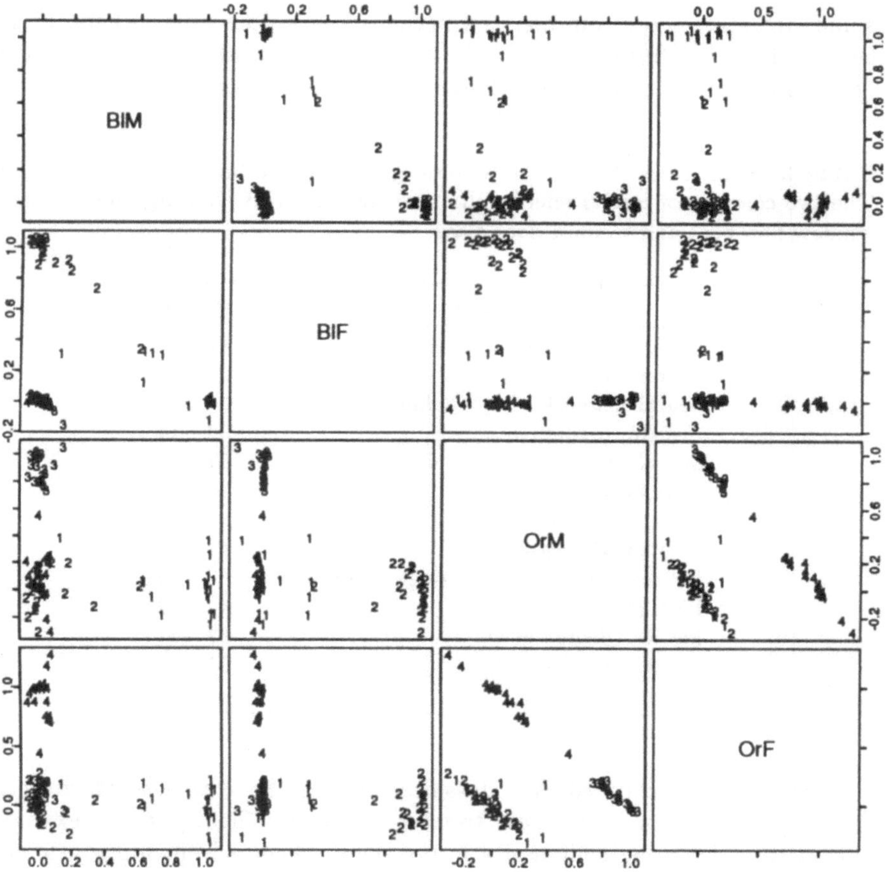

Fig. 2. Scatterplots of the outputs from a neural-network regression fitted to the training set of the crabs data. The groups labelled as 1 to 4 are in the order of the labels on the diagonal, blue males, blue females, orange males and orange females.

linear discriminant analysis. The whole dataset was split randomly, resulting in a training set of size 89 and a test set of size 96. The analysis here overlaps that in Ripley (1994a) and uses the same training and test sets.

The results are given in table 2. The estimated lower bound for the Bayes risk was 11%, which no method comes close to achieving. (Of course, the bound may be too conservative.) The main neural network results used softmax and maximum-likelihood estimation. (They are averaged over 5 runs using different random initial weights.) Using neural network regression on the class indicators and post-processing by discriminant analysis took about twice as long, since the weight estimation for the network was slower. (The results were also considerably more variable than the log-linear fits.) As some errors are more common and perhaps less serious than others, in the second figure confusion between the two types of window glass is allowed. (Differences of 4% or less are not significant[1]; see section 6.)

Table 2. Error rates (%) for the forensic glass example for a test set of size 96. The two columns of results refer to all errors and to errors ignoring those between window non-float and window float glass.

methods	error rate %	
linear discriminant	41	22
nearest neighbour	26	17
neural network with 2 hidden	38	16
ditto, predictive	38	14
neural network with 6 hidden	33	16
ditto, predictive	28	12
ditto logistic outputs	39	17
ditto, via regression	41	19
PP regression (5 and 2 ridge functions)	40	19
BRUTO	42	22
MARS (degree = 1)	37	17
MARS (degree = 2)	31	19
classification tree	28	15

It is sometimes claimed that classification trees have an ease of interpretation. Figure 3 is none too easy to interpret. One difficulty in this example is that there is strong collinearity in the chemical measurements which sum to approximately 100%; it might be better to use a perceptron tree method (such as CART) but I do not have access to suitable software.

The predictive results are based on 10,000 random samples from Gaussians about the peaks found in 20 optimization runs; in fact many fewer would have sufficed. Although for two hidden units all 20 runs gave the same confusion matrix, the cases in error differed from run to run.

[1] Here and elsewhere the conventional significance level of 5% is assumed.

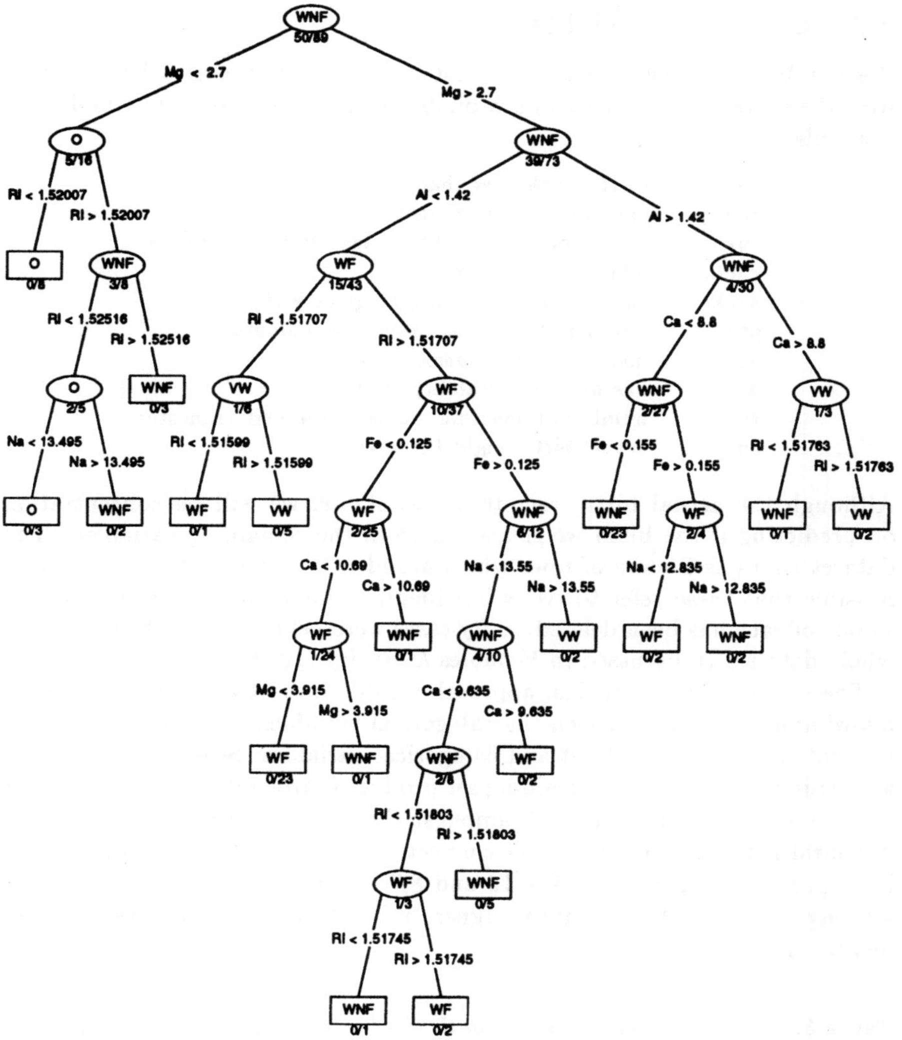

Fig. 3. Classification tree for the forensic glass example. At each node the majority classification is given, together with the error rate amongst training-set cases reaching that node.

5.3 Low birth weights

Hosmer & Lemeshow (1989) give a dataset on 189 births at a US hospital, with the main interest being in low birth weight. The following variables are available:

`low`	birth weight less than 2.5kg
`age`	age of mother in years
`lwt`	weight of mother (lbs) at last menstrual period
`race`	white / black / other
`smoke`	smoking status during pregnancy (0/1)
`ptl`	number of previous premature labours
`ht`	history of hypertension (0/1)
`ui`	has uterine irritability (0/1)
`ftv`	number of physician visits in the first trimester
`bwt`	actual birthweight (grams)

Although the actual birth weights are available, we will be concentrating on predicting if the birth weight is low from the remaining variables. The dataset contains 5 pairs of rows which are identical apart from the ID; it is possible that these refer to twins but identical birth weights seem unlikely, so one of each has been deleted. Fifty cases were held back as a test set. The whole data set is discussed in Venables & Ripley (1994).

The conventional statistical approach would be to fit a logistic regression, allowing interactions between the categorical variables, and between the numerical variable age and lwt and categorical variables. Selecting and fitting a logistic regression on the training set produced error rates of 6/13 amongst the low-weight births and 5/37 amongst the normal births in the test set. A neural network with skip-layer connections and two and six hidden units both produced error rates of 4/13 and 8/37 in the two groups. Note that although the overall error rate is higher, more of the risk group are correctly identified.

Table 3. Error rates (%) for the low birth weight data. That of the normal group is given first, then the low weight group. Values in parentheses are standard errors.

methods	raw rate	smoothed
logistic regression	14 (6), 46 (14)	27 (4), 56 (8)
neural net (2 hidden)	22 (7), 31 (13)	28 (5), 34 (9)
multiple minima (2 hidden)	24 (7), 31 (13)	33 (4), 38 (8)
plus local averaging	24 (7), 38 (14)	34 (4), 36 (6)
neural net (6 hidden)	22 (7), 31 (13)	24 (5), 28 (11)

These numbers are too small to be reliable estimates of error rates. We can use the predicted posterior probability outputs from the models to produce better estimates (see section 6). As table 3 shows, these reveal that on this occasion we are lucky; there are several posterior error probabilities between 0.4 and 0.5 but none between 0.5 and 0.6.

The actual birthweights are available in this dataset. It might be thought desirable to train a regression to predict the actual birth weight and then threshold the result. In fact this proved to be worse. A regression model with interactions had error rates of 7/13 and 6/37, and a neural network had error rates of 8/13 and 4/37.

Predictive approach

We can also consider the predictive approach. For the logistic regression it will make little difference to the eventual classification, as the only non-linear element is the logistic itself, and that is linear around $x = 0.5$. Thus averaging over an (approximate) Gaussian distribution for the parameter estimates will bring in slightly the extreme estimates of posterior probabilities, but has a negligible effect on the estimated error rates.

For the neural networks this is no longer the case, not least because the optimization procedure finds many local minima. We experimented with 2 hidden units. Each of 20 runs produced a separate local minimum, and the weights given to each were 43%, 17%, 9%, 8%, 7%, 6%, 4%, ... The effect of local averaging is also shown, based on a total of 1000 samples of weight sets.

The results here are too variable to draw useful conclusions about the value of attempting the integrations of the predictive approach.

6 Statistical Analysis of Comparative Experiments

Comparative experiments such as those in section 5 are very common - throughout the neural networks literature and in related fields (e.g. Weiss & Kulikowski, 1991). It emerged at Les Arcs that the statistical techniques to design and analyse such experiments were much less well known to the participants.

The design and analysis of comparative experiments has been developed over most of this century, originally for agricultural experiments in the 1920's and 1930's and more recently for industrial and medical experiments. (Medical experiments are known as clinical trials.) An excellent basic reference is Box, Hunter & Hunter (1978). Experiments in our field are computer experiments and have much in common with work in the field of simulation; Kleijnen & van Groenendaal (1992) provide a non-technical introduction in that context which is amplified in Kleijnen (1987). Important ideas from that field include importance sampling and stratified sampling, both of which can be used to design 'difficult' test sets and to compensate for the increased difficulty in estimating error rates. For example, we might arrange the rare patterns to be well-represented in the test set, but down-weighted (e.g. Candela & Chellappa, 1993).

It should always be possible to give some idea of the variability of a quoted performance estimate. For example, if the error rate is (as usual) found by counting R errors in a test set of size N, then R has a binomial(N, P) distribution, and we can estimate the standard error of $\hat{p} = R/N$ by $\sqrt{\hat{p}(1-\hat{p})/N}$. This can be quoted in terms of error bars, for example as in Ng & Lippmann (1991) (shown by Dr. Lippmann at the ASI). The convention in statistics is to quote approximate 95% confidence intervals, that is plus and minus *twice* the standard error. However, the crucial observation is that since the *same* test set was used for each method, the comparisons between methods are usually much more accurate than the error bars suggest. (In the terminology of the design of experiments we have a paired comparison, or a blocked experiment if there are more than two methods.) Consider the first two lines of table 1. As frequently happens, the 4 errors made in the second line are also made in the first line, so the difference in error rates is 4/120. Its standard error would be estimated as $\sqrt{(4-120/30^2)}/120 \approx 2/120$ so the difference is just significant. On the other hand the standard error of the unpaired difference between 4/120 and 8/120 is $\sqrt{0.0163^2+0.0227^2} \approx 3.37/120$ so the Ng-Lippmann approach would conclude no significant difference. A general version of this argument is to compare R_1/N to R_2/N and to assume that R_2 contains all R_1 errors. The paired standard error for $R_2 - R_1$ is then approximately $\sqrt{R_2 - R_1}$, so we can find a significant difference only with $|R_2 - R_1| \geq 4$, and this applies only if the worse method makes all the errors of the better method. This should be borne in mind in assessing tables 1 and 2.

The analysis of the last paragraph is approximate, in particular depending on approximating binomial distributions by normals. More precise methods are available, such as *McNemar's test* (Fleiss, 1981; Kotz *et al.*, 1985). Let n_A and n_B be the number of errors made by method A and not method B, and *vice versa*. Then McNemar's test (with continuity correction) refers

$$\frac{|n_A - n_B| - 1}{\sqrt{n_A + n_B}}$$

to a $N(0,1)$ distribution, and an exact test refers n_A to a binomial $(n_A + n_B, 1/2)$ distribution. This suggests that we need $|R_2 - R_1| \geq 5$ for a significant difference.

One pitfall to be avoided is to give too much emphasis to statistically significant results. In an experiment in which method A with error rate 29.8% is significantly better than method B with error rate 30.1%, it is clear that the difference is extremely unlikely to be of practical importance, especially if we estimate the Bayes risk as 6%.

It is often possible to provide more accurate estimates of the true error rate than the observed error rate on the test set. The true error rate is given by

$$E\left[1-\max_j p(j \mid \mathbf{X})\right]$$

If the classification method provides estimated posterior probabilities $\hat{p}(j \mid \mathbf{x})$ then

$$B = \frac{1}{\text{size of test set}} \sum_{p \in \text{test set}} [1 - \max_j \hat{p}(j \mid \mathbf{x}_p)]$$

provides an approximately unbiased estimator of the error rate if the posterior probabilities are accurate estimates. These estimates will be less variable because they average over the distribution of Y given $\mathbf{X} = \mathbf{x}$; see table 3. Devijver & Kittler (1982, §10.7) call this the *risk-averaging approach.* and McLachlan (1992, §10.5) refers to *smoothing of the error rate.* The smoothed versions are particularly well-suited to paired comparisons and to use in bootstrapping. It is necessary to check that the model for the posterior probabilities is *well calibrated,* so that, say, about 70% of events given probability 0.7 occur. (Techniques for checking calibration are given by Dawid, 1982, 1986.)

If the performance has to be estimated from the training set, there are a number of ways to estimate and (approximately) remove the bias of the observed error rate (or B) evaluated at the training set. McLachlan (1992, Chapter 10) discusses cross-validation, the jackknife, the bootstrap and refinements such as the double bootstrap and the '0.632 estimator'. If these are used in comparative experiments, there is some danger that their biases will differ between methods and so bias the comparisons.

The major difficulty with statistical studies is selection bias, sometimes known as the 'bottom-drawer effect'. Statistically significant events do occur by chance, and if enough are tried one will occur. It is hard to estimate how much is tried and discarded, especially from published studies. (It is often the case that the example in the paper is the only successful one of those the author tried!) Another danger is that some methods are 'tuned' more assiduously than others. The competitions which are beginning to emerge avoid some of these effects, but maybe we need to test methods with average rather than expert users to reflect their 'real-world' performance levels.

Acknowledgements

All of the examples were computed using the statistical system S-Plus. The code for BRUTO and MARS was from the S library `fda` available by ftp from `statlib@lib.stat.cmu.edu`. I am grateful to Trevor Hastie and Rob Tibshirani for providing a pre-release copy of their code and for illuminating discussions. Discussions with David MacKay encouraged me to include the numerical results on the predictive approach.

The final preparation of this paper was done whilst visiting the *Isaac Newton Institute for the Mathematical Sciences* in Cambridge, England.

References

My earlier papers Ripley (1993a,b, 1994a) explore these and other issues in greater depth with examples. Ripley & Hjort (1994) will cover this ground in depth.

Berger, J. O. (1985) *Statistical Decision Theory and Bayesian Analysis.* New York: Springer.

Bishop, C. (1991) Improving the generalization properties of radial basis function neural networks. *Neural Computation* **3**, 579–588.

Bishop, C. (1993) Curvature-driven smoothing: a learning algorithm for feedforward networks. *IEEE Trans. Neural Networks.*

Box, G. E. P., Hunter, W. G. and Hunter, J. S. (1978) *Statistics for Experimenters: an Introduction to Design, Data Analysis and Model Building.* New York: Wiley.

Breiman, L. (1991) The Π–method for estimating multivariate functions from noisy data. *Technometrics* **33**, 125–160.

Breiman, L. (1993) Hinging hyperplanes for regression, classification and function approximation. *Trans. IEEE IT* **3**, 999–1013.

Breiman, L., Friedman, J. H., Olshen, R. A. and Stone, C. J. (1984) *Classification and Regression Trees.* Monterey: Wadsworth and Brooks/Cole.

Breiman, L. and Ihaka, R. (1984) Nonlinear discriminant analysis via ACE and scaling. Technical Report #40, U.C. Berkeley Statistics Department.

Brent, R. P. (1991) Fast training algorithms for multilayer neural nets. *IEEE Trans. Neural Networks* **2**, 346–354.

Bridle, J. S. (1989) Probabilistic interpretation of feedforward classification network outputs, with relationships to statistical pattern recognition. In *Neurocomputing: Algorithms, Architectures and Applications* eds F. Fogleman-Soulie and J. Hérault. New York: Springer.

Bridle, J. S. (1990) Training stochastic model recognition algorithms as networks can lead to maximum mutual information estimation of parameters. In *Advances in Neural Information Processing Systems 2* (ed. D. S. Touretzky) pp. 211–217. San Mateo, CA: Morgan Kaufmann.

Buntine, W. L. (1992) Learning classification trees. *Statistics and Computing* **2**, 63–73.

Buntine, W. L. and Weigend, A. S. (1991) Bayesian back-propagation. *Complex Systems* **5**, 603–643.

Campbell, N. A. and Mahon, R. J. (1974) A multivariate study of variation in two species of rock crab of genus *Leptograpsus. Aust. J. Zool.* **22**, 417–425.

Candela, G. T and Chellappa, R. (1993) Comparative performance of classification methods for fingerprints. US National Institute of Standards and Technology report NISTIR 5163.

Chou, P. A. (1991) Optimal partitioning for classification and regression trees. *IEEE Trans. PAMI* **13**, 340–354.

Chou, P. A., Lookabaugh, T. and Gray, R. M. (1989) Optimal pruning with applications to tree-structured source coding and modeling. *IEEE Trans. Inf. Theory* **35**, 299–315.

Coomans, D. and Broeckaert, I. (1986) *Potential Pattern Recognition.* Letchworth: Research Studies Press.

Copas, J. B. (1988) Binary regression models for contaminated data (with discussion). *J. Roy. Statistic. Soc. B* **50**, 225-265.

Crawford, S. L. (1989) Extensions to the CART algorithm. *Int. J. Man-Machine Studies* **31**, 197–217.

Cybenko, G. (1989) Approximation by superpositions of a sigmoidal function. *Math. Control Systems Signals* **2**, 303–314.

Dawid, A. P. (1976) Properties of diagnostic data distributions. *Biometrics* **32**, 647–658.

Dawid, A. P. (1982) The well-calibrated Bayesian (with discussion). *J. Amer. Statist. Assoc.* **77**, 605–613.

Dawid, A. P. (1986) Probability forecasting. In *Encyclopedia of Statistical Sciences* eds S. Kotz, N. L. Johnson & C. B. Read, pp. 210–218. New York: Wiley.

Devijver, P. A. and Kittler, J. (1982) *Pattern Recognition. A Statistical Approach.* Englewood Cliffs, NJ: Prentice-Hall.

Diaconis, P. and Shahshahani, M (1984) On non-linear functions of linear combinations. *SIAM J. Sci. Statist. Comput.* **5**, 175–191.

Dietterich, T. G. (1990) Machine learning. *Annual Review of Computer Science* **4**, 255–306.

Efron, B. (1975) The efficiency of logistic regression compared to normal discriminant analysis. *J. Amer. Statist. Assoc.* **70**, 892–898.

Fisher, R. A. (1936) The use of multiple measurements in taxonomic problems. *Annals of Eugenics* **7**, 179–188.

Fleiss, J. L. (1981) *Statistical Methods for Rates and Proportions.* Second Edition. New York: Wiley.

Friedman, J. H. (1991) Multivariate adaptive regression splines (with discussion). *Annals of Statistics* **19**, 1–141.

Friedman, J. H. and Stuetzle, W. (1981) Projection pursuit regression. *J. Amer. Statist. Assoc.* **78**, 817–823.

Fukunaga, K. (1990) *Introduction to Statistical Pattern Recognition.* 2nd edition. London: Academic Press.

Gelfand, S. B. and Delp, E. J. (1991) On tree structured classifiers. In Sethi & Jain (1991) pp. 51–70.

Geman, S., Bienenstock, E. and Doursat, R. (1992) Neural networks and the - bias/variance dilemma. *Neural Computation* **4**, 1–58.

Girosi, F. and Poggio, T. (1990) Networks and the best approximation property. *Biological Cybernetics* **63**, 169–176.

Gish, H. (1990) A probabilistic approach to the understanding and training of neural network classifiers. In *Proc. 1990 IEEE Conf. Acoustics, Speech and Signal Proc., Albuquerque* pp. 1361–1364. New York: IEEE Press.

Guo, H. and Gelfand, S. B. (1992) Classification trees with neural network feature extraction. *IEEE Trans. Neural Networks* **3**, 923–933.

Hampshire, J. B. and Pearlmutter, B. A. (1990) Equivalence proofs for multi-layer perceptron classifiers and the Bayesian discriminant function. In *Proceedings of the 1990 Connectionist Models Summer School* eds D. S. Touretzky, Elman, T. Sejnowski & G. Hinton, San Mateo, CA: Morgan Kaufmann.

Hand, D. J. (1982) *Kernel Discriminant Analysis.* Letchworth: Research Studies Press.

Hastie, T. J. and Tibshirani, R. J. (1990) *Generalized Additive Models.* London: Chapman and Hall.

Henrichon, E. G. Jr and Fu, K. S. (1969) A nonparametric partitioning procedure for pattern classification. *IEEE Trans. Comput.* **18**, 614–624.

Hinton, G. E. (1989) Connectionist learning procedures. *Artificial Intelligence* **40**, 185–234.

Hosmer, D. W. and Lemeshow, S. (1989) *Applied Logistic Regression*. New York: Wiley.

Hwang, J.-N., Lay, S.-R., Maechler, M., Martin, D. and Schimert, J. (1993) Regression modeling in back-propagation and projection pursuit learning. *IEEE Trans. Neural Networks*.

Hwang, J.-N., Li, D., Maechler, M., Martin, D. and Schimert, J. (1992) Projection pursuit learning networks for regression. *Engineering Applications Artificial Intelligence* **5**, 193-204.

Jones, L. K. (1990) Constructive approximations for neural networks by sigmoidal functions. *Proc. IEEE* **78**, 1586–1589.

Kleijnen, J. P. C. (1987) *Statistical Tools for Simulation Practioners*. New York: Marcel Dekker.

Kleijnen, J. P. C. and van Groenendaal, W. (1992) *Simulation: A Statistical Perspective*. Chichester: Wiley.

Kotz, S., Johnson, N. L. and Read, C.B. (1985) *Encyclopedia of Statistical Sciences*. Volume 5. New York: Wiley.

MacKay, D. J. C. (1992a) Bayesian interpolation. *Neural Computation* **4**, 415–447.

MacKay, D. J. C. (1992b) A practical Bayesian framework for backprop networks. *Neural Computation* **4**, 448–472.

MacKay, D. J. C. (1992c) The evidence framework applied to classification networks. *Neural Computation* **4**, 720–736.

McLachlan, G. J. (1992) *Discriminant Analysis and Statistical Pattern Recognition*. New York: Wiley.

Miller, J. W., Goodman, R. and Smyth, P. (1993) On loss functions which minimize to conditional expected values and posterior probabilities. *IEEE Trans. Inf. Theory*.

Murphy, P. M., & Aha, D. W. (1992). *UCI Repository of Machine Learning Databases* [Machine-readable data repository]. Irvine, CA: University of California, Department of Information and Computer Science. Available by anonymous ftp from `ics.uci.edu` in directory `pub/machine-learning-databases`.

Neal, R. (1993) Bayesian learning via stochastic dynamics. In *Advances in Neural Information Processing Systems 5*, eds C. L. Giles, S. J. Hanson, and J. D. Cowan, pp. 475–482, San Mateo, CA: Morgan Kaufmann.

Ng, K and Lippmann, R. P. (1991) A comparative study of the practical characteristics of neural network and conventional pattern classifiers. In *Advances in Neural Information Processing Systems 3*, eds R. P. Lippmann, J. E. Moody and D. S. Touretzky, pp. 970–976, San Mateo, CA: Morgan Kaufmann.

van Ooyen, A. and Nienhuis, B. (1992) Improving the convergence of the backpropagation algorithm. *Neural Networks* **5**, 465–471.

Park, J. and Sandberg, I. W. (1991) Universal approximation using radial-basis-function networks. *Neural Computation* **3**, 246–257.

Park, J. and Sandberg, I. W. (1993) Approximation and radial-basis-function networks. *Neural Computation* **5**, 305–316.

Poggio, T. and Girosi, F. (1990) Networks for approximation and learning. *Proc. IEEE* **78**, 1481–1497.

Quinlan, J. R. (1986) Induction of decision trees. *Machine Learning* **1**, 81–106.

Quinlan, J. R. (1990) Decision trees and decision making. *IEEE Trans. SMC* **20**, 339–346.

Quinlan, J. R. (1993) *C4.5: Programs for Machine Learning.* San Mateo, CA: Morgan Kaufmann.

Richard, M. D. and Lippmann, R. P (1991) Neural network classifiers estimate Bayesian *a posteriori* probabilities. *Neural Computation* **3**, 461–483.

Ripley, B. D. (1993a) Statistical aspects of neural networks. In *Networks and Chaos – Statistical and Probabilistic Aspects* (eds O. E. Barndorff-Nielsen, J. L. Jensen and W. S. Kendall), pp. 40–123. London: Chapman & Hall.

Ripley, B. D. (1993b) Neural networks and flexible regression and discrimination. In *Statistics and Images* ed. K. V. Mardia. *Advances in Applied Statistics*, Abingdon: Carfax.

Ripley, B. D. (1994a) Neural networks and related methods for classification (with discussion). *J. Roy. Statist. Soc. B* **56**.

Ripley, B. D. (1994b) Comment on: 'Neural networks: a review from a statistical perspective'. *Statistical Science* **9**.

Ripley, B. D. and Hjort, N. L. (1984) *Pattern Recognition and Neural Networks – A Statistical Approach.* Cambridge: Cambridge University Press.

Rousseeuw, P. J. and van Zomeren, B. C. (1990). Unmasking multivariate outliers and leverage points (with discussion). *J. Amer. Statist. Assoc.* **85**, 633–651.

Ruck, D. W., Rogers, S. K., Kabrisky, M., Oxley, M. E. and Suter, B. W. (1990) The multilayer perceptron as an approximation to a Bayes optimal discriminant function. *IEEE Trans. Neural Networks* **1**, 296–298.

Safavian, S. R and Landgrebe, D. (1991) A survey of decision tree classifier methodology. *IEEE Trans. SMC* **21**, 660-674.

Sethi, I. K. (1990) Entropy nets: from decision trees to neural networks. *Proc. IEEE* **78**, 1605–1613.

Sethi, I. K. (1991) Decision tree performance enhancement using an artificial neural network implementation. In Sethi & Jain (1991) pp. 71–88.

Sethi, I. K. and Jain, A. K. eds (1991) *Artificial Neural Networks and Statistical Pattern Recognition. Old and New Connections.* Amsterdam: North Holland.

Smyth, P. (1993) Probability density estimation and local basis function neural networks. In *Computational Learning Theory and Natural Learning Systems 2* eds T. Petsche, M. Kearns, S. Hanson and R. Rivest. Cambridge. MA: The MIT Press.

Solla, S. A., Levin, E. and Fleisher, M. (1988) Accelerated learning in layered neural networks. *Complex Systems* **2**, 625–639.

Spackman, K. A. (1992) Maximum likelihood training of connectionist models: comparison with least-squares back propagation and logistic regression. *Proceedings of the 15th Annual Symposium on Computer Applications in Medical Care, Nov. 1991*, pp. 285–289. New York: IEEE Press.

Specht D. F. (1990) Probabilistic neural networks. *Neural Networks* **3**, 109–118.

Staudte, R. G. and Sheather, S. J. (1990). *Robust Estimation and Testing.* New York: Wiley.

Strömberg, J. E., Zrida, J. and Isaksson, A. (1991) Neural trees—using neural nets in a tree classifier structure. *IEEE Int. Conf. Acoustics, Speech and Signal Processing*, pp. 137–140. IEEE Press.

Titterington, D. M., Smith, A. F. M. and Makov, U. E. (1985) *Statistical Analysis of Finite Mixture Distributions*. Chichester: Wiley.

Venables, W. N. and Ripley, B. D. (1994) *Statistics with S*. New York: Springer.

Wahba, G. (1990) *Spline Models for Observational Data*. Philadelphia: SIAM.

Wasserman, P. D. (1993) *Advanced Methods in Neural Computing*. New York: Van Nostrand Reinhold.

Weiss, S. M. and Kulikowski, C. A. (1991) *Computer Systems that Learn: Classification and Prediction Methods from Statistics, Neural Nets, Machine Learning and Expert Systems*. San Mateo, CA: Morgan Kaufmann.

Parametric Statistical Estimation with Artificial Neural Networks: A Condensed Discussion

Halbert White

Department of Economics and Institute for Neural Computation
University of California, San Diego, CA 92093-0508

Abstract. Learning in artificial neural networks is a process by which experience arising from exposure to measurements of empirical phenomena is converted to knowledge, embodied in network weights. This process can be viewed formally as statistical estimation of the parameters of a parametrized probability model. We exploit this formal viewpoint to give a unified theory of learng in artificial neural networks. The theory encompasses both supervised and unsupervised learning in either feedforward or recurrent networks. We begin by describing various objects appropriate for learning, such as conditional means, variances or quantiles, or conditional densities. We then show how artificial neural networks can be viewed as parametric statistical models directed toward these objects of interest. We show how a probability density can be associated with the output of any network, and use this density to define network weights indexing an information-theoretically optimal approximation to the object of interest. We next study statistical properties of quasi-maximum likelihood estimators consistent for the optimal weights, including issues associated with statistical inference about the optimal weights. Finally, we consider computational methods for obtaining these estimators, with special attention to extensions of the method of back-propagation.

1 Data Generating Processes as Objects of Learning

We begin with a description of how the observed data are generated.

Assumption A.1: The observed data are the realization of a stochastic process $\{Z_t : \Omega \to I\!R^v,\ t = 1, 2, \ldots\}$, $v \in I\!N$, on the complete probability space $(\Omega, \mathcal{F}, P_o)$. For convenience and without loss of generality, we take $\Omega = I\!R^{v\infty} \equiv \times_{t=1}^{\infty} I\!R^v$, $\mathcal{F} = \mathcal{B}^{v\infty} \equiv \mathcal{B}(I\!R^{v\infty})$ (i.e., the Borel σ-field generated by $I\!R^{v\infty}$) and let $\{ Z_t \}$ be the "coordinate variable process": for $\omega = \{ z_t \} \in I\!R^{v\infty}$, we have $Z_t(\omega) = z_t$, $t = 1, 2, \ldots$. □

In practice, we observe finite sequences of data, not infinite sequences. The behavior of a finite sequence $\{ Z_t : t = 1, \ldots, n \}$, $n \in \mathbb{N}$, is governed by the probability measure P_o^n on $(\mathbb{R}^{vn}, \mathcal{B}^{vn})$, where $\mathbb{R}^{vn} \equiv \times_{t=1}^n \mathbb{R}^v$, $\mathcal{B}^{vn} \equiv \mathcal{B}(\mathbb{R}^{vn})$. P_o^n is also called the "distribution" of $Z^n \equiv (Z_1, \ldots, Z_n)$ and is defined as

$$P_o^n(A^n) = P_o[A^n \times \mathbb{R}^v \times \mathbb{R}^v \times \ldots], A^n \in \mathcal{B}^{vn}, n = 1, 2, \ldots .$$

An equivalent characterization of the distribution of Z^n is given by its probability density function $g^n : \mathbb{R}^{vn} \to \mathbb{R}^+$, defined implicitly by

$$P_o^n(A^n) = \int_{A^n} g^n(z^n) \nu^n(dz^n), A^n \in \mathcal{B}^{vn}, n = 1, 2, \ldots ,$$

where the integral is taken in the sense of Lebesgue, and ν^n is a σ-finite measure (i.e., there exists a sequence $\{ B_i \in \mathcal{B}^{vn}, i = 1, 2, \ldots \}$ for which $\mathbb{R}^{vn} = \cup_{i=1}^{\infty} B_i$ and $\nu^n(B_i) < \infty, i = 1, 2, \ldots$), such that ν^n "dominates" P_o^n, i.e., if $B \in \mathcal{B}^{vn}$ and $\nu^n(B) = 0$ then $P_o^n(B) = 0$. Under these conditions on ν^n, the existence of g^n is guaranteed by the Radon-Nikodým theorem. We write $g^n = dP_o^n / d\nu^n$; g^n is called the Radon-Nikodým derivative or the Radon-Nikodým density

In many cases, however, knowledge of g^n is more than one wants. The reason is that g^n embodies all relationships between the measured quantities jointly, while interest often attaches instead solely to the relationship between certain target variables, an $l \times 1$ subvector Y_t of Z_t, say, and the remaining components of Z_t, say X_t (so that $Z_t = (Y_t', X_t')'$). In time-series contexts, preceding values Z^{t-1} may also be relevant in understanding the behavior of Y_t. Everything that can possibly be known about the relationship of Y_t to $\ddot{Z}^{t-1} \equiv (Z^{t-1}, X_t)$ can be expressed in terms of the conditional probability distributions of Y_t given $\ddot{Z}^{t-1}$, or as in the case of the joint probability distribution of Z^n, in terms of an appropriate conditional density function.

Such conditional densities can be expressed as

$$g_t(y_t \mid \ddot{z}^{t-1}) \equiv g^t(z^t) / \ddot{g}^{t-1}(\ddot{z}^{t-1}),$$

where $\ddot{g}^t = d\ddot{P}_o^t / d\ddot{\nu}^t$ is the probability density function of $\ddot{Z}^t$, i.e., the Radon-Nikodým derivative of $\ddot{P}_o^t$, the distribution of $\ddot{Z}^t$, with respect to a σ-finite measure $\ddot{\nu}^t$ dominating $\ddot{P}_o^t$. When a suitable σ-finite measure ν_t exists on $(\mathbb{R}^l, \mathcal{B}^l)$, conditional probabilities are given by

$$P_o[Y_t \in C \mid \ddot{Z}^{t-1} = \ddot{z}^{t-1}] = \int_C g_t(y \mid \ddot{z}^{t-1}) \nu_t(dy), \quad C \in \mathcal{B}^l, t = 1, 2, \ldots .$$

An appropriate assumption in this context is the following:

Assumption A.2: For P_o^t and $\ddot{P}_o^t$ as defined above, and given σ-finite measures ν^t, $\ddot{\nu}^t$ such that ν^t dominates P_o^t and $\ddot{\nu}^t$ dominates $\ddot{P}_o^t$, there exists a σ-finite measure ν_t such that $\nu^t = \nu_t \otimes \ddot{\nu}^{t-1}$. □

Even g_t may be more than one really cares about. Frequently, only certain aspects of the conditional distribution are of direct interest, such as the conditional mean of Y_t given $\ddot{Z}^{t-1}$,

$$\mu_t(\ddot{Z}^{t-1}) = E(Y_t \mid \ddot{Z}^{t-1}) \equiv \int_{I\!R^l} y\, g_t(y \mid \ddot{Z}^{t-1}) v_t(dy)\,,$$

or the conditional variance of Y_t given $\ddot{Z}^{t-1}$ (with Y_t a scalar),

$$\sigma_t^2(\ddot{Z}^{t-1}) = E([Y_t - \mu_t(\ddot{Z}^{t-1})]^2 \mid \ddot{Z}^{t-1}) \equiv \int_{I\!R} [y - \mu_t(\ddot{Z}^{t-1})]^2 g_t(y \mid \ddot{Z}^{t-1}) v_t(dy)\,.$$

Instead of conditional means and variances, interest may attach to conditional quantiles of the distribution of Y_t given $\ddot{Z}^{t-1}$, such as the conditional median, or the conditional quartiles. Taking Y_t to be a scalar for simplicity, the conditional pth quantile of Y_t given $\ddot{Z}^{t-1}$ is given by a function $Q_{p,t}$ such that

$$P_o[Y_t \le Q_{p,t}(\ddot{Z}^{t-1}) \mid \ddot{Z}^{t-1}] = p \quad 0 \le p \le 1\,.$$

The conditional median $Q_{.5,t}(\ddot{Z}^{t-1})$ provides a minimum mean absolute error prediction of Y_t given $\ddot{Z}^{t-1}$. The interquartile range $Q_{.75,t}(\ddot{Z}^{t-1}) - Q_{.25,t}(\ddot{Z}^{t-1})$ is a measure of the uncertainty attaching to prediction of Y_t based on $\ddot{Z}^{t-1}$.

2 Artificial Neural Networks and Parametric Models

A leading example of the networks under consideration is the standard hidden layer feedforward network, with output given by

$$f(x,\theta) = \beta_0 + \sum_{j=1}^{q} G(\tilde{x}'\gamma_j)\beta_j\,,$$

where x represents an $r \times 1$ vector of real-valued network inputs, $\tilde{x} \equiv (1,x')'$ is the augmented input vector containing inputs x together with a unit bias input, γ_j is an $(r+1) \times 1$ vector of real-valued weights (connection strengths) from the input layer to hidden unit j, $j = 1, \ldots, q$ (q is the number of hidden units), G is the common hidden unit activation function (e.g., the logistic, $G(a) = 1/[1+\exp(-a)]$), β_j is a real-valued hidden to output unit weight, $j = 1, \ldots, q$, and β_0 is the hidden to output bias. We represent the entire vector of network weights as θ. For simplicity, we sometimes work with a single output.

Assumption A.3: Network architecture is such that for each $t = 1, 2, \ldots$, network output is given by $f_t : I\!R^{vt} \times \Theta \to I\!R^k$, $k \in I\!N$, where Θ is a compact subset of $I\!R^s$, $s \in I\!N$. Further, for each z^t in $I\!R^{vt}$, $f_t(z^t, \cdot)$ is continuous on Θ, and for each θ in Θ, $f_t(\cdot, \theta)$ is measurable-$\mathcal{B}^{vt}$, $t = 1, 2, \ldots$. □

Note that we permit network output to depend on the entire history of inputs and targets. This permits treatment of recurrent networks. Also note that the number of network outputs is k, which need not equal the number of targets, l. The opportunities afforded by this flexibility are discussed in Section 3.

3 Associating Conditional Densities With Network Models

Fundamental to our unification of network learning within the framework of parametric statistical estimation is the association of a conditional probability density with any network output function. We do this by making use of a sequence of function $\{\phi_t\}$ satisfying the following condition.

Assumption A.4: Let $k, l \in I\!N$ be given. $\{\phi_t : I\!R^l \times I\!R^k \to I\!R^+\}$ is a sequence of functions such that: for each y in $I\!R^l$ we have that $\phi_t(y, \cdot)$ is continuous on $I\!R^k$; for each $\tau \in I\!R^k$ we have that $\phi_t(\cdot, \tau)$ is measurable-$\mathcal{B}^l$; and for some σ-finite measure ζ_t on $(I\!R^l, \mathcal{B}^l)$

$$\int \phi_t(y, f_t(z^t, \theta))\zeta_t(dy) = 1 \tag{3.1}$$

for all $z^t = (y, \ddot{z}^{t-1})$ in $I\!R^{vt}$ and all θ in Θ, $t = 1, 2, \ldots$. □

With Assumption A.4, the function h_t defined as

$$h_t(z^t, \theta) \equiv \phi_t(y, f_t(z^t, \theta))$$

is the desired density associated with f_t. It is a conditional density function for Y_t given $\ddot{Z}^{t-1}$ for all θ in Θ because by construction, it is non-negative and integrates to 1 over $I\!R^l$ for every $\ddot{z}^{t-1} \in I\!R^{vt-1}$ and every θ in Θ. The function $\theta \to h_t(z^t, \theta)$ is called a "(conditional) likelihood function," and $h_t(z^t, \theta)$ is called "the conditional likelihood of y given $\ddot{z}^{t-1}$ at θ," or simply "the likelihood."

For the remainder of the discussion, we restrict attention to the case in which f_t does not depend on y. We henceforth write $f_t(\ddot{z}^{t-1}, \theta)$ in place of $f_t(z^t, \theta)$. This is appropriate for supervised training of feedforward and recurrent networks. Unsupervised training of such networks is possible, but for brevity will not be discussed here. See White (1994) for discussion of this possibility.

3.1 Location Families

Most applications of feedforward and recurrent networks have either implicitly or explicitly focused attention on the conditional expectation of Y_t, in which case it is appropriate to choose $\phi(y, \cdot)$ as a location family of densities, with τ the location parameter. A leading example is the standard normal location family, for which $\phi(y, \tau) = (2\pi)^{-1/2}\exp[-(y-\tau)^2/2]$, $\tau \in I\!R$. Replacing τ with $f_t(\ddot{z}^{t-1}, \theta)$ gives likelihood

$$h_t(z^t, \theta) = (2\pi)^{-1/2}\exp[-(y - f_t(\ddot{z}^{t-1}, \theta))^2/2] .$$

This choice leads directly to familiar back-propagation learning.

Another important and useful location family is the linear exponential family

$$\phi(y,\tau)=\exp[a(\tau)+b(y)+y'c(\tau)]\ ,$$

with functions a , b and c chosen so that for some σ-finite measure ζ

$$\int\phi(y,\tau)\zeta(dy)=1$$

and

$$\int y\phi(y,\tau)\zeta(dy)=\tau\ .$$

A potentially serious drawback of the exponential location family is its extreme sensitivity to outliers. This sensitivity is measured by the "influence function" (Hampel 1968, 1974; Huber 1981, Section 1.5). It can be shown that the influence function is proportional to $-\partial\log\phi(y,\tau)/\partial\tau$ (with y and τ now scalar for simplicity). For the exponential family

$$\partial\log\phi(y,\tau)/\partial\tau=\partial a(\tau)/\partial\tau+y\partial c(\tau)/\partial\tau\ .$$

The restriction that $\int y\phi(y,\tau)\zeta(dy)=\tau$ can be shown to imply that $\partial a(\tau)/\partial\tau=-\tau\partial c(\tau)/\partial\tau$ (e.g. White 1993, Lemma 6.7) so that

$$\partial\log\phi(y,\tau)/\partial\tau=(\partial c(\tau)/\partial\tau)(y-\tau)\ .$$

This function is unbounded in y, with the implication (as discussed by Hampel 1968, 1974, and Huber 1981) that the results of learning based on this family can be grossly affected by just a few outliers.

By picking ϕ in such a way that the influence function is bounded, one can achieve "robust" learning procedures that are affected much less adversely by outliers. Huber (1981, p. 71) gives some location families that lead to more robust learning:

$$\phi(y,\tau)=\exp[-(y-\tau)]/(1+\exp[-(y-\tau)])^2$$

$$\phi(y,\tau)=1/[\pi(1+(y-\tau)^2)]$$

$$\begin{aligned}\phi(y,\tau)&=c\exp[-(y-\tau)^2/2] & |y-\tau|&=<c\\ &=c\exp[-|y-\tau|]+c^2/2 & |y-\tau|&>c\ ,\end{aligned}$$

where c is now a constant chosen so that $\phi(\cdot,\tau)$ integrates to 1 over $\mathbb{R}$.

To this list we add Student's t-distribution with d degrees of freedom,

$$\phi(y,\tau)=(d\pi)^{-1/2}(\Gamma[(d+1)/2]/\Gamma(d/2))(1+(y-\tau)^2/d)^{-(d+1)/2}\ ,$$

where $\Gamma(\cdot)$ denotes the standard gamma function. The t-distribution links the Cauchy and normal distributions, as d = 1 gives the Cauchy, while $d=\infty$ gives the normal. The influence function is bounded for all $d<\infty$.

3.2 Location-Scale Families

Consideration of conditional variance is important in such applications as quality control, where the variance measures the variability of a production process, or in financial market applications, where the variance measures the riskiness of an asset. In such cases the same approach applies. The idea is to complement an l-output network focused on describing the conditional location of an l-variate target with a network focused on describing the conditional dispersion (e.g., variance) of the target. With multiple targets, the complementary network measures the conditional co-dispersion (e.g., the conditional covariance) of the targets. In this case, $k = l + l(l+1)/2$.

Specifically, suppose network 1 produces output $f_t^1(\ddot{z}^{t-1}, \theta_1)$, while network 2 produces output $f_t^2(\ddot{z}^{t-1}, \theta_2)$, where θ_1 and θ_2 are weight vectors associated with each of the two separate networks. If network one has l outputs devoted to hitting a target Y_t of l components, then network 2 will have $l(l+1)/2$ outputs (targeted for example of the non-redundant elements of $(Y_t - f_t^1(\ddot{Z}^{t-1}, \theta_1))(Y_t - f_t^1(\ddot{Z}^{t-1}, \theta_1))'$) to capture the co-dispersion among the targets.

To associate a conditional density h_t with these output functions, it suffices first to specify any location-scale family of probability densities using $\phi(\cdot, \tau)$, where now $\tau' = (\mu', \sigma^{2\prime}), \sigma^2 \equiv \text{vech}\, \Sigma$, with vech denoting the "vec half" operator that puts the upper triangle of an $l \times l$ symmetric matrix Σ into an $l(l+1)/2$ column vector.

We replace μ by $f_t^1(\ddot{z}^{t-1}, \theta_1)$ and σ^2 by $f_t^2(\ddot{z}^{t-1}, \theta_2)$ to obtain likelihood

$$h_t(z^t, \theta) = \phi(y, f_t^1(\ddot{z}^{t-1}, \theta_1), f_t^2(\ddot{z}^{t-1}, \theta_2)),$$

with $\theta = (\theta_1', \theta_2')'$.

For example, the multivariate normal family (with y an $l \times 1$ vector)

$$\phi(y, \tau) = (2\pi)^{-l/2} (\det \Sigma)^{-1/2} \exp[-(y-\mu)' \Sigma^{-1} (y-\mu)/2]$$

delivers likelihood

$$h_t(z^t, \theta) = (2\pi)^{-l/2} (\det \text{vech}_l^{-1} f_t^2(\ddot{z}^{t-1}, \theta_2))^{-1}$$

$$\times \exp[(y_t - f_t^1(\ddot{z}^{t-1}, \theta_1))' [\text{vech}_l^{-1} f_t^2(\ddot{z}^{t-1}, \theta_2)]^{-1} (y_t - f_t^1(\ddot{z}^{t-1}, \theta_2))/2],$$

where vech_l^{-1} is the inverse of vech, creating a symmetric $l \times l$ matrix Σ from an $l(l+1)/2 \times 1$ vector σ^2. Note that care may be needed to ensure that f_t^2 takes on admissible values: if $\Sigma = \text{vech}_l^{-1} f_t^2 = [\sigma_{ij}]$, it is necessary that $\sigma_{ii} \geq 0$, $\sigma_{ij} \leq \sigma_{ii}^{1/2} \sigma_{jj}^{1/2}$. This may be accomplished by suitable restriction of Θ_2 (the parameter space containing θ_2) and/or suitable choice of output activation functions.

More robust learning methods can be achieved by associating network output with a multivariate Student's t density with d degrees of freedom,

$$\phi(y, \tau) = (d)^{d/2} (d/(d-2))^{-l/2} (\det \Sigma)^{-1/2} (\Gamma[(d+l)/2]\, \Gamma(d/2))$$

$$\times [d + (y-\mu)' \Sigma^{-1} (y-\mu)(d/(d-2))]^{-(l-d)/2}.$$

3.3 A Quantile Family

When interest attaches to conditional quantiles $Q_{p,t}$, it can be shown (White 1991, 1993) that an appropriate choice for $\phi(y, \tau)$ is of the form $\phi(y, \tau)$

$$= c \exp[-|y-\tau|(p1[y-\tau \geq 0]+(1-p)1[y-\tau < 0])],$$

where c is a constant ensuring integration to one in (3.1). As in the location case, $f_t(\ddot{z}^{t-1}, \theta)$ replaces τ in $\phi(y, \tau)$ to obtain the density h_t. Conditional quantiles are useful in providing interval predictions (i.e. upper and lower bounds) that will contain the target being predicted with specified probability.

4 Information Theory and Learning

Let $(\Omega, \mathcal{F})$ be a measurable space and let P and Q be candidate data generating processes (i.e., probability measures) on $(\Omega, \mathcal{F})$.

Suppose we want to determine which of P or Q is responsible for generating a given realization $\omega \in \Omega$. Suppose that P and Q are both dominated by a σ-finite measure ν (this can always be ensured by taking $\nu=(P+Q)/2$), and let $g=dP/d\nu$ and $h=dQ/d\nu$ be the associated (Radon-Nikodým) density functions. Let $\omega \in \Omega$. Kullback and Leibler (1951) define the log density ratio $\log[g(\omega)/h(\omega)]$ as the *information in* ω *for discriminating between* P *and* Q. This quantity is fundamental in statistics, where it is known as the log-likelihood ratio, and is known to be optimal in a variety of senses for discriminating between P and Q (Neyman and Pearson 1933, Bahadur and Raghavachari 1970).

If the data (ω) are in fact generated by P then the expected value of $\log[g(\omega)/h(\omega)]$,

$$I(g:h) \equiv \int \log(g/h)\, g d\nu ,$$

represents the expected information for discriminating between P and Q (equivalently, g and h). The quantity $I(g:h)$ is called the *Kullback - Liebler Information Criterion* (KLIC). It is an information theoretic measure of the surprise experienced on average when we believe the world is described by h, and are then informed that in fact the world is described by g.

The KLIC is a generalization of the Shannon-Wiener (Shannon 1948; Wiener 1948) information (entropy). When P is dominated by Q, the density $p=dP/dQ$ is defined. The Shannon-Wiener entropy of p is

$$\int p \log p \, dQ .$$

The sense in which the KLIC generalizes Shannon-Wiener entropy is given by the following result.

Proposition 4.1: *Let* $(\Omega, \mathcal{F})$ *be a measurable space, let* P *and* Q *be probability measures on* $(\Omega, \mathcal{F})$ *such that* P *is dominated by* Q*, and let* ν *be a* σ*-finite measure on* $(\Omega, \mathcal{F})$ *dominating both* P *and* Q*. Let* $S_P \equiv \operatorname{supp} P$ *(the support of* P*), and let* $p = dP/dQ$, $g = dP/d\nu$*, and* $h = dQ/d\nu$*. Then*

$$\int_{S_P} p \log p \, dQ = I(g:h) \equiv \int_{S_P} g \log(g/h) \, d\nu . \quad \square$$

The proofs of this and subsequent results may be found in White (1994).

The following well-known result establishes a crucial property of the KLIC, namely that the information $I(g:h)$ is positive, except in the case that $g = h$, in which case the information $I(g:h)$ is zero. Formally we have

Theorem 4.2: *Let* $(\Omega, \mathcal{F})$ *be a measurable space, let* P *and* Q *be probability measures on* $(\Omega, \mathcal{F})$ *and let* ν *be a* σ*-finite measure on* $(\Omega, \mathcal{F})$ *dominating* P *and* Q*. Put* $g = dP/d\nu$ *and* $h = dQ/d\nu$*. Then* $I(g:h) \equiv \int \log(g/h) g \, d\nu \geq 0$ *and* $I(g:h) = 0$ *if and only if* $g = h$ *almost everywhere* $-\nu$. $\square$

We saw in the preceding section that a density can be associated with the output function of any network indexed by weights θ. For the present discussion, let this density be denoted h_θ. With ν properly chosen, one can define a probability measure Q_θ as $Q_\theta(F) = \int_F h_\theta d\nu$ for $F \in \mathcal{F}$. The collection of all such measures,

$$\mathcal{Q} \equiv \{ Q_\theta : \theta \in \Theta \} ,$$

will be called the "parametric probability model generated by the network" or, more briefly, the "network probability model."

If, as can generally be arranged, the σ-finite measure ν dominates P and every member of $\mathcal{Q}$, then the KLIC $I(g:h_\theta)$ is defined for each $\theta \in \Theta$ and obeys Theorem 4.2. It follows that a choice for network weights with an appealing information-theoretic interpretation is the value θ^* solving the problem

$$\min_{\theta \in \Theta} I(g:h_\theta) .$$

The information-theoretically optimal network gives h_{θ^*}, as h_{θ^*} causes us the least expected surprise when we are informed of the true density g.

We can write

$$\begin{aligned} I(g:h_\theta) &= \int \log(g/h_\theta) g d\nu \\ &= \int (\log g) g d\nu - \int (\log h_\theta) g d\nu \\ &= E(\log g) - E(\log h_\theta) , \end{aligned}$$

where E denotes expectation with respect to the data generating measure P. Because the first term does not involve θ, minimization of $I(g:h_\theta)$ is equivalent to maximization of

$$\mathcal{L}(\theta) \equiv E(\log h_\theta)\,,$$

the "expected log-likelihood." By virtue of the law of large numbers, the expectation operator E can be approximated by an average of suitable observations $\{h_{t\theta}\}$, enabling us to approximate θ^* by a solution $\hat{\theta}_n$ to the problem

$$\max_{\theta\in\Theta} \hat{\mathcal{L}}_n(\theta) = n^{-1} \sum_{t=1}^{n} \log h_{t\theta}\,.$$

The "empirical log-likelihood" $\hat{\mathcal{L}}_n(\theta)$ is computable; therefore, the remaining issues are statistical (What are the properties of a solution $\hat{\theta}_n$?) and computational (What methods are available to obtain $\hat{\theta}_n$?). We take up statistical issues in Section 5 and computational issues in Section 6.

To bring this discussion to bear on the specific setup of Sections 1-3, put $(\Omega, \mathcal{F}) = (\mathbb{R}^{vn}, \mathcal{B}^{vn})$, take $g = g^n = dP_o^n / dv^n$ and $h_\theta = h_\theta^n = \Pi_{t=1}^n h_{t\theta}\ddot{g}_t$, with $h_{t\theta} = h_t(\cdot, \theta)$ (as discussed at the end of Section 3) and $\ddot{g}_t$ denoting the conditional density of X_t given Z^{t-1}. Optimally informative weights θ_n^* solve the problem

$$\min_{\theta\in\Theta} I^n(g^n : h_\theta^n) \equiv \int (\log g^n / h_\theta^n) g^n dv^n\,,$$

or the equivalent problem

$$\max_{\theta\in\Theta} \mathcal{L}_n(\theta) \equiv E(\log h_\theta^n)\,,$$

or the equivalent problem

$$\max_{\theta\in\Theta} \bar{\mathcal{L}}_n(\theta) \equiv n^{-1} \sum_{t=1}^{n} E(\log h_{t\theta})\,. \tag{4.1}$$

5 Statistical Estimation

If $\{h_{t\theta}\}$ is a sequence of suitably behaved random variables, then the law of large numbers guarantees that

$$\lim_{n\to\infty} n^{-1} \sum_{t=1}^{n} [\log h_{t\theta} - E(\log h_{t\theta})] = 0 \quad a.s. - P_o\,,$$

where $a.s. - P_o$ stands for "almost surely in P_o-probability;" that is,

$$P_o\{\omega : n^{-1} \sum_{t=1}^{n} [\log h_{t\theta}(\omega) - E(\log h_{t\theta}(\cdot))] \to 0 \text{ as } n \to \infty\} = 1\,,$$

where $h_{t\theta}(\omega) \equiv h_t(Z^t(\omega), \theta)$. This says that while it can happen that one could observe a realized sequence $\{h_{t\theta}(\omega)\}$ for which convergence fails, the probability of this occurrence is zero. It is more likely that the book you are now reading will disappear by the time you finish this sentence, as this disappearance has non-zero (albeit negligible) probability.

Heuristically, then, a "quasi-maximum likelihood estimator" (QMLE) $\hat{\theta}_n$ solving the problem

$$\min_{\theta \in \Theta} \hat{L}_n(\theta) \equiv n^{-1} \sum_{t=1}^{n} \log h_{t\theta} \tag{5.1}$$

ought to provide a good approximation to the solution θ_n^* to the problem

$$\max_{\theta \in \Theta} \bar{L}_n(\theta) \equiv n^{-1} \sum_{t=1}^{n} E(\log h_{t\theta}) ,$$

and therefore to the problem of minimizing the KLIC.

5.1 Existence and Consistency

Existence of a solution to the problem (5.1) is guaranteed by the first result of this section.

Theorem 5.1: *Suppose that Assumptions A.1, A.3 and A.4 hold. Then for each* $n = 1, 2, \ldots$, *there exists a measurable function* $\hat{\theta}_n : \Omega \to \Theta$ *such that* $\hat{\theta}_n$ *solves the problem* $\max_{\theta \in \Theta} \hat{L}_n(\theta)$. □

We now add assumptions that permit statement of a convergence (consistency) result.

Assumption A.5: The sequence $\{ h_t : \Omega \times \Theta \to I\!R^+ \}$ is such that

(a) $E(\log h_{t\theta})$ exists and is finite for all $\theta \in \Theta$, $t = 1, 2, \ldots$;

(b) $\bar{L}_n(\theta) = n^{-1} \sum_{t=1}^{n} E(\log h_{t\theta})$ defines a function continuous on Θ uniformly in n; and

(c) $\sup_{\theta \in \Theta} | n^{-1} \sum_{t=1}^{n} \log h_{t\theta} - E(\log h_{t\theta}) | \to 0$ *a.s.* $-P_o$. □

Assumption A.6: $\{ \Theta_n^* \}$ is identifiable, where $\Theta_n^* = \{\theta^* \in \Theta \mid \bar{L}_n(\theta^*) \geq \bar{L}_n(\theta)$ for all $\theta \in \Theta\}$. $\{ \Theta_n^* \}$ is "identifiable" in the sense that $\{\bar{L}_n\}$ is such that $\rho(\theta, \Theta_n^*) \geq \delta > 0$ implies that for some $\varepsilon_\delta > 0$

$$\limsup_n \sup_{\theta^* \in \Theta_n^*} \bar{L}_n(\theta) - \bar{L}_n(\theta^*) < -\varepsilon_\delta ,$$

where ρ denotes the Euclidean metric on $I\!R^s$. □

Theorem 5.2: *Suppose that Assumptions A.1, A.3-A.5 and A.6 hold. Then* $\rho(\hat{\theta}_n, \Theta_n^*) \to 0$ *a.s.* $-P_o$. *In addition,* $\hat{L}_n(\hat{\theta}_n) - \bar{L}_n(\theta_n^*) \to 0$ *a.s.* $-P_o$ *for any sequence* $\{\theta_n^* \in \Theta_n^*\}$. □

In other words, network weights that solve the problem (5.1) are arbitrarily close to network weights that maximize $\bar{L}_n(\theta)$ for all n sufficiently large, with probability one. The weights maximizing $\bar{L}_n(\theta)$ have a fundamental information theoretic interpretation by virtue of the following result.

Theorem 5.3: *Suppose Assumptions A.1-A.6 hold and that for all $\theta \in \Theta$ we have $E(\log g_t / h_{t\theta}) < \infty$, $t=1,2,\ldots$. Then $\rho(\hat{\theta}_n, \Theta_n^\dagger) \to 0$ a.s. $-P_o$, where*

$$\Theta_n^* = \Theta_n^\dagger \equiv \{\theta^\dagger \in \Theta \mid I^n(g^n : h_{\theta^\dagger}^n) \leq I^n(g^n : h_\theta^n) \text{ for all } \theta \in \Theta\} \quad \square$$

5.2 Convergence in Distribution and Statistical Inference

Because $\hat{\theta}_n$ is a random vector, its behavior is described completely by its probability distribution. This distribution is usually complicated to obtain for given n, but can often be well approximated when n is large, i.e., in large samples. This approximation permits statistical inference to be conducted with approximate control exercised over the probability of committing the error of wrongly rejecting the null hypothesis (Type I error).

We add further assumptions appropriate for obtaining the desired large sample approximations.

Assumption A.6′: θ_n^* is the unique identifiable interior maximizer of $\bar{L}_n(\theta) = n^{-1} \sum_{t=1}^n E(\log h_{t\theta})$ on Θ, $n=1,2,\ldots$. $\square$

Assumption A.7:

(a) $h_t(Z^t, \cdot)$ is twice continuously differentiable on Θ a.s. $-P_o$.

(b) The elements of $|\nabla \log h_t(Z^t, \theta)|$ and $|\nabla^2 \log h_t(Z^t, \theta)|$ are each dominated by a function $d_t(Z^t)$ such that $E(d_t(Z^t)) < \infty$. $\square$

Assumption A.8:

(a) $\nabla^2 \bar{L}_n$ is continuous on Θ uniformly in n.

(b) $\sup_{\theta \in \Theta} n^{-1} \Sigma_{t=1}^n \nabla^2 \log h_{t\theta} - E(\nabla^2 \log h_{t\theta}) \to 0$ a.s. $-P_o$. $\square$

Assumption A.9: $A_n^* \equiv \nabla^2 \bar{L}_n(\theta_n^*)$ is non-singular uniformly in n. $\square$

Assumption A.10: $B_n^{*-1/2} \sqrt{n} \nabla \hat{L}_n(\theta_n^*) = B_n^{*-1/2} n^{-1/2} \Sigma_{t=1}^n \nabla \log h_t(Z^t, \theta_n^*) \xrightarrow{d} N(0, I_s)$, where $\{B_n^* \equiv E([\sqrt{n} \nabla \hat{L}_n(\theta_n^*)] [\sqrt{n} \nabla \hat{L}_n(\theta_n^*)]')\}$ is bounded and non-singular uniformly in n.

Theorem 5.4: *Suppose Assumptions A.1, A.3-A.5 and A.6′-A.10 hold. Then*

(a) $\sqrt{n}(\hat{\theta}_n - \theta_n^*) = A_n^{*-1} n^{-1/2} \sum_{t=1}^{n} \nabla \log h_t(Z^t, \theta_n^*) + o_{P_o}(1)$;

(b) $B_n^{*-1/2} A_n^* \sqrt{n}(\hat{\theta}_n - \theta_n^*) \xrightarrow{d} N(0, I_s)$. □

This knowledge makes it possible in principle to conduct statistical inference on the information-theoretically optimal weights θ_n^*. In particular, it will often be of interest to know whether or not certain elements of θ_n^* are zero, as when certain inputs are hypothesized to be irrelevant in influencing a given target.

Such hypotheses can be tested using the theory of inference for misspecified models developed by White (1982, 1992) and Gallant and White (1988). Formally, one tests the null hypothesis

$$H_o : r(\theta_n^*) = 0$$

against the alternative hypothesis

$$H_a : r(\theta_n^*) \neq 0 ,$$

where $r:\Theta \rightarrow I\!R^p$ is a (possibly nonlinear) function expressing the restrictions of interest. It follows from Theorem 5.4 and standard properties of the normal distribution that the test statistic

$$\mathcal{W}_n^* = n\, r(\hat{\theta}_n)'[R(\hat{\theta}_n) A_n^{*-1} B_n^* A_n^{*-1} R(\hat{\theta}_n)']^{-1} r(\hat{\theta}_n)$$

converges in distribution under H_o to the χ_p^2 distribution (chi-squared with p degrees of freedom), while $\mathcal{W}_n^* \rightarrow \infty$ almost surely under H_a, where $R(\theta)$ is the $p \times s$ Jacobian matrix of r with respect to θ.

A practical difficulty in implementing this procedure is that A_n^* and B_n^* are unknown. However, they can often be estimated sufficiently well by computable estimators, say $\hat{A}_n$ and $\hat{B}_n$. Replacing A_n^* and B_n^* with $\hat{A}_n$ and $\hat{B}_n$ in $\mathcal{W}_n^*$ leads to the statistic

$$\hat{\mathcal{W}}_n = n r(\hat{\theta}_n)'[R(\hat{\theta}_n) \hat{A}_n^{-1} \hat{B}_n \hat{A}_n^{-1} R(\hat{\theta}_n)']^{-1} r(\hat{\theta}_n)$$

which has the same properties as $\mathcal{W}_n^*$. An appropriate choice for $\hat{A}_n$ is

$$\hat{A}_n = n^{-1} \sum_{t=1}^{n} \nabla^2 \log h_t(Z^t, \hat{\theta}_n) .$$

An appropriate choice for $\hat{B}_n$ depends on P_o and the relationship between P_o and the network probability model. In certain contexts (e.g. $\{ Z_t \}$ i.i.d.), the choice

$$\hat{B}_n = n^{-1} \sum_{t=1}^{n} (\nabla \log h_t(Z^t, \hat{\theta}_n))\, (\nabla \log h_t(Z^t, \hat{\theta}_n))'$$

is appropriate. In other cases, more complicated estimators are required.

6 Computation

The results of the previous section justify seeking network weights that deliver an approximate solution to the problem

$$\max_{\theta\in\Theta} \hat{L}_n(\theta)=n^{-1}\sum_{t=1}^{n}\log h_{t\theta} . \tag{6.1}$$

Any method for solving this problem will do; because of its inherent nonlinearity, the range of possible approaches is especially broad. Possibilities include simulated annealing (e.g. Kirkpatrick, Gelatt and Vecchi 1983, Cerny 1985, Hajek 1985, 1988), the genetic algorithm (e.g. Holland 1975, David 1987, Goldberg 1989), multi-start methods (Rinnooy Kan, Boender and Timmer 1985) and a variety of other possibilities (e.g. Baba 1989, Styblinski and Tang 1990, etc.).

In this section we show how back-propagation-like methods can be used to find an approximate solution to the first order conditions necessary for an interior solution to (6.1),

$$\nabla\hat{L}_n(\theta)=n^{-1}\sum_{t=1}^{n}\nabla\log h_{t\theta}=0 .$$

When $\nabla\log h_{t\theta}$ depends only on a finite length (say $r\times 1$) subvector of Z^t, which we denote W_t (for "whatever"), we have a "Markov" case. For simplicity, suppose that h_t is well behaved enough that for some function ψ, $\psi(W_t,\theta)=\nabla\log h_t(Z^t,\theta)$ (Note that this rules out the recurrent network case; a treatment of this case is given in White 1994.)

The first order conditions are now

$$\begin{aligned}\nabla\hat{L}_n(\theta)&=n^{-1}\sum_{t=1}^{n}\psi(W_t,\theta)\\ &=\int\psi(w,\theta)\hat{Q}_n(dw)=0 ,\end{aligned} \tag{6.2}$$

where $\hat{Q}_n$ represents the empirical distribution of W_t, $t=1,\dots,n$:

$$\hat{Q}_n(w)\equiv(\#\text{ of times } W_t\leq w)/n.$$

As pointed out by White (1987), back-propagation is an application of the method of stochastic approximation (SA) proposed by Robbins and Monro (1951) for attempting to solve equations of the form (6.2). The SA algorithm has the form

$$\ddot{\theta}_{m+1}=\ddot{\theta}_m+a_m\psi(\ddot{W}_{m+1},\ddot{\theta}_m)\quad m=1,2,\dots, \tag{6.3}$$

where $\{\ddot{W}_m\}$ is a sequence of random variables drawn from the distribution $\hat{Q}_n$ and $\{a_m\}$ is an appropriately chosen (scalar) sequence of learning rates. The dependence properties of $\{\ddot{W}_m\}$ can be fairly general without destroying the convergence results we seek; however, it is feasible and very convenient to draw $\{ \ddot{W}_m \}$ independently.

In practice, this means that observations on $\ddot{W}_m$ are obtained by drawing from the observed values $w_1, \dots, w_n$ independently and with replacement. This can be formally expressed as

$$\ddot{W}_m = W_{T_m}(\omega),$$

where T_m is a random integer drawn from the set $\{ 1, \dots, n \}$ independently of other draws and with each possible value having probability $1/n$. When $\ddot{W}_m$ is selected in this manner, we refer to (6.3) as "re-sampled stochastic approximation", or "re-sampled back-propagation."

The next result describes the behavior of the recursion (6.3) in a general setting.

Theorem 6.1: *Let $(\Omega', \mathcal{F}', P')$ be a complete probability space such that the sequence of random variables $\{W_m: \Omega' \to \mathbb{R}^r\}$ is i.i.d. with distribution Q (so that $Q(B) = P'[W_n \in B]$ for all $B \in \mathcal{B}^r$, $n = 1, 2, \dots$).*

Let $\psi: \mathbb{R}^r \times \mathbb{R}^s \to \mathbb{R}^s$ be a measurable mapping such that for a given compact subset Θ of $\mathbb{R}^s$: (i) there exist functions $b: \Theta \to \mathbb{R}^+$, $c_1: \mathbb{R}^r \to \mathbb{R}^+$, $c_2: \mathbb{R}^r \to \mathbb{R}^+$ with b continuous on Θ, c_1 and c_2 measurable such that

$$| \psi(w, \theta) | \le b(\theta) c_1(dw) + c_2(w)$$

for all (w, θ) in $\mathbb{R}^r \times \Theta$; and (ii) there exist functions $\gamma_1: \mathbb{R}^+ \to \mathbb{R}^+$ and $c_3: \mathbb{R}^r \to \mathbb{R}^+$ such that $\gamma_1(u) \to 0$ as $u \to 0$, c_3 is measurable, and for each (w, θ_1, θ_2) in $\mathbb{R}^r \times \Theta \times \Theta$

$$| \psi(w, \theta_1) - \psi(w, \theta_2) | \le \gamma_1(|\theta_1 - \theta_2|) c_3(w),$$

where $|\cdot|$ denotes the Euclidean norm.

Suppose in addition that $\int (c_1(w) + c_2(w)) Q(dw) < \infty$, and for the sequence $\{a_m\}$ of positive real numbers such that $\sum_{m=1}^{\infty} a_m = \infty$ and $\sum_{m=0}^{\infty} a_m^2 < \infty$, define the sequence

$$\ddot{\theta}_{m+1} = \ddot{\theta}_m + a_m \psi(W_{m+1}, \ddot{\theta}_m), \; m = 0, 1, \dots;$$

the interpolated sequence

$$\theta^0(\tau) = (\tau_{m+1} - \tau) \ddot{\theta}_m / a_m + (\tau - \tau_m) \ddot{\theta}_{m+1} / a_m, \tau \in [\tau_m, \tau_{m+1}) \; m = 0, 1, \dots,$$

with $\tau_m \equiv \sum_{i=0}^{m-1} a_i$, $\tau_0 \equiv 0$; and the leftward shifts of θ^0,

$$\theta^m(\tau) = \theta^0(\tau + \tau_m), \quad \tau \ge 0, \quad m = 0, 1, \dots.$$

Let $\pi: \mathbb{R}^s \to \Theta$ be a projection mapping ($\pi(\theta) = \theta$ for $\theta \in \Theta$) and for simplicity, *let* $\ddot{\theta}_m$ *denote the projected sequence* $\pi(\ddot{\theta}_m)$ *and let* θ^0 *and* θ^m *denote the interpolation and leftward shift of the projected sequence respectively. Then*

(a) *There exists a* P'*-null set* Ω_0' *such that for* $\omega \notin \Omega_0'$, $\{\theta^m(\cdot)\}$ *is bounded and equicontinuous on bounded intervals, and* $\{\theta^m(\cdot)\}$ *has a convergent subsequence whose limit* $\theta(\cdot)$ *satisfies the ODE* $\dot{\theta} = \pi[\Psi(\theta)]$, $\Psi(\theta) \equiv \int \psi(w,\theta)Q(dw)$.

Let $\Theta^\dagger$ *be the set of locally asymptotically stable (in the sense of Liapounov) equilibria in* Θ *for this ODE with domain of attraction* $D(\Theta^\dagger) \subseteq \mathbb{R}^k$.

(b) *if* $\Theta \subseteq D(\Theta^\dagger)$, *then* $\ddot{\theta}_m \to \Theta^\dagger$ as $m \to \infty$ *a.s.* $-P'$.

(c) *If* Θ *is not contained in* $D(\Theta^\dagger)$ *but for each* $\omega \notin \Omega_0$, $\ddot{\theta}_m(\omega)$ *enters a compact subset of* $D(\Theta^\dagger)$ *infinitely often, then* $\ddot{\theta}_m \to \Theta^\dagger$ as $m \to \infty$ *a.s.* $-P'$.

(d) *Given the conditions in (c), if* $\Theta^\dagger$ *contains only finitely many points, there exists a measurable function* $\theta^\dagger : \Omega \times \Theta \to \Theta^\dagger$ *such that* $\ddot{\theta}_m(\omega') - \theta^\dagger(\omega', \ddot{\theta}_0) \to 0$ *as* $m \to \infty$ *for all* $\omega' \in F'$, $P'(F') = 1$. □

To apply this result, we add further suitable assumptions.

Assumption A.4′: Assumption A.4 holds, $h_t(Z^t, \cdot)$ is continuously differentiable *a.s.* $-P_o$, and there exists a sequence $\{\xi_t : \mathbb{R}^{vt} \to \mathbb{R}^r\}$ and a function $\psi : \mathbb{R}^r \times \Theta \to \mathbb{R}^s$ such that $\psi(\xi_t(z^t), \theta) = \nabla \log h_t(z^t, \theta)$, for all $z^t \in \mathbb{R}^{vt}$, $\theta \in \Theta$, $t = 1, 2, \ldots$, and ψ satisfies conditions (i) and (ii) of Theorem 6.1 with $E(c_1(W_t) + c_2(W_t)) < \infty$, $W_t \equiv \xi_t(Z^t)$, $t = 1, 2, \ldots$. □

Assumption B.1: For each $n = 1, 2, \ldots$, $\{\ddot{W}_{nm}, m = 1, 2, \ldots\}$ is a sequence of random variables independently and identically distributed as $\hat{Q}_n$. □

Assumption B.2: $\{a_m\}$ is a sequence of positive real numbers such that $\sum_{m=0}^{\infty} a_m = \infty$ and $\sum_{m=0}^{\infty} a_m^2 < \infty$. □

We now have sufficient structure to state the following result describing the convergence of re-sampled back-propagation.

Corollary 6.2: *Given Assumptions A.1, A.3, A.4′, B.1 and B.2, for each* $n = 1, 2, \ldots$ *and each* ω *in* Ω *the conclusions of Theorem 6.1 hold with the limit sequence* $\theta_n(\cdot, \omega)$ *of* $\{\theta_n^m(\cdot, \omega)\}$ *satisfying the ODE*

$$\dot{\theta} = \pi(\hat{\Psi}_n(\theta)), \; \hat{\Psi}_n(\theta) = \int \psi(w, \theta)\hat{Q}_n(dw) = n^{-1} \sum_{t=1}^{n} \nabla \log h_t(Z^t(\omega), \theta).$$

Further, if the conditions of Theorem 6.1(b), (c) or (d) hold, then for any sequence $\{\varepsilon_n > 0\}$ *there exists a sequence of integers* $\{m_n\}$, $m_n \to \infty$ *as* $n \to \infty$, *such that with* $\tilde{\theta}_n \equiv \ddot{\theta}_{n,m_n}$ *we have* $|\tilde{\theta}_n(\omega, \cdot) - \hat{\theta}_n^{\dagger}(\omega, \cdot, \ddot{\theta}_{n,0})| < \varepsilon_n$ *for all* n *sufficiently large a.s.* $-P'$, *where* $\hat{\theta}_n^{\dagger}(\omega, \cdot, \cdot): \Omega' \times \Theta \to \Theta_n^{\dagger}(\omega)$, *the set of solutions to* $\hat{\Psi}_n(\theta) = 0$. *When* $\hat{\theta}_n^{\dagger}(\omega, \omega', \ddot{\theta}_{n,0})$ *is the solution to (6.1), and Assumptions A.5 and A.6 also hold, then* $\rho(\tilde{\theta}_n(\omega, \omega'), \Theta_n^*) \to 0$. □

Although we shall not go into the details here, if $\{ a_m \}$ and $\{ m_n \}$ are properly chosen and some additional regularity conditions hold, then it can be shown that $\sqrt{n}(\tilde{\theta}_n - \theta_n^*) = \sqrt{n}(\hat{\theta}_n - \theta_n^*) + o_{P_o P'}(1)$, which implies that the conclusions of Theorem 5.4(ii) hold for $\sqrt{n}(\tilde{\theta}_n - \theta_n^*)$. For example, the choice $a_m \propto m^{-1}$ and $m_n \propto n^{1+\delta}$, $\delta > 0$ (together with the appropriate regularity conditions) suffice for $\varepsilon_n = o(n^{-1/2})$.

Another important use of $\tilde{\theta}_n$ is as a starting value for Newton iterations of the form

$$\hat{\theta}_n^{k+1} = \hat{\theta}_n^k + \hat{H}_n^k \hat{\Psi}_n(\hat{\theta}_n^k), \quad k = 0, 1, \ldots,$$

where $\hat{\theta}_n^0 = \tilde{\theta}_n$ and $\{ \hat{H}_n^k \}$ is an appropriately chosen sequence of negative definite matrices.

7 Practical Matters

7.1 When to Stop Training

For a network of given size, the previous discussion makes clear that from a statistical standpoint our ultimate goal must be to obtain $\hat{\theta}_n$. As the results on resampled back-propagation show, $\ddot{\theta}_m$ may converge to $\hat{\theta}_n$ as $m \to \infty$, so training can in principle continue indefinitely in pursuit of our goal. The same is true if one uses Newton (e.g. Gauss-Newton) methods in pursuit of $\hat{\theta}_n$. Thus in this statistical context, there is no such thing as "overtraining," because the closer one gets to $\hat{\theta}_n$, the better. The widespread concern in the artificial neural network literature about overtraining is irrelevant in the present context because for a network of fixed complexity, $\hat{\theta}_n$ is what one really is after. Concern about overtraining may in part result from confusion with the very real danger of overfitting. Overfitting is the subject of the next subsection, and statistically speaking, is a completely separate issue.

Given that overtraining is not a concern for us, we must still answer the question of when to stop training. The answer depends on the method of training, but because of the typically non-concave nature of $\hat{L}_n(\theta)$, it is sensible only to consider multistart searches. The general multistart procedures has the following steps: (1) draw a random weight vector θ_i from the uniform distribution on Θ; (2) carry out local search from θ_i until a local stopping rule is enforced; (3) keep the result of (2) if it is the best so far; (4) iterate (1)-(3) until a global stopping rule is enforced.

Now consider the local stopping rule. One possibility is to periodically examine the magnitude of $\nabla \hat{L}_n(\hat{\theta}^k)$, where $\hat{\theta}^k$ is the weight vector for the current (kth) "epoch" (e.g., a Gauss-Newton step or a resampling epoch of size n), and to stop training when $\nabla \hat{L}_n(\hat{\theta}^k)$ is sufficiently close to zero in some suitable metric, because $\nabla \hat{L}_n(\theta) = 0$ is a necessary condition for a local maximum interior to Θ. When the number of weights s is large, this can be a costly operation.

Instead, it is usually cheap and effective to monitor $\hat{\Delta}_n^k = \exp \hat{L}_n(\hat{\theta}^k) - \exp \hat{L}_n(\hat{\theta}^{k-1})$, where $\hat{\theta}^k$ is the weight vector at the end of epoch k, and to stop local search when

$$c^k = \hat{\Delta}_n^k / [1 + \exp \hat{L}_n(\hat{\theta}^k)]$$

is small. When $\exp \hat{L}_n(\hat{\theta}^k)$ is close to zero, c^k is small when $\hat{\Delta}_n^k$ is small absolutely, while when $\exp \hat{L}_n(\hat{\theta}^k)$ is large, c^k is small when $\hat{\Delta}_n^k$ is small relative to $\exp \hat{L}_n(\hat{\theta}^k)$. While not foolproof, this procedure at least provides reasonable insurance against useless wheel-spinning.

7.2 When To Stop Growing

An essential feature of artificial neural networks is the considerable flexibility provided by varying the number of intermediate (non-input/non-output) units. When there is only a finite amount of data available, care must be taken to use a network of appropriate complexity: too complex a network will overfit the data and provide poor generalization, while too simple a network can fail to extract useful regularities from the data.

Let $\hat{L}_n(\hat{\theta}_n, s)$ denote the best empirical log-likelihood for a network with s weights. By itself, $\hat{L}_n(\hat{\theta}_n, s)$ gives us no useful guidance about the appropriateness of a particular network complexity. Larger networks can always fit the data better than smaller networks, so if we have done a good job of finding $\hat{\theta}_n$ for a given complexity, $\hat{L}_n(\hat{\theta}_n, s)$ will essentially always be larger for larger networks than for smaller networks. The problem is that $\hat{L}_n(\hat{\theta}_n, s)$ is a biased (over-optimistic) measure $\bar{L}_n(\hat{\theta}_n^*, s)$, which represents expected performance from an optimal network with s weights, for data outside the training set.

A variety of theoretical approaches exists for estimating the bias of $\hat{L}_n(\hat{\theta}_n, s)$. Each of these approaches leads to a penalty for network complexity of the form

$$\pi(s, n) = s\rho_n / n ,$$

where ρ_n takes different forms for the different approaches. Three leading possibilities, in order of their conservativism, are the Schwarz Information Criterion (SIC) with $\rho_n = (\tfrac{1}{2}) \log n$ (Schwarz 1978), the Hannan-Quinn Information Criterion (HQIC) with $\rho_n = \log \log n$ (Hannan and Quinn 1979), and the Akaike Information Criterion (AIC), with $\rho_n = 1$ (Akaike 1973).

Use of these criteria leads to choosing the network for which the complexity-penalized empirical log-likelihood

$$\hat{\mathcal{L}}_n(\hat{\theta}_n, s) - s p_n / n$$

is greatest.

Direct methods for computing unbiased measures of expected performance are generally variants of the method of cross-validation (Stone 1973, Wahba 1974). The basic idea is simple: calculate an estimate of $\bar{\mathcal{L}}_n(\theta_n^*, s)$ from data not used to obtain $\hat{\theta}_n$. An easy way to do this is to split the available data set randomly into two parts: a training set, and a cross-validation set. The random allocation is important for ensuring that the same data relationships exist in each data set. Let the training set have n observations $t = 1, \ldots, n$ and let the cross-validation set have m observations, $t = n+1, \ldots, n+m$. Then a relatively unbiased estimate of $\bar{\mathcal{L}}_n(\theta_n^*, s)$ can be computed as

$$\ddot{\mathcal{L}}_n(\hat{\theta}_n, s) = m^{-1} \sum_{t=n+1}^{n+m} \log h_{t\hat{\theta}_n}(s),$$

where $h_{t\theta}(s)$ indicates the likelihood associated with a network having s weights. Note that the t index in the sum above runs over observations in the cross-validation dataset, while the weights used are those from the training dataset.

8 Summary

Putting together all of the methods described in the preceding sections gives a practical and comprehensive framework for network learning including supervised and unsupervised methods for feedforward and recurrent networks. For reasons of brevity we have focused on the supervised training case, and in Section 7 restricted attention to feedforward networks. Discussion of more general possibilities can be found in White (1994). Further useful background is available in White (1993).

In Section 1 we describe various objects appropriate for learning, and in Section 2, we showed how artificial neural networks can be viewed as parametric statistical models directed toward these objects of interest. In Section 3, we saw how a probability density can be associated with the output of any network, and in Section 4, we showed how these density functions can be used to define weights θ_n^* indexing an information-theoretically optimal approximation to the object of interest. In Section 5 we studied statistical properties of the network quasi-maximum likelihood estimator $\hat{\theta}_n$ which approximates θ_n^*. Computational methods for obtaining $\hat{\theta}_n$ are described in Section 6, including re-sampled back-propagation. Section 7 contains some recommendations useful for practical implementation of the methods studied here.

While the methods described here cover a lot of ground, they still leave out of account a variety of useful approaches to network learning. Still, we hope that our theory may provide a starting point and useful frame of reference for enhancing and further extending the theory and practice of artificial neural network learning.

Acknowledgements

Support from IBM Corporation and the National Science Foundation under grants SES-8921382 and SES-9209023 is gratefully acknowledged. The author wishes to thank Max Stinchcombe for helpful discussions.

References

Akaike, H. (1973), "Information Theory and an Extension of the Maximum Likelihood Principle," in B.N. Petrov and F.Csaki, eds., *Second International Symposium on Information Theory*. Budapest: Akademiai Kiado, pp. 267-281.

Baba, N (1989), "A New Approach for Finding the Global Minimum of Error Function of Neural Networks," *Neural Networks* 2, 367-374.

Bahadur, and Raghavachari (1970), "Some Asymptotic Properties of Likelihood Ratios on General Spaces," *Proceeding of the Sixth Berkeley Symposium on Mathematical Statistics and Probability*, vol. 1. Berkeley: University of California Press, pp. 129-152.

Cerny, V. (1985), "Thermodynamical Approach to the Traveling Salesman Problem: An Efficient Simulation Algorithm, I" *Journal of Optimization Theory and Applications* 45, 41-51.

Gallant, A.R. and H. White (1988). *A Unified Theory of Estimation and Inference for Nonlinear Dynamic Models*. Oxford: Basil Blackwell.

Goldberg, D. (1989). *Genetic Algorithms in Search, Optimization and Machine Learning*. Reading, MA: Addison-Wesley.

Hajek, B. (1985), "A Tutorial Survey of Theory and Applications of Simulated Annealing," in *Proceedings of the 24th IEEE Conference on Decision and Control*, pp. 755-760.

Hajek, B. (1988), "Cooling Schedules for Optimal Annealing," *Mathematics of Operations Research* 13, 311-329.

Hampel, F. (1968), "Contributions to the Theory of Robust Estimation," University of California, Berkeley, Ph.D. Dissertation.

Hampel, F. (1974), "The Influence Curve and its Role in Robust Estimation," *Journal of the American Statistical Association* 62, 1179-1186.

Hannan, E.J. and B.G. Quinn (1979), "The Determination of the Order of an Autoregression," *Journal of the Royal Statistical Society, Series* B 41, 190-195.

Huber, P. (1981), *Robust Statistics*. New York: Wiley.

Kirkpatrick, S., C.D. Gelatt, Jr. and M.P. Vecchi (1983), "Optimization by Simulated Annealing," *Science* 220, 671-680.

Kullback, L. and R.A. Leibler (1951), "On Information and Sufficiency," *Annals of Mathematical Statistics* 22, 79-86.

Neyman, J. and E.S. Pearson (1933), "On the Problem of the Most Efficient Tests of Statistical Hypotheses," *Philosophical Transactions of the Royal Society* A 236, 333-380.

Rinnooy Kan, A.G.H., C.G.E. Boender and G.Th. Timmer (1985), "A Stochastic Approach to Global Optimization," in K. Schittkowski, e.d., *Computational Mathematical Programming*, NATO ASI Series F15. Berlin: Springer-Verlag, pp. 281-308.

Robbins, H. and S. Monro (1951) "A Stochastic Approximation Method," *Annals of Mathematical Statistics* 22, 400-407.

Schwarz, G. (1978), "Estimating the Dimension of a Model, " *The Annals of Statistics* 6, 461-464.

Shannon, C.E. (1948), "A Mathematical Theory of Communication," *Bell System Technical Journal* 27, 379-423, 623-656.

Stone, M. (1974), "Cross-Validitory Choice and Assessment of Statistical Predictions," *Journal of the Royal Statistical Society, Series B* 36, 111-133.

Styblinski, M.A. and T.-S. Tang (1990), "Experiments in Nonconvex Optimization: Stochastic Approximation with Function Smoothing and Simulated Annealing," *Neural Networks*, 3, 467-483.

Wahba, G. (1975), "Smoothing Noisy Data with Spline Functions," *Numerical Mathematics* 24, 383-393.

White, H. (1982), "Maximum Likelihood Estimation of Misspecified Models," *Econometrica*, 50, 1-25.

White, H. (1987), "Some Asymptotic Results for Back-Propagation," in *Proceedings of the IEEE First International Conference on Neural Networks*, San Diego. New York: IEEE Press, pp. III:261-266.

White, H. (1991), "Nonparametric Estimation of Conditional Quantiles Using Neural Networks," in C. Page and R. LePage eds., *Proceedings of the Twenty-Second Symposium on the Interface*. New York: Springer-Verlag, pp. 190-199.

White, H. (1993), *Estimation, Inference and Specification Analysis*. New York: Cambridge University Press (in press).

White, H. (1994), "Parametric Statistial Estimation With Artificial Neural Networks," in P. Smolensky, M.C. Mozer and D.E. Rumelhart, eds., *Mathematical Perspectives on Neural Networks*. Hilldale, NJ: L. Erlbaum Associates (to appear).

Wiener, N. (1948), *Cybernetics*. New York: Wiley.

Prediction Risk and Architecture Selection for Neural Networks

John Moody

Oregon Graduate Institute, Department of Computer Science and Engineering, P.O. Box 91000, Portland, OR 97291–1000, Email: moody@cse.ogi.edu

Abstract. We describe two important sets of tools for neural network modeling: prediction risk estimation and network architecture selection. Prediction risk is defined as the expected performance of an estimator in predicting new observations. Estimated prediction risk can be used both for estimating the quality of model predictions and for model selection. Prediction risk estimation and model selection are especially important for problems with limited data. Techniques for estimating prediction risk include data resampling algorithms such as *nonlinear cross–validation (NCV)* and algebraic formulae such as the *predicted squared error (PSE)* and *generalized prediction error (GPE)*. We show that exhaustive search over the space of network architectures is computationally infeasible even for networks of modest size. This motivates the use of *heuristic* strategies that dramatically reduce the search complexity. These strategies employ directed search algorithms, such as selecting the number of nodes via *sequential network construction (SNC)* and pruning inputs and weights via *sensitivity based pruning (SBP)* and *optimal brain damage (OBD)* respectively.

Keywords. prediction risk, network architecture selection, cross–validation (CV), nonlinear cross–validation (NCV), predicted squared error (PSE), generalized prediction error (GPE), effective number of parameters, heuristic search, sequential network construction (SNC), pruning, sensitivity based pruning (SBP), optimal brain damage (OBD).

1 Introduction and Motivation

This paper describes two important sets of tools for neural network modeling: prediction risk estimation and network architecture selection. Prediction risk is defined as the expected performance of an estimator in predicting new observations. While estimating prediction risk is important in its own right for providing a means of estimating the expected error for predictions made by a network, it is also an important tool for model selection.

In this section, we motivate the need for neural network architecture selection techniques and survey various selection criteria. Section 2 introduces prediction risk, while sections 3 and 4 present prediction risk estimation techniques, including test set validation, *nonlinear cross-validation (NCV)*, the *predicted squared error (PSE)*, and the *generalized prediction error (GPE)*. Section 5 describes architecture selection for perceptron architectures and the complexity and impossibility of exhaustive search over the space of architectures. Section 6 describes some computationally feasible heuristic search strategies, including determining the number of nodes via *sequential network construction (SNC)*, *sensitivity based pruning (SBP)* of inputs, and *optimal brain damage (OBD)* pruning of weights.

1.1 Nonparametric Modeling with Limited Data

Many data modeling problems are characterized by two difficulties: (1) the absence of a complete *a priori* model of the data generation process (such as the models frequently available in physics) and (2) by a limited quantity of data. When constructing statistical models for such applications, the issues of model selection and estimation of generalization ability or *prediction risk* are crucial and must be addressed in order to construct a near optimal model.

When a complete *a priori* model for the data generation process does not exist, one often adopts a *nonparametric modeling* approach. In nonparametric modeling, elements of a class of functions known to have good approximation properties, such as smoothing splines (for one or two dimensional problems) or neural networks (for higher dimensional problems), are used to fit the data. An element of this class (e.g., a particular neural network) is then chosen which "best fits" the data.

The notion of "best fits" can be precisely defined via an objective criterion, such as *maximum a posteriori probability (MAP)*, minimum *Bayesian information criterion (BIC)* (Akaike, 1977; Schwartz, 1978), *minimum description length (MDL)* (Rissanen, 1978), or *minimum prediction risk (P)*. In this paper, we focus on the prediction risk as our selection criterion for two reasons. First, it is straightforward to compute, and second, it provides more information than selection criteria like MAP, BIC, or MDL, since it tells us how much confidence to put in predictions produced by our best model.

The restriction of limited data makes the model selection and prediction risk estimation problems more difficult. A limited training set results in a more severe bias / variance (or underfitting vs overfitting) tradeoff (see for example Geman, Bienenstock and Doursat (1992)), so the model selection problem is both more challenging and more crucial. In particular, it is easier to overfit a small training set, so care must be taken not to select a model which is too large.

The expected training and test errors and the bias / variance tradeoff for finite training samples as a function of model size are illustrated in Figure 1.

Also, limited data sets make prediction risk estimation more difficult if there is not enough data available to hold out a sufficiently large independent test sample. In these situations, one must use alternative approaches that enable the estimation of prediction risk from the training data alone, such as data resampling and algebraic estimation techniques. Data resampling methods include nonlinear refinements of *v–fold cross–validation (NCV)* and *bootstrap estimation* (see section 3.3),

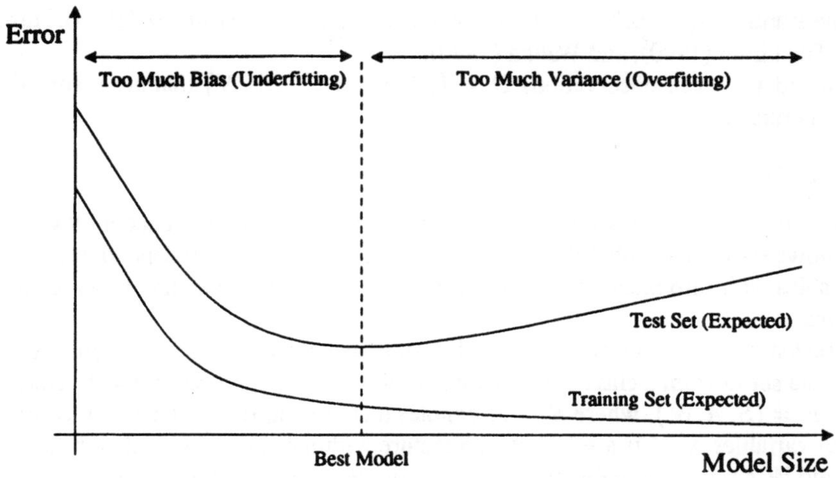

Figure 1: Idealized depiction of the expected training error and expected test error (prediction risk) versus model size for models trained on a fixed finite training sample. Note the regions of underfitting (high model bias) and overfitting (high model variance). Model selection techniques attempt to find the optimal tradeoff between bias and variance. The optimal model corresponds to a global minimum of the expected test error or prediction risk curve. Since the prediction risk can not be computed directly, it must be estimated. Examples of actual (not expected) training error, test error, and estimated prediction risk curves can be found in Utans and Moody (1991), Moody and Utans (1992), and Moody and Yarvin (1992).

while algebraic estimates in the regression context include various formulae derived for linear models, for example *generalized cross-validation (GCV)* (Craven and Wahba, 1979; Golub, Heath and Wahba, 1979), Akaike's *final prediction error (FPE)* (Akaike, 1970), Akaike's *information criterion A (AIC)* (Akaike, 1973), and *predicted squared error (PSE)* (see discussion in Barron (1984)), and the recently proposed *generalized prediction error (GPE)* for nonlinear models (Moody (1991; 1992; 1994)).

2 Prediction Risk

2.1 Prediction Risk for Squared Error Loss

The notion of generalization ability can be defined precisely as the *prediction risk*, the expected performance of an estimator is predicting new observations. We present here a brief, simplified description for the most typical case: a signal plus noise data generation model with a squared error loss function. (We present more general formulations in Moody (1992) and Moody (1994).) For comprehensive discussions of the standard approaches to prediction risk estimation, see Eubank (1988), Hastie and Tibshirani (1990), and Wahba (1990).

Consider a set of observations $D = \{(\vec{x}_j, t_j); j = 1 \ldots N\}$ that are assumed to be generated as

$$t_j = \mu(x_j) + \epsilon_j \tag{1}$$

where $\mu(x)$ is an unknown function, the inputs x_j are drawn independently with an unknown stationary probability density function $p(x)$, the ϵ_j are independent random variables with zero mean ($\bar{\epsilon} = 0$) and variance σ_ϵ^2, and the t_j are the observed target values.

The learning or regression problem is to find an estimate $\hat{\mu}_\lambda(x; D)$ of $\mu(x)$ given the data set D from a class of predictors or models $\mu_\lambda(x)$ indexed by λ. In general, $\lambda \in \Lambda = (S, A, W)$, where $S \subset X$ denotes a chosen subset of the set of available input variables X, A is a selected architecture within a class of model architectures $\mathcal{A}$, and W are the adjustable parameters (weights) of architecture A. Here we make explicit the dependence of $\hat{\mu}$ on the available data D used for training. $\hat{\mu}$ also depends on the architecture class $\mathcal{A}$ which is chosen independently of the data set D and its size N.

The *prediction risk* $P(\lambda)$ is defined as the expected performance on future data:

$$P(\lambda) = \int dx\; p(x)[\mu(x) - \hat{\mu}(x)]^2 + \sigma_\epsilon^2 \,. \tag{2}$$

(Here, we have used the squared error, but $P(\lambda)$ can be defined for other loss functions as well.) This can be approximated by the expected performance on a finite test set:

$$P(\lambda) \approx E\{\frac{1}{N}\sum_{j=1}^{N}(t_j^* - \hat{\mu}_\lambda(x_j^*))^2\} \,, \tag{3}$$

where (x_j^*, t_j^*) are new observations that were not used in constructing $\hat{\mu}_\lambda(x)$. In what follows, we shall use $P(\lambda)$ as a measure of the generalization ability of a model.

Our strategy is to choose an architecture λ in the model space Λ which minimizes an estimate of the prediction risk $P(\lambda)$. The set of networks considered is determined by the heuristic search strategies described in Section 6.

2.2 Prediction Risk for Nonlinear Models

The training error functions of nonlinear models, such as two layer perceptrons, often contain many local minima (see Figure 2). Each minimum should be viewed as defining a different predictor. In order to seek out good local minima, a good learning procedure must therefore include both a gradient-based optimization algorithm and a technique like random restart which enables sampling of the space of minima.

Since the models we use as predictors are trained to a particular "good" local minimum in weight space, we are interested in estimating the generalization ability

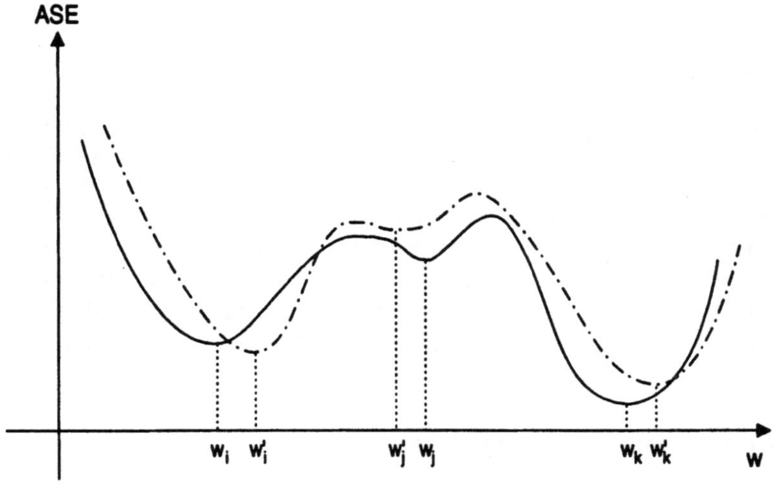

Figure 2: A nonlinear model can have many local minima in the error function. Each local minimum $\mathbf{w}_i$, $\mathbf{w}_j$ and $\mathbf{w}_k$ (solid curve) corresponds to a different set of parameters and thus to a different model. Training on a different finite sample of data or retraining on a subsample, as in nonlinear cross-validation, gives rise to a slightly different error curve (dashed) and perturbed minima $\mathbf{w}'_i$, $\mathbf{w}'_j$ and $\mathbf{w}'_k$. Variations due to data sampling in error curves and their minima are termed *model variance.*

or prediction risk associated with that minimum and not others. This point is important for the estimation procedures described in the next section.

Note that different finite training samples of fixed size will result in slightly different error surfaces in weight space. This is illustrated in Figure 2 by the difference between the solid and dashed curves. Note that the minima of the dashed curve differ slightly from the minima of the solid curve. This effect gives rise to *model variance.*

2.3 Estimates of the Prediction Risk

Since it is not possible to exactly calculate the prediction risk P_λ given only a finite sample of data, we have to estimate it. The standard method based on test–set validation is not advisable when the data set is small.

Cross-validation (CV) is a sample re–use method for estimating prediction risk; it makes maximally efficient use of the available data. We have developed a nonlinear refinement refinement of CV called NCV. Algebraic estimates, such as generalized cross–validation (GCV), the final prediction error (FPE), the predicted squared error (PSE), and the generalized prediction error (GPE), combine the average training squared error (*ASE*) with a measure of the model complexity. These will be discussed in the next sections.

3 Test-Set Validation and Cross-Validation

3.1 Test-Set Validation

If enough data is available, it is possible to use only part of the data for training the network. The remaining exemplars form a test-set that can be used to estimate the prediction risk. The obvious disadvantage of this method is that not all data is used for training. Even in cases where the data set is large, one would like to use as much data as possible for training, since the estimation error associated with model variance becomes worse as the training set size is reduced. However, if the test-set is too small, an accurate estimate of the prediction risk cannot be obtained. Test-set validation becomes practical only if the data-sets are very large or new data can be generated cheaply.

3.2 Cross-Validation: General Formulation

Cross–Validation is a method that makes minimal assumptions on the statistics of the data. The idea of cross-validation can be traced back to Mosteller and Tukey (1968). For reviews, see Stone (1974; 1978), Geisser (1975), Eubank (1988), Hastie and Tibshirani (1990), and Wahba (1990). For our presentation of the general method in this section, we follow Eubank. We then present a refinement of the method for nonlinear models called NCV in Section 3.3.

Denoting a predictor trained on all N data samples by $\hat{\mu}_\lambda(x)$, let $\hat{\mu}_{\lambda(j)}(x)$ be a predictor trained using all observations except (x_j, t_j) such that $\hat{\mu}_{\lambda(j)}(x)$ minimizes

$$ASE_j = \frac{1}{(N-1)} \sum_{k \neq j} \left(t_k - \hat{\mu}_{\lambda(j)}(x_k)\right)^2 \ . \tag{4}$$

For $\hat{\mu}_{\lambda(j)}(x)$ we can treat the jth omitted datum as a test set, and repeat this for all j. Then, an asymptotically unbiased estimator for the prediction risk $P(\lambda)$ of the model trained on *all* N *exemplars* $\hat{\mu}_\lambda(x)$ is the *cross-validation average squared error*

$$CV(\lambda) = \frac{1}{N} \sum_{j=1}^{N} \left(t_j - \hat{\mu}_{\lambda(j)}(x_j)\right)^2 \ . \tag{5}$$

This form of $CV(\lambda)$ is known as *leave–one–out* cross–validation.

However, $CV(\lambda)$ in (5) is expensive to compute for neural network models; it involves constructing an additional N networks, each trained with $N-1$ patterns. For the work described in this paper we therefore use a variation of the method, *v-fold cross–validation*, that was introduced by Geisser (1975) and Wahba and Wold (1975). Instead of leaving out only one observation for the computation of the sum in (5), we delete larger subsets of D.

Let the data D be divided into v randomly selected disjoint subsets D_j of roughly equal size: $\cup_{j=1}^{v} D_j = D$ and $\forall i \neq j,\ D_i \cap D_j = \emptyset$. Let N_j denote the number of observations in subset D_j. Let $\hat{\mu}_{\lambda(D_j)}(x)$ be an estimator trained on all data except

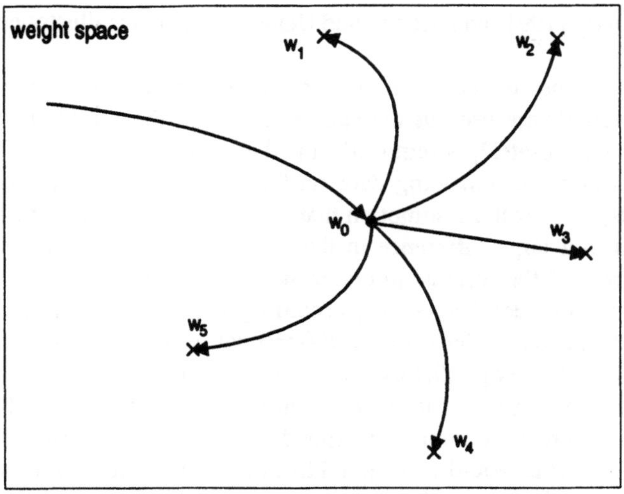

Figure 3: Illustration of the computation of 5–fold *nonlinear cross-validation (NCV)*. First, the network is trained on all data to obtain $\mathbf{w}_0$ which is used as starting point for the cross-validation. Each subset $D_i, i = 1 \ldots 5$ is removed from the training data D in turn. The network is trained, starting at $\mathbf{w}_0$, using the remaining data. This "perturbs" the weights to obtain $\mathbf{w}_i$. The test error of the "perturbed model" w_i is computed on the hold-out sample D_i. The average of these errors is the 5-fold CV estimate of the prediction risk for the model with weights w_0.

for $(x, t) \in D_j$. Then, the cross-validation average squared error for subset j is defined as

$$CV_{D_j}(\lambda) = \frac{1}{N_j} \sum_{(x_k, t_k) \in D_j} \left(t_k - \hat{\mu}_{\lambda(D_j)}(x_k)\right)^2 . \tag{6}$$

These are averaged over j to obtain the v-fold cross-validation estimate of prediction risk:

$$CV(\lambda) = \frac{1}{v} \sum_j CV_{D_j}(\lambda) . \tag{7}$$

Typical choices for v are 5 and 10. Note that leave–one–out CV is obtained in the limit $v = N$. Note that CV is a nonparametric estimate of the prediction risk that relies only on the available data.

3.3 NCV: Cross-Validation for Nonlinear Models

The frequent occurrence of multiple minima in nonlinear models (see Figure 2), each of which represents a different predictor, requires a refinement of the cross-validation procedure. This refinement, *nonlinear cross-validation (NCV)*, was implemented by

Utans and Moody (1991) and Moody and Utans (1992) and is illustrated in Figure 3 for $v = 5$.

A network is trained on the entire data set D to obtain a model $\hat{\mu}_\lambda(x)$ with weights $\mathbf{w}_0$. These weights are used as the starting point for the v-fold cross–validation procedure. Each subset D_j is removed from the training data in turn. The network is re-trained using the remaining data starting at $\mathbf{w}_0$ (rather than using random initial weights). Under the assumption that deleting a subset from the training data does not lead to a large difference in the locally-optimal weights, the retraining from $\mathbf{w}_0$ "perturbs" the weights to obtain $\mathbf{w}_i, i = 1 \ldots v$. The $CV(\lambda)$ computed for the "perturbed models" $\hat{\mu}_{\lambda(D_j)}(x)$ according to Equation (7) thus estimates the prediction risk for the model with locally-optimal weights $\mathbf{w}_0$ as desired, and not the performance of other predictors at other local minima.

If the network is trained from random initial weights for each subset, it could converge to a different minimum corresponding to $\mathbf{w}_i$ different from the one corresponding to $\mathbf{w}_0$. This would correspond to a different model. Thus, starting from $\mathbf{w}_0$ assures us that the cross-validation estimates the prediction risk for a particular model in question corresponding to $\mathbf{w} \approx \mathbf{w}_0$.

In Figure 2, the unperturbed model could be associated with one of the minima of the solid error curve (say w_k), and a perturbed model would be associated with the corresponding minimum of the dashed curve with weights w'_k. Our NCV algorithm attempts to avoid finding a "wrong" perturbed model (e.g., with weights w'_i). NCV has the additional benefit of having much less computational load than would be incurred by retraining from random initial weights.

Note that the same perturbation procedure described here yields nonlinear refinements of the bootstrap and jackknife algorithms as well. (See for example Efron and Gong (1983).)

4 Algebraic Estimates of Prediction Risk

4.1 Predicted Squared Error for Linear Models

For linear regression models with the squared error loss function, a number of useful algebraic estimates for the prediction risk have been derived. These include the well known *generalized cross–validation (GCV)* (Craven and Wahba, 1979; Golub *et al.*, 1979) and Akaike's *final prediction error (FPE)* (Akaike, 1970) formulas:

$$GCV(\lambda) = ASE(\lambda)\frac{1}{\left(1 - \frac{Q(\lambda)}{N}\right)^2} \qquad FPE(\lambda) = ASE(\lambda)\left(\frac{1 + \frac{Q(\lambda)}{N}}{1 - \frac{Q(\lambda)}{N}}\right) . \tag{8}$$

$Q(\lambda)$ denotes the number of weights of model λ. Note that although GCV and FPE are slightly different for small sample sizes, they are asymptotically equivalent for large N:

$$GCV(\lambda) \approx FPE(\lambda) \approx ASE(\lambda)\left(1 + 2\frac{Q(\lambda)}{N}\right) \tag{9}$$

A more general expression of *predicted squared error (PSE)* is:

$$PSE(\lambda) = ASE(\lambda) + 2\widehat{\sigma}^2 \frac{Q(\lambda)}{N}, \tag{10}$$

where $\widehat{\sigma}^2$ is an estimate of the noise variance in the data. Estimation strategies for (10) and its statistical properties have been analyzed by Barron (1984). FPE is obtained as special case of PSE by setting $\widehat{\sigma}^2 \equiv ASE(\lambda)/(N-Q(\lambda))$. See Eubank (1988), Hastie and Tibshirani (1990) and Wahba (1990) for tutorial treatments.

It should be noted that that PSE, FPE and GCV are asymptotically unbiased estimates of the prediction risk for the neural network models considered here under certain conditions. These are: (1) the noise ϵ_j in the observed targets t_j is independent and identically distributed, (2) the resulting model is unbiased, (3) weight decay is not used, and (4) the nonlinearity in the model can be neglected. For PSE, we further require that an asymptotically unbiased estimate of $\widehat{\sigma}^2$ is used. In practice, however, essentially all neural network fits to data will be biased and/or have significant nonlinearity.

Although PSE, FPE and GCV are asymptotically unbiased only under the above assumptions, they are much cheaper to compute than NCV since no retraining is required.

4.2 Generalized Prediction Error (GPE) for Nonlinear Models

The predicted squared error PSE, and therefore the final prediction error FPE, are special cases of the *generalized prediction error GPE* (Moody (1991; 1992; 1994)). We present an abbreviated description here.

GPE estimates prediction risk for biased nonlinear models which may use general loss functions and include regularizers such as weight decay. The algebraic form is

$$GPE(\lambda) \equiv \mathcal{E}_{\text{train}}(\lambda) + \frac{2}{N} \operatorname{tr} \widehat{V}\widehat{G}(\lambda) \ , \tag{11}$$

where $\mathcal{E}_{\text{train}}(\lambda)$ is the training set error (average value of loss function on training set), $\widehat{V}$ is a nonlinear generalization of the estimated *noise covariance matrix* of the observed targets, and $\widehat{G}(\lambda)$ is the estimated *generalized influence matrix*, a nonlinear analog of the standard influence or hat matrix.

GPE can be expressed in an equivalent form as:

$$GPE(\lambda) = \mathcal{E}_{\text{train}}(\lambda) + 2\,\widehat{\sigma}^2_{eff} \frac{\widehat{Q}_{eff}(\lambda)}{N}, \tag{12}$$

where $\widehat{Q}_{eff} \equiv \operatorname{tr}\widehat{G}$ is the estimated *effective* number of model parameters, and $\widehat{\sigma}^2_{eff} \equiv (\operatorname{tr}\widehat{V}\widehat{G})/(\operatorname{tr}\widehat{G})$ is the estimated effective noise variance in the data. For nonlinear and/or regularized models, $\widehat{Q}_{eff}(\lambda)$ is generally not equal to the number of weights $Q(\lambda)$.

When the noise in the target variables is assumed to be independent with uniform variance and the squared error loss function is used, (12) simplifies to:

$$GPE(\lambda) = ASE(\lambda) + 2\widehat{\sigma}^2 \frac{\widehat{Q}_{eff}(\lambda)}{N} \ . \tag{13}$$

Note that replacing $\widehat{Q}_{eff}(\lambda)$ with $Q(\lambda)$ gives the expression for PSE. Various other special cases of (11) and (13) have been derived by other authors and can be found in Eubank (1988), Hastie and Tibshirani (1990) and Wahba (1990). Larsen (1992) has extended (11) to autoregressive time series models, and Liu (1993) and Moody (1994) have shown that N-fold cross validation is equivalent to $O(1/N)$ to the general form of GPE in equation (11).

5 Neural Network Architecture Selection

For the discussion of architecture selection in this paper, we focus on the most widely used neural network architecture, the two-layer *perceptron* (or *backpropagation*) network. The response function $\hat{\mu}_\lambda(x)$ for such a network with I_λ input variables, H_λ internal (hidden) neurons, and a single output neuron is:

$$\hat{\mu}_\lambda(x) = f(\,v_0 + \sum_{\alpha=1}^{H_\lambda} v_\alpha\, g(w_{\alpha 0} + \sum_{\beta=1}^{I_\lambda} w_{\alpha\beta}\, x_\beta))\ . \tag{14}$$

Here, x_β are the input variables, f and g are typically sigmoidal nonlinearities, the $w_{\alpha\beta}$ and $w_{\alpha 0}$ are input weights and thresholds, the v_α and v_0 are the second layer weights and threshold, and the index λ is an abstract label for the specific two layer perceptron network architecture. While we consider for simplicity this restricted class of perceptron networks in this paper, our approach can be easily generalized to networks with multiple outputs and multiple layers.

For two layer perceptrons, the *architecture selection problem* is to find a good (hopefully near-optimal) architecture λ for modeling a given data set. The architecture λ is characterized by

- the number of hidden units H_λ,
- the number of input variables I_λ,
- and the subset of weights v_α and $w_{\alpha\beta}$ that are non-zero.

If all of the v_α and $w_{\alpha\beta}$ are non-zero, the network is referred to as *fully connected*. If many of the input weights $w_{\alpha\beta}$ are zero, the network is *sparsely connected*, while setting to zero one of the v_α (or all $w_{\alpha\beta}$ for fixed α) corresponds to removing a hidden unit.

Note that for brevity of exposition in the sequel, we denote weights and biases in either layer of the network generically by w.

5.1 Complexity of Exhaustive Search

If we consider a set of two layer perceptrons up to some maximal size determined by $I_{\max}$ and $H_{\max}$, then the maximal fully connected network has

$$M_{\max} = 1 + H_{\max}(I_{\max} + 2)$$

weights. All smaller two layer networks can be obtained from the maximal network by setting weights and thresholds to zero. The total number of resulting network topologies (treating the ordering of the hidden units as unique and thus not considering permutations of them) is

$$N_{max} = 2^{M_{max}}$$

For example, a set of networks with $I_{max} = 10$ and $H_{max} = 12$ yields $N_{max} = 2^{145} \approx 4.46 \times 10^{43}$. Even though the maximal network in this example is modest in size, N_{max} is a prohibitively large number of network topologies to search exhaustively. If each of the N_{max} networks could be trained and tested in one microsecond of CPU time, the total time required to train and test all N_{max} networks in this example would be 1.41×10^{30} years or roughly 10^{20} times the age of the universe.

Even if exhaustive search for an optimum (as measured by a selection criterion) were computationally feasible, it would likely prove to be pointless, since based on our experience, many network architectures are likely to provide similar performance. (See, for example, Figure 3 of Moody and Yarvin (1992).) Moreover, the model variance for networks trained on small, noisy data sets will make the near-optimal models indistinguishable from the asymptotically optimal model.[1]

Thus, we are compelled to consider restricted search strategies over the space of network architectures. This is the subject of Section 6.

6 Heuristic Search over the Space of Perceptron Architectures

Given the futility of exhaustively sampling the space of possible networks in search of an optimum, we present efficient heuristic search algorithms. These were developed while building a model for corporate bond rating prediction. Brief descriptions of the original work can be found in Utans and Moody (1991) and Moody and Utans (1992). A more detailed description of the bond rating problem and our empirical results is presented in Moody and Utans (1994).

First, a locally-optimal number of internal units is selected from a sequence of fully connected networks with increasing number of hidden units. An efficient algorithm, *sequential network construction (SNC)*, is used for training the networks in this sequence. Then, using the optimal fully connected network, input variables are pruned via *sensitivity based pruning (SBP)* and weights are pruned via *optimal brain damage (OBD)*.

Figure 4 depicts two search strategies. After selecting the number of hidden units H_λ, input removal and weight elimination can be carried out in parallel (A) or sequentially (B). The first strategy (A), which was used for the bond rating simulations described in Utans and Moody (1991) and Moody and Utans (1992), allows a comparison of the results of the input and weight pruning steps but requires a final step of combining the resulting networks to obtain the final network architecture. On the other hand, the sequential approach (B) is less costly to implement since for

[1] The term *asymptotic* refers to the limit of infinite training set size.

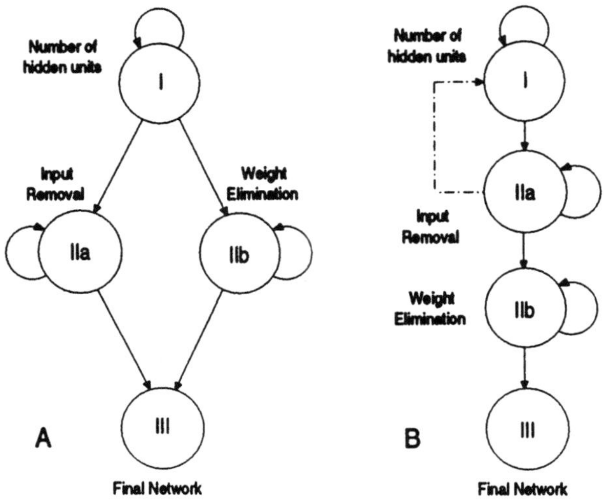

Figure 4: Heuristic Search Strategies: After selecting the number of hidden units H_λ, the input removal and weight elimination can be carried out in parallel (A) or sequentially (B). In (B), the selection of the number of hidden units and removal of inputs may be iterated (dashed line).

the weight elimination stage, the network is already reduced in size by removing inputs. This alternative corresponds to a *coarse to fine* strategy: pruning inputs removes groups of weights while the final weight elimination is concerned with individual weights. A refinement of the sequential approach is to re-determine the optimal number of hidden units after a good set of input variables has been selected or after the removal of each unnecessary input variable. This results in an iterative procedure (dashed line in Figure 4 (B)).

6.1 Selecting the Number of Hidden Units

For determining the number of hidden units, we construct and train a nested set of models, using an efficient algorithm which we call *sequential network construction (SNC).*

Before proceeding, we would like to note that many authors have independently proposed iterative network construction algorithms. Probably the best known of these is the cascade correlation algorithm (Fahlman and Lebiere, 1990). Cascade correlation was preceded by Ash (1989); see also Moody (1989). We have not attempted to exhaustively review this area, nor do we claim that SNC is necessarily unique or optimal.

6.1.1 The SNC Algorithm

The SNC algorithm constructs a sequence of networks, each of which is fully connected and uses all input variables, differing only in the number of hidden units. The sequence is built as follows: First a network with a small number of hidden units is trained, using random initial weights. Larger networks are obtained iteratively, by adding units in clumps of size C to the largest net in the sequence. This continues until a network of some predetermined maximum size has been produced.

When a larger network, of size $H_\lambda + C$, is constructed, it is trained as follows:

1. The weights of the previous network are used as initial weights for the first H_λ units of the new network. The weights of the newly added clump of C units are initialized to small random values.

2. The weights of the new clump are trained to a local optimum while keeping the weights of the first H_λ units fixed.

3. Finally, all weights are allowed to vary, and are trained until a local optimum for the entire network is reached.

The SNC algorithm is designed to solve two problems. First, it substantially reduces computation time compared to what would be required if larger networks were trained from scratch. Secondly, the sequence of networks constructed comprise a *nested set*.

6.1.2 Nested Models and Inverse Pruning

In general, a nonlinear network has many local minima, and each local minimum corresponds to a different set of parameters and thus to a different model (see Figure 2). The SNC algorithm, on the other hand, provides some continuity in model space by constructing a nested sequence in which larger networks contain the smaller networks.

The sequential construction accomplishes this nesting as follows. As larger networks are constructed, the features discovered by the smaller network's hidden units will continue to be used by the larger networks. In effect this means that as the sequence grows, the networks are trained to learn corrections to the mappings discovered so far. Moreover, we have found that the effect on existing hidden units of adding a new hidden unit once the model is big enough is likely to be small.

Because of the resulting continuity in model space, SNC can be thought of as an *inverse pruning* procedure. Since the most recently added clump of units serves only to correct a mapping learned already, it is highly likely that a node pruning method would prune these units first. Also, it is clearly less expensive computationally to construct a sequence of networks from small to large than it is to first train large networks and prune from large to small.

Three advantages are obtained by constructing a nested set of models. First, the sequence will have monotonically decreasing (or non-increasing) training error. Secondly, the sequence is likely to have an easily identifiable minimum of prediction risk. Thirdly, architecture selection via prediction risk has a formal connection to the hypothesis testing approach to pruning when the set of models is nested (see for example the discussion in Akaike (1974)). The *inverse pruning* approach allows the theory and techniques of hypothesis testing to be applied to models trained via SNC.

Note that in spite of these advantages of SNC, it is possible that pruning nodes from a larger network may give rise to a better fit to the data and better generalization for a given final number of nodes. This is not to say, however, that a larger network obtained via SNC might not perform as well or better. Resolving the issue of whether SNC or node pruning is more effective in general requires a systematic study.

Finally, for each network in the sequence produced by SNC, an estimate of the prediction risk is computed. The network selected at this stage for further refinement via input and weight pruning is the one with the smallest estimated prediction risk.

6.2 Pruning Inputs and Weights via Directed Search

After the number of hidden units of the fully connected network with all available input variables is determined, the next step of our heuristic search is to select input variables and remove individual weights from the network.

As before, we evaluate a candidate network architecture by computing an estimate of the prediction risk. In order to avoid searching over the very large range of architectures obtained by considering all possible combinations of inputs and all possible connection structures, we propose a directed search strategy using the *sensitivity-based input pruning (SBP)* and *optimal brain damage (OBD)* algorithms.

With these algorithms, candidate architectures are constructed by evaluating the effect of removing an input variable or an individual weight from the fully connected network. These are ranked in order of increasing training error. Inputs and weights are then removed following a "Best First" strategy, i.e. selecting the input or weight that, when removed, increases the training error least. The candidate architecture is obtained by retraining the remaining weights, starting from their previous values, to find a new minimum in weight space. Note that we assume that the weights obtained after making a small modification to the network, such as removing a single input variable or a single weight, brings us closer to a good solution.

Note that the weight elimination stage can reduce the number of hidden units if all weights to or from a particular hidden unit are eliminated. For example, for the model considered here with a single output unit, eliminating a weight from a hidden unit to the output unit effectively removes that hidden unit from the network. Pruning units this way is more costly computationally than choosing a good number of hidden units in the first place (as is the purpose of our SNC and unit selection algorithm). However, both methods can complement each other.

6.2.1 Pruning of Input Variables via Sensitivity Analysis

In Moody and Utans (1992) and Utans and Moody (1991), we proposed a simple *sensitivity-based pruning* method for input variables *(SBP)*. The SBP algorithm computes a *sensitivity measure* S_i to evaluate the change in training error that would result if input x_i were removed from the network. The sensitivity of the network model to variable i is defined as:

$$S_i = \frac{1}{N} \sum_j S_{ij} \ , \tag{15}$$

where S_{ij} is the sensitivity computed for exemplar x_j. Since there are usually many fewer inputs than weights, a direct evaluation of S_i is feasible:

$$S_{ij} = SE(\overline{x}_i, w_\lambda) - SE(x_{ij}, w_\lambda) \qquad \text{with} \qquad \overline{x}_i = \frac{1}{N} \sum_{j=1}^{N} x_{ij} \ . \tag{16}$$

S_i measures the effect on the training squared error (*SE*) of replacing the ith input x_i by its average $\overline{x}_i$ for all exemplars. Replacement of a variable by its average value removes its influence on the network output.

Note that in computing S_i, no retraining is done in evaluating $SE(\overline{x}_i, w_\lambda)$. Also note that it is not sufficient to just set $x_{ij} = 0 \ \forall \ j$, because the value of the bias of each hidden unit was determined during training and would not be offset properly by setting the input arbitrarily to zero. Of course, if the inputs are normalized to have zero mean prior to training, then setting an input variable to zero is equivalent to replacing it by its mean.

If the number of input variables I_λ is large, S_i is expensive to compute and can be approximated. For a small change of the ith input of the jth exemplar, dx_{ij},

$$dSE = \sum_i \frac{\partial SE}{\partial x_{ij}} dx_{ij} + \frac{1}{2} \sum_{i_1 i_2 j} \frac{\partial^2 SE}{\partial x_{i_1 j} \partial x_{i_2 j}} dx_{i_1 j} dx_{i_2 j} + O(||x_{ij}||^3) \ . \tag{17}$$

The linear term in Equation (17) approximates S_{ij} as

$$\hat{S}_{ij} = \frac{\partial SE}{\partial x_{ij}} dx_{ij} \qquad \text{with} \qquad dx_{ij} = \overline{x}_i - x_{ij} \ , \tag{18}$$

and the derivative information can be efficiently computed as a minor extension to the backpropagation algorithm used for training.

Note that the SBP algorithm neglects possible correlations between inputs. An improvement of the method would be to first orthogonalize the inputs (for example by a KL transform) and perform the sensitivity analysis using the transformed inputs. The pruning would be performed on input eigennodes rather than the actual input variables. This approach has been explored recently by Levin, Leen and Moody (1994).

A related input pruning algorithm based on a different approximation of the sensitivity measure has been proposed by Refenes, Francis and Zapranis (1994).

6.2.2 Weight Pruning via "Optimal Brain Damage"

Optimal Brain Damage (OBD) was introduced by LeCun, Denker and Solla (1990) as a method to reduce the number of weights in a neural network to avoid overfitting.

OBD is designed to select those weights in the network whose removal will have a small effect on the training average squared error (*ASE*). Assuming that the original network is too large, removing these weights and retraining the now smaller network should improve the generalization performance.

The method approximates *ASE* at a minimum $\mathbf{w} = \mathbf{w}^*$ in weight space by a diagonal quadratic expansion. The change in *ASE* caused by a small change $d\mathbf{w}$ from $\mathbf{w}^*$ is

$$dASE = \sum_k \frac{\partial ASE}{\partial w_k} dw_k + \frac{1}{2} \sum_{kl} \frac{\partial^2 ASE}{\partial w_k \partial w_l} dw_k dw_l + O(||w_k||^3) \ , \tag{19}$$

where for simplicity of notation w_k represents any weight in any layer of the network.

Since the approximation is taken at a minimum in weight space, the first term in Equation (19) vanishes. In addition, terms higher order than quadratic are ignored. Thus, Equation (19) reduces to

$$dASE = \frac{1}{2} \sum_k \frac{\partial^2 ASE}{\partial w_k \partial w_k} dw_k dw_l \ . \tag{20}$$

The evaluation of the Hessian becomes prohibitively expensive for large networks. By approximating the Hessian by considering only diagonal terms $\partial^2 ASE / \partial w_k^2$, we assume that weights can be removed individually without influencing each other. The *saliency* defined as

$$s_k = \frac{1}{2} \frac{\partial^2 ASE}{\partial w_k \partial w_k} w_k^2 \tag{21}$$

is a measure (in the diagonal approximation) of the change of *ASE* when weight w_k is removed from the network by setting its value to zero. Note that the saliency must be computed after training has stopped at a local minimum. The second derivatives required for s_k can be efficiently computed by a method similar to the backpropagation of first derivatives for weight updates during training (LeCun *et al.*, 1990).

The procedure for eliminating weights as described by LeCun *et al.* (1990) consists of ranking the weights in the network according to increasing s_k, removing first one weight or a few weights, then retraining the network, and repeating an arbitrary number of times. In contrast, we accept a network modification only if the expected performance on the test set is improved as measured by a decrease in the estimate of the prediction risk $\widehat{P}(\lambda)$.

6.3 Final Remarks on Pruning

6.3.1 Multiple Minima of Prediction Risk

Note that since the networks are trained to minimize the training error *ASE* and not $P(\lambda)$, the prediction risk need not be a monotonically decreasing function of the number of inputs or weights eliminated, and there can be multiple minima in the sequence of networks considered. Since the SBP and OBD procedures start with a fully connected network, it is not sufficient to stop removing weights when $\widehat{P}(\lambda)$ first increases. This is particularly true given that both SBP and OBD are greedy algorithms, and they neglect interactions between multiple inputs and weights. Thus, removing additional inputs or weights even after $\widehat{P}(\lambda)$ first increases can lead to a further reduction of the prediction risk and thus yield a smaller final network.

6.3.2 Other Pruning Methods

A number of other pruning methods besides those we have described here are potentially effective and should be considered when constructing neural network models. These include the *irrelevant hidden unit* and *irrelevant input* hypothesis tests (White, 1989), pruning of units via skeletonization (Mozer and Smolensky, 1990), *optimal brain surgeon OBS* (Hassibi and Stork, 1993), and *principal components pruning PCP* (Levin *et al.*, 1994). It is important to note that all these methods, along with OBD and our method of input pruning via SBP, are closely related to the Wald hypothesis testing procedure (see for example Buse (1982)). In fact, the saliencies used in OBD, OBS, and SBP are special cases of the Wald test statistic.

Acknowledgements

The author thanks Joachim Utans for help in preparing this manuscript and Steve Rehfuss and Eric Wan for careful proof readings. The author is responsible for any remaining errors. This work was supported by the Advanced Research Projects Agency under grant N00014-92-J-4062.

References

Akaike, H. (1970), 'Statistical predictor identification', *Ann. Inst. Statist. Math.* **22**, 203–217.

Akaike, H. (1973), Information theory and the extension of the maximum likelihood principle, Akademia Kiado, Budapest, pp. 267–810.

Akaike, H. (1974), 'A new look at the statistical model identification', *IEEE Transactions on Automatic Control* **AC-19**(6), 716–723.

Akaike, H. (1977), On entropy maximization principle, *in* P. R. Krishnaiah, ed., 'Applications of Statistics', North-Holland Publishing Company, pp. 27–41.

Ash, T. (1989), 'Dynamic node creation in backpropagation neural networks', *Connection Science* **1**(4), 365–375.

Barron, A. (1984), Predicted squared error: a criterion for automatic model selection, *in* S. Farlow, ed., 'Self–Organizing Methods in Modeling', Marcel Dekker, New York.

Buse, A. (1982), 'The likelihood ratio, wald, and lagrange multiplier test: An expository note', *The American Statistician* **36**(3), 153–157.

Craven, P. and Wahba, G. (1979), 'Smoothing noisy data with spline functions: Estimating the correct degree of smoothing by the method of generalized cross-validation', *Numer. Math.* **31**, 377–403.

Efron, B. and Gong, G. (1983), 'A leisurely look at the bootstrap, the jackknife and cross-validation', *The American Statistician* 37(1), 36–48.

Eubank, R. L. (1988), *Spline Smoothing and Nonparametric Regression*, Marcel Dekker, Inc.

Fahlman, S. E. and Lebiere, C. (1990), The cascade-correlation learning algorithm, *in* D. S. Touretzky, ed., 'Advances in Neural Information Processing Systems 2', Morgan Kaufmann Publishers, San Mateo, CA, pp. 525–532.

Geisser, S. (1975), 'The predictive sample reuse method with applications', *Journal of The American Statistical Association* 70(350).

Geman, S., Bienenstock, E. and Doursat, R. (1992), 'Neural networks and the bias/variance dilemma', *Neural Computation* 4(1), 1–58.

Golub, G., Heath, H. and Wahba, G. (1979), 'Generalized cross validation as a method for choosing a good ridge parameter', *Technometrics* 21, 215–224.

Hassibi, B. and Stork, D. G. (1993), Second order derivatives for network pruning: Optimal brain surgeon, *in* S. J. Hanson, J. D. Cowan and C. L. Giles, eds, 'Advances in Neural Information Processing Systems 5', Morgan Kaufmann Publishers, San Mateo, CA, pp. 164–171.

Hastie, T. J. and Tibshirani, R. J. (1990), *Generalized Additive Models*, Vol. 43 of *Monographs on Statistics and Applied Probability*, Chapman and Hall.

Larsen, J. (1992), A generalization error estimate for nonlinear systems, *in* 'Proceedings of the 1992 IEEE Workshop on Neural Networks for Signal Processing', IEEE Service Center, Piscataway, NJ, pp. 29–38.

LeCun, Y., Denker, J. S. and Solla, S. A. (1990), Optimal brain damage, *in* D. S. Touretzky, ed., 'Advances in Neural Information Processing Systems 2', Morgan Kaufmann Publishers.

Levin, A. U., Leen, T. K. and Moody, J. E. (1994), Fast pruning using principal components, *in* J. Cowan, G. Tesauro and J. Alspector, eds, 'Advances in Neural Information Processing Systems 6', Morgan Kaufmann Publishers, San Francisco, CA.

Liu, Y. (1993), Neural network model selection using asymptotic jackknife estimator and cross-validation method, *in* S. J. Hanson, J. D. Cowan and C. L. Giles, eds, 'Advances in Neural Information Processing Systems 5', Morgan Kaufmann Publishers, San Mateo, CA, pp. 599–606.

Moody, J. E. (1989), Fast learning in multi-resolution hierarchies, *in* D. S. Touretzky, ed., 'Advances in Neural Information Processing Systems 1', Morgan Kaufmann Publishers, San Mateo, CA.

Moody, J. E. (1991), Note on generalization, regularization and architecture selection in nonlinear learning systems, *in* B. H. Juang, S. Y. Kung and C. A. Kamm, eds, 'Neural Networks for Signal Processing', IEEE Signal Processing Society, pp. 1–10.

Moody, J. E. (1992), The effective number of parameters: an analysis of generalization and regularization in nonlinear learning systems, *in* J. E. Moody, S. J. Hanson and R. P. Lippmann, eds, 'Advances in Neural Information Processing Systems 4', Morgan Kaufmann Publishers, San Mateo, CA, pp. 847–854.

Moody, J. E. (1994), 'The *effective* number of parameters and generalized prediction error for nonlinear regression.', *To appear* .

Moody, J. E. and Utans, J. (1992), Principled architecture selection for neural networks: Application to corporate bond rating prediction, *in* J. E. Moody, S. J. Hanson and R. P. Lippmann, eds, 'Advances in Neural Information Processing Systems 4', Morgan Kaufmann Publishers, San Mateo, CA, pp. 683–690.

Moody, J. E. and Yarvin, N. (1992), Networks with learned unit response functions, *in* J. E. Moody, S. J. Hanson and R. P. Lippmann, eds, 'Advances in Neural Information Processing Systems 4', Morgan Kaufmann Publishers, San Mateo, CA, pp. 1048–55.

Moody, J. and Utans, J. (1994), Architecture selection strategies for neural networks: Application to corporate bond rating prediction, *in* A. N. Refenes, ed., 'Neural Networks in the Captial Markets', John Wiley & Sons.

Mosteller, F. and Tukey, J. W. (1968), Data analysis, including statistics, *in* G. Lindzey and E. Aronson, eds, 'Handbook of Social Psychology, Vol. 2', Addison–Wesley. (first edition 1954).

Mozer, M. C. and Smolensky, P. (1990), Skeletonization: A technique for trimming the fat from a network via relevance assessment, *in* D. S. Touretzky, ed., 'Advances in Neural Information Processing Systems 1', Morgan Kaufmann Publishers, San Mateo, CA.

Refenes, A. N., Francis, G. and Zapranis, A. D. (1994), 'Stock performance modeling using neural networks: A comparative study with regression models', *Neural Networks* . accepted June 1993.

Rissanen, J. (1978), 'Modeling by shortest data description', *Automatica* **14**, 465–71.

Schwartz, G. (1978), 'Estimating the dimension of a model', *Ann. Stat.* **6**, 461–4.

Stone, M. (1974), 'Cross–validatory choice and assessment of statistical predictions', *Roy. Stat. Soc.* **B36**, 111–147.

Stone, M. (1978), 'Cross–validation: A review', *Math. Operationsforsch. Statist., Ser. Statistics* **9**(1).

Utans, J. and Moody, J. (1991), Selecting neural network architectures via the prediction risk: Application to corporate bond rating prediction, *in* 'Proceedings of the First International Conference on Artificial Intelligence Applications on Wall Street', IEEE Computer Society Press, Los Alamitos, CA.

Wahba, G. (1990), *Spline Models for Observational Data*, Vol. 59 of *Regional Conference Series in Applied Mathematics*, SIAM Press, Philadelphia.

Wahba, G. and Wold, S. (1975), 'A completely automatic french curve: Fitting spline functions by cross–validation', *Communications in Statistics* **4**(1), 1–17.

White, H. (1989), 'Learning in artificial neural networks: A statistical perspective', *Neural Computation* **1**, 425–464.

Regularization Theory, Radial Basis Functions and Networks

Federico Girosi

Artificial Intelligence Laboratory, M.I.T., Cambridge, 02139 MA, USA

Abstract. This paper consists of two parts. In the first part we consider the problem of learning from examples in the setting of the theory of the approximation of multivariate functions from sparse data. We first will show how an approach based on *regularization theory* leads to develop a family of approximation techniques, including Radial Basis Functions, and some tensor product and additive splines. Then we will show how this fairly classical approach has to be extended in order to cope with special features of the problem of learning of examples, such as high dimensionality and strong anisotropies. Furthermore, the same extension that leads from Radial Basis Functions (RBF) to Hyper Basis Functions (HBF) also leads from additive models to ridge approximation models, such as some forms of Projection Pursuit Regression.

In the second part we consider the problem of estimating the complexity of the approximation problem. We first briefly discuss the problem of degree of approximation, that is related to the number of parameters that are needed in order to guarantee a generalization error smaller than a certain amount. Then we consider certain Radial Basis Functions techniques, and, using a lemma by Jones (1992) and Barron (1991, 1993) we show that it is possible to define function spaces and basis functions for which the rate of convergence to zero of the error is $O(\frac{1}{\sqrt{n}})$ *in any number of dimensions*. The apparent avoidance of the "curse of dimensionality" is due to the fact that these function spaces are more and more constrained as the dimension increases. Examples include spaces of the Sobolev type, in which the number of weak derivatives is required to be larger than the number of dimensions.

Keywords. Approximation theory, regularization theory, Radial Basis Functions, ridge regression, neural networks, curse of dimensionality, rates of convergence.

1 Architectures

In recent years approximation theory has found interesting applications in the fields of Artificial Intelligence and Computer Science. For instance, a problem that fits very naturally in the framework of approximation theory is the problem of learning to perform a particular task from a set of examples. The examples are sparse data points in a multidimensional space, and learning means to reconstruct a surface that fits the data. Since the problem of approximating a surface from sparse data points is ill-posed, regularization theory (Tikhonov, 1963; Tikhonov and Arsenin, 1977; Morozov, 1984; Bertero, 1986) seems to be an appropriate mathematical framework for learning from examples. The regularization approach consists in finding, among the infinite number of functions that interpolate or approximate the data, the function that best satisfies a smoothness constraint, whose specific form depends on the a priori knowledge we have on the class of functions we want to approximate. The solution to the approximation problem is therefore found as the function that minimizes a functional consisting of two parts: one is the mean square error over the data, and the other is a smoothness functional, usually called *stabilizer* (Wahba, 1977, 1990; Bertero, 1986). Depending on the choice of the stabilizer, different approximation techniques can be obtained, such as the multidimensional splines of Duchon (1977) and Meinguet (1979), the more general Radial Basis Functions (Powell, 1987, 1990; Franke, 1982, 1987; Micchelli, 1986; Kansa, 1990; Madych and Nelson, 1991; Dyn, 1987, 1991; Hardy, 1990), and certain tensor product and additive splines (Hastie and Tibshirani, 1987, 1990; Buja, Hastie and Tibshirani, 1989; Whaba, 1990).

In many practical cases, however, the regularization approach cannot be applied in a straightforward manner. In order to overcome these difficulties, some extensions of the standard regularization approach has been proposed, and applied to the Radial Basis Functions (RBF) technique (Poggio and Girosi, 1990; Girosi, 1992), deriving the so-called Hyper Basis Function (HBF) approximation scheme. Interestingly, it turned out (Girosi, Jones and Poggio, 1993) that the extension that leads from RBF to HBF can also be applied to additive models, leading to ridge approximation techniques, of the type of Projection Pursuit Regression (PPR) (Friedman and Stuezle, 1981; Huber, 1985).

Noticing that all these techniques can be represented in terms of neural networks with one layer of hidden units, we therefore conclude that many neural network architectures, called Generalized Regularization Networks (GRN) (Girosi, Jones and Poggio, 1993), correspond to different classes of smoothness functionals in a classical regularization principle. Three broad classes are a) Radial Basis Functions that generalize into Hyper Basis Functions, b) some tensor product splines, and c) additive splines that generalize into schemes of the type of ridge approximation.

In the second part of this paper we consider the problem of estimating the complexity of the approximation problem. We first briefly discuss the general problem of degree of approximation, that is related to the number of parameters that are needed in order to guarantee a generalization error smaller than a certain amount. Then we consider a specific Radial Basis

Functions technique and we show that it is possible to define a function space for which the rate of convergence to zero of the error is $O(\frac{1}{\sqrt{n}})$ *in any number of dimensions* (Girosi and Anzellotti, 1992; Girosi, 1993). Results of this type have been obtained by other authors for neural networks and ridge function approximation schemes (Jones, 1992; Barron, 1991, 1993; Breiman, 1992; Mhaskar, 1993). The apparent avoidance of the "curse of dimensionality" is due to the fact that these function spaces are more and more constrained as the dimension increases.

1.1 The regularization approach to the approximation problem

Suppose that the set $D = \{(\mathbf{x}_i, y_i) \in R^d \times R\}_{i=1}^N$ of data has been obtained by random sampling a function f, belonging to some space of functions X defined on R^d, in the presence of noise, and suppose we are interested in recovering the function f, or an estimate of it, from the set of data D. The regularization approach (Tikhonov, 1963; Tikhonov and Arsenin, 1977; Morozov, 1984; Bertero, 1986; Wahba, 1990; Poggio and Girosi, 1989, 1990) consists in choosing as a solution of the approximation problem the function that minimizes the following functional:

$$H[f] = \sum_{i=1}^{N} (f(\mathbf{x}_i) - y_i)^2 + \lambda \phi[f] \ . \tag{1}$$

where λ is a positive number that is usually called the *regularization parameter*, and $\phi[f]$ is a *smoothness functional*, that penalizes functions with oscillatory and "non smooth" behaviour. It can be shown that, for a wide class of functionals ϕ, the solutions of the minimization of the functional (1) all have the same form (see the appendix in [26] for a sketch of the proof). In this section we just present a family of smoothness functionals and the corresponding solutions of the variational problem. We refer the reader to the current literature for the mathematical details (Wahba, 1990; Madych and Nelson, 1990; Dyn, 1987, 1991).

The class of smoothness functionals we consider is of the following form:

$$\phi[f] = \int_{R^d} ds \, \frac{|\tilde{f}(\mathbf{s})|^2}{\tilde{G}(\mathbf{s})} \tag{2}$$

where $\tilde{}$ indicates the Fourier transform, $\tilde{G}$ is some positive function that falls off to zero as $\|\mathbf{s}\| \rightarrow \infty$. It is clear that such a functional penalizes functions whose spectrum has high frequency content, and therefore has the property of measuring the smoothness of the function. For a well defined class of functions G (Madych and Nelson, 1990; Dyn, 1991) this functional is a semi-norm, with a finite dimensional null space $\mathcal{N}$. The next section will be devoted to giving examples of the possible choices for the stabilizer ϕ. For the moment we just assume that it can be written as in eq. (2), and make the additional assumption that $\tilde{G}$ is symmetric, so that its Fourier transform G is real and symmetric. In this case it is possible to show (see the appendix in [26] for a sketch of the proof) that the function that minimizes the functional (1) has the form:

$$f(\mathbf{x}) = \sum_{i=1}^{N} c_i G(\mathbf{x} - \mathbf{x}_i) + \sum_{\alpha=1}^{k} d_\alpha \psi_\alpha(\mathbf{x}) \tag{3}$$

where $\{\psi_\alpha\}_{\alpha=1}^{k}$ is a basis in the k dimensional null space $\mathcal{N}$ and the coefficients d_α and c_i satisfy the following linear system:

$$(G + \lambda I)\mathbf{c} + \Psi^T \mathbf{d} = \mathbf{y}$$

$$\Psi \mathbf{c} = 0$$

where I is the identity matrix, and we have defined

$$(\mathbf{y})_i = y_i \ , \quad (\mathbf{c})_i = c_i \ , \quad (\mathbf{d})_i = d_i \ ,$$
$$(G)_{ij} = G(\mathbf{x}_i - \mathbf{x}_j) \ , \quad (\Psi)_{\alpha i} = \psi_\alpha(\mathbf{x}_i)$$

The approximation scheme of eq. form (3) has a simple interpretation in terms of a network with one layer of hidden units, which we call a *Regularization Network* (RN) (Girosi, Jones and Poggio, 1993).

1.2 Classes of stabilizers

In this section, following (Girosi, Jones and Poggio, 1993), we discuss three different types of stabilizers belonging to the class (2). Each of them corresponds to different *a priori* assumptions about the smoothness of the function that must be approximated.

1.2.1 Radial stabilizers

Most of the commonly used stabilizers have radial symmetry, and the corresponding approximation technique is known as Radial Basis Functions (Powell, 1987, 1990; Franke, 1982, 1987; Micchelli, 1986; Kansa, 1990; Madych and Nelson, 1991; Dyn, 1987, 1991; Hardy, 1990). The class of admissible Radial Basis Functions is the class of conditionally positive definite functions of any order, since it has been shown (Madych and Nelson, 1991; Dyn, 1987, 1991) that in this case the functional of eq. (2) is a semi-norm, and the associated variational problem is well defined. All the Radial Basis Functions can therefore be derived in this framework. We explicitly give two important examples.

Duchon multivariate splines

Duchon (1977) considered measures of smoothness of the form

$$\phi[f] = \int_{R^d} ds\ \|\mathbf{s}\|^{2m} |\tilde{f}(\mathbf{s})|^2 \ .$$

In this case $\tilde{G}(\mathbf{s}) = \frac{1}{\|\mathbf{s}\|^{2m}}$, corresponding basis function is:

$$G(\mathbf{x}) = \begin{cases} \|\mathbf{x}\|^{2m-d} \ln \|\mathbf{x}\| & \text{if } 2m > d \text{ and } d \text{ is even} \\ \|\mathbf{x}\|^{2m-d} & \text{otherwise.} \end{cases} \tag{4}$$

and the null space of $\phi[f]$ is the vector space of polynomials of degree at most m in d variables. These basis functions are radial and conditionally positive definite, so that they represent just particular instances of the well known Radial Basis Functions technique (Micchelli, 1986; Wahba, 1990). In two dimensions, for $m = 2$, eq. (4) yields the so called "thin plate" basis function $G(\mathbf{x}) = \|\mathbf{x}\|^2 \ln \|\mathbf{x}\|$ (Harder and Desmarais, 1972).

The Gaussian

A stabilizer of the form

$$\phi[f] = \int_{R^d} ds\ e^{\frac{\|\mathbf{s}\|^2}{\beta}} |\tilde{f}(\mathbf{s})|^2 \ ,$$

where β is a fixed positive parameter, has $\tilde{G}(\mathbf{s}) = e^{-\frac{\|\mathbf{s}\|^2}{\beta}}$ and as basis function the Gaussian function. The Gaussian function is positive definite, and it is well known from the theory of reproducing kernels (Aronszajn, 1950) that positive definite functions can be used to define *norms* of the type (2). Since $\phi[f]$ is a norm, its null space contains only the zero element, and the additional null space terms of eq. (3) are not needed, unlike in Duchon splines. A disadvantage of the Gaussian is the appearance of the scaling parameter β, while Duchon splines, being homogeneous functions, do not depend on any scaling parameter. However, it is possible to devise good heuristics that give sub-optimal, but still good, values of β, or good starting points for cross-validation procedures.

Other Basis Functions

Here we give a list of other functions that can be used as basis functions in the Radial Basis Functions technique, and that are therefore associated with the minimization of some functional. In the following table we indicate as "p.d." the positive definite functions, which do not need any polynomial term in the solution, and as "c.p.d. k" the conditionally positive definite functions of order k, which need a polynomial of degree k in the solution.

$G(r) = e^{-\beta r^2}$	Gaussian, p.d.
$G(r) = \sqrt{r^2 + c^2}$	multiquadric, c.p.d. 1
$G(r) = \frac{1}{\sqrt{c^2+r^2}}$	inverse multiquadric, p.d.
$G(r) = r^{2n+1}$	multivariate splines, c.p.d. n
$G(r) = r^{2n} \ln r$	multivariate splines, c.p.d. n

1.2.2 Tensor product stabilizers

An alternative to choosing a radial function $\tilde{G}$ in the stabilizer (2) is a *tensor product* type of basis function, that is a function of the form

$$\tilde{G}(\mathbf{s}) = \Pi_{j=1}^{d} \tilde{g}(s_j) \tag{5}$$

where s_j is the j-th coordinate of the vector $\mathbf{s}$, and $\tilde{g}$ is an appropriate one-dimensional function. When g is positive definite the functional $\phi[f]$ is clearly a norm and its null space is empty. In the case of a conditionally positive definite function the structure of the null space can be more complicated and we do not consider it here. Stabilizers with $\tilde{G}(\mathbf{s})$ as in equation (5) have the form

$$\phi[f] = \int_{R^d} ds \, \frac{|\tilde{f}(\mathbf{s})|^2}{\Pi_{j=1}^{d} \tilde{g}(s_j)}$$

which leads to a *tensor product* basis function

$$G(\mathbf{x}) = \Pi_{j=1}^{d} g(x_j)$$

where x_j is the j-th coordinate of the vector $\mathbf{x}$ and $g(x)$ is the Fourier transform of $\tilde{g}(s)$. An interesting example is the one corresponding to the choice:

$$\tilde{g}(s) = \frac{1}{1+s^2} \, ,$$

which leads to the basis function:

$$G(\mathbf{x}) = \Pi_{j=1}^{d} e^{-|x_j|} = e^{-\sum_{j=1}^{d} |x_j|} = e^{-\|\mathbf{x}\|_{L_1}} \, .$$

This basis function is interesting from the point of view of VLSI implementations, because it requires the computation of the L_1 norm of the input vector $\mathbf{x}$, which is usually easier to compute than the Euclidean norm L_2. However, this basis function in not very smooth, and its performance in practical cases should be tested experimentally.

1.2.3 Additive stabilizers

We have seen in the previous section how some tensor product approximation schemes can be derived in the framework of regularization theory. We now will see that is also possible to derive the class of *additive approximation* schemes in the same framework, where by additive approximation we mean an approximation of the form

$$f(\mathbf{x}) = \sum_{\mu=1}^{d} f_\mu(x^\mu) \tag{6}$$

where x^μ is the μ-th component of the input vector $\mathbf{x}$ and the f_μ are one-dimensional functions that will be defined as the *additive components* of f (from now on Greek letter indices will be used in association with components of the input vectors). Additive models are well known in statistics (Hastie and Tibshirani, 1986, 1987, 1990; Buja, Hastie and Tibshirani, 1989; Whaba, 1990) and can be considered as a generalization of linear models. They are appealing because, being essentially a superposition of one-dimensional functions, they have a low complexity, and they share with linear models the feature that the effects of the different variables can be examined separately.

The simplest way to obtain such an approximation scheme is to choose a stabilizer that corresponds to an additive basis function:

$$G(\mathbf{x}) = \sum_{\mu=1}^{n} \theta_\mu g(x^\mu) \tag{7}$$

where θ_μ are certain fixed parameters. Such a choice, in fact, leads to an approximation scheme of the form (6) in which the additive components f_μ have the form:

$$f_\mu(x) = \theta_\mu \sum_{i=1}^{N} c_i G(x^\mu - x_i^\mu) \tag{8}$$

Notice that the additive components are not independent at this stage, since there is only one set of coefficients c_i. We postpone the discussion of this point to section (1.3.2).

We would like to write stabilizers corresponding to the basis function (7) in the form (2), where $\tilde{G}(\mathbf{s})$ is the Fourier transform of $G(\mathbf{x})$. We notice that the Fourier transform of an additive function like the one in equation (7) is not well behaved, since it involves a delta function. For example, in two dimensions we obtain

$$\tilde{G}(\mathbf{s}) = \theta_x \tilde{g}(s_x)\delta(s_y) + \theta_y \tilde{g}(s_y)\delta(s_x) \tag{9}$$

and the interpretation of the reciprocal of this expression is delicate. However, *almost* additive basis functions can be obtained if we approximate the delta functions in eq. (9) with Gaussians of very small variance. Consider, for example in two dimensions, the stabilizer:

$$\phi[f] = \int_{R^d} ds\, \epsilon \frac{|\tilde{f}(\mathbf{s})|^2}{\theta_x \tilde{g}(s_x) e^{-(\frac{s_y}{\epsilon})^2} + \theta_y \tilde{g}(s_y) e^{-(\frac{s_x}{\epsilon})^2}} \tag{10}$$

This corresponds to a basis function of the form:

$$G(x,y) = \theta_x g(x) e^{-\epsilon^2 y^2} + \theta_y g(y) e^{-\epsilon^2 x^2} . \tag{11}$$

In the limit of ϵ going to zero the denominator in expression (10) approaches eq. (9), and the basis function (11) approaches a basis function that is the sum of one-dimensional basis functions. In this paper we do not discuss this limit process in a rigorous way. Instead we outline another way to obtain additive approximations in the framework of regularization theory.

Let us assume that we know *a priori* that the function f that we want to approximate is additive, that is:

$$f(\mathbf{x}) = \sum_{\mu=1}^{d} f_\mu(x^\mu)$$

We then apply the regularization approach and impose a smoothness constraint, not on the function f as a whole, but on each single additive component, through a regularization functional of the form:

$$H[f] = \sum_{i=1}^{N} (y_i - \sum_{\mu=1}^{d} f_\mu(x_i^\mu))^2 + \lambda \sum_{\mu=1}^{d} \frac{1}{\theta_\mu} \int_R ds\, \frac{|\tilde{f}_\mu(s)|^2}{\tilde{g}(s)}$$

where θ_μ are given positive parameters which allow us to impose different degrees of smoothness on the different additive components. The minimizer of this functional is easily found, and skipping null space terms, it has the usual form

$$f(\mathbf{x}) = \sum_{i=1}^{N} c_i G(\mathbf{x} - \mathbf{x}_i) \tag{12}$$

where

$$G(\mathbf{x} - \mathbf{x}_i) = \sum_{\mu=1}^{d} \theta_\mu g(x^\mu - x_i^\mu) ,$$

as in eq. (7).

We notice that the additive component of eq. (12) can be written as

$$f_\mu(x^\mu) = \sum_{i=1}^{N} c_i^\mu g(x^\mu - x_i^\mu)$$

where we have defined

$$c_i^\mu = \frac{c_i}{\theta_\mu} \ .$$

The additive components are therefore not independent because the parameters θ_μ are fixed. If the θ_μ were free parameters, the coefficients c_i^μ would be independent, as well as the additive components.

Notice that the two ways we have outlined for deriving additive approximation from regularization theory are equivalent. They both start from a prior assumption of additivity and smoothness of the class of functions to be approximated. In the first technique the two assumptions are both in the choice of the stabilizer, (eq. 10); in the second they are made explicit and exploited sequentially.

1.3 Extensions: from regularization networks to generalized regularization networks

In this section we will first review some extensions of regularization networks, and then will apply them to Radial Basis Functions and to additive splines.

A fundamental problem in almost all practical applications in learning and pattern recognition is the choice of the relevant variables. It may happen that some of the variables are more relevant than others, that some variables are just totally irrelevant, or that the relevant variables are linear combinations of the original ones. It can therefore be useful to work not with the original set of variables $\mathbf{x}$, but with a linear transformation of them, $\mathbf{W}\mathbf{x}$, where $\mathbf{W}$ is a possibily rectangular matrix. In the framework of regularization theory, this can be taken into account by making the assumption that the approximating function f has the form $f(\mathbf{x}) = F(\mathbf{W}\mathbf{x})$ for some smooth function F. The smoothness assumption is now made directly on F, through a smoothness functional $\phi[F]$ of the form (2). The regularization functional is now expressed in terms of F as

$$H[F] = \sum_{i=1}^{N}(y_i - F(\mathbf{z}_i))^2 + \lambda\phi[F]$$

where $\mathbf{z}_i = \mathbf{W}\mathbf{x}_i$. The function that minimizes this functional is clearly, accordingly to the results of section (1.1), of the form:

$$F(\mathbf{z}) = \sum_{i=1}^{N} c_i G(\mathbf{z} - \mathbf{z}_i) \ .$$

(plus eventually a polynomial in $\mathbf{z}$). Therefore the solution for f is:

$$f(\mathbf{x}) = F(\mathbf{W}\mathbf{x}) = \sum_{i=1}^{N} c_i G(\mathbf{W}\mathbf{x} - \mathbf{W}\mathbf{x}_i) \qquad (13)$$

This argument is exact for given and known $\mathbf{W}$, as in the case of classical Radial Basis Functions. Usually the matrix $\mathbf{W}$ is unknown, and it must be estimated from the examples. Estimating both the coefficients c_i and the matrix $\mathbf{W}$ by least squares is probably not a good idea, since we would end up trying to estimate a number of parameters that is larger than the number of data points (though one may use regularized least squares). Therefore, it has been proposed to replace the approximation scheme of eq. (13) with a similar one, in which he basic shape of the approximation scheme is retained, but the number of basis functions is decreased. The resulting approximating function that we call the *Generalized Regularization Network* (GRN) is:

$$f(\mathbf{x}) = \sum_{\alpha=1}^{n} c_\alpha G(\mathbf{W}\mathbf{x} - \mathbf{W}\mathbf{t}_\alpha) \ . \tag{14}$$

where $n < N$ and the *centers* $\mathbf{t}_\alpha$ are chosen according to some heuristic (Moody and Darken, 1989; Broomhead and Lowe, 1988), or are considered as free parameters (Poggio and Girosi, 1989, 1990). The coefficients c_α and the elements of the matrix $\mathbf{W}$ are estimated accordingly to a least squares criterion. The elements of the matrix $\mathbf{W}$ could also be estimated through cross-validation, which may be a formally more appropriate technique.

In the special case in which the matrix $\mathbf{W}$ and the centers are kept fixed, the resulting technique is one originally proposed by Broomhead and Lowe (1988), and the coefficients satisfy the following linear equation:

$$G^T G\mathbf{c} = G^T \mathbf{y} \ ,$$

where we have defined the following vectors and matrices:

$$(\mathbf{y})_i = y_i \ , \quad (\mathbf{c})_\alpha = c_\alpha \ , \quad (G)_{i\alpha} = G(\mathbf{x}_i - \mathbf{t}_\alpha) \ .$$

This technique, which has become quite common in the neural network community, has the advantage of retaining the form of the regularization solution, while being less complex to compute. A complete theoretical analysis has not yet been given, but some results, in the case in which the matrix $\mathbf{W}$ is set to identity, are already available (Sivakumar and Ward, 1991).

The next sections discuss approximation schemes of the form (14) in the cases of radial and additive basis functions.

1.3.1 Extensions of Radial Basis Functions

In the case in which the basis function is radial, the approximation scheme of eq. (14) becomes:

$$f(\mathbf{x}) = \sum_{\alpha=1}^{n} c_\alpha G(\|\mathbf{x} - \mathbf{t}_\alpha\|_{\mathbf{W}})$$

where we have defined the weighted norm:

$$\|\mathbf{x}\|_{\mathbf{W}} \equiv \mathbf{x} \cdot \mathbf{W}^T \mathbf{W} \mathbf{x} \ . \tag{15}$$

The basis functions of eq. (14) are not radial anymore, or, more accurately, they are radial in the metric defined by eq. (15). This means that the level curves of the basis functions are not circles, but ellipses, whose axes do not need to be aligned with the coordinate axis. Notice that in this case what is important is not the matrix $\mathbf{W}$ itself, but rather the product matrix $\mathbf{W}^T\mathbf{W}$. Therefore, by the Cholesky decomposition, it is sufficient to take $\mathbf{W}$ upper triangular. The approximation scheme defined by eq. (14) has been discussed in detail in (Poggio and Girosi, 1990; Girosi, 1992), so we do will not discuss it further, and will consider, in the next section, its analogue in the case of additive basis functions.

1.3.2 Extensions of additive splines

In the previous sections we have seen an extension of the classical regularization technique. In this section we derive the form that this extension takes when applied to additive splines (as in Girosi, Jones and Poggio, 1993). The resulting scheme is very similar to Projection Pursuit Regression (Friedman and Stuezle, 1981; Huber, 1985).

We start from the "classical" additive spline, derived from regularization in section (1.2.3):

$$f(\mathbf{x}) = \sum_{i=1}^{N} c_i \sum_{\mu=1}^{d} \theta_\mu G(x^\mu - x_i^\mu) \tag{16}$$

In this scheme the smoothing parameters θ_μ should be known, or can be estimated by cross-validation. An alternative to cross-validation is to consider the parameters θ_μ as *free parameters*, and estimate them with a least square technique together with the coefficients c_i. If the parameters θ_μ are free, the approximation scheme of eq. (16) becomes the following:

$$f(\mathbf{x}) = \sum_{i=1}^{N} \sum_{\mu=1}^{d} c_i^\mu g(x^\mu - x_i^\mu)$$

where the coefficients c_i^μ are now independent. Of course, now we must estimate $N \times d$ coefficients instead of just N, and we are likely to encounter the overfitting problem. We then adopt the same idea presented in section (1.3), and consider an approximation scheme of the form

$$f(\mathbf{x}) = \sum_{\alpha=1}^{n} \sum_{\mu=1}^{d} c_\alpha^\mu G(x^\mu - t_\alpha^\mu) \ , \tag{17}$$

in which the number of centers is smaller than the number of examples, reducing the number of coefficients that must be estimated. We notice that eq. (17) can be written as

$$f(\mathbf{x}) = \sum_{\mu=1}^{d} f_\mu(x^\mu)$$

where each additive component has the form:

$$f_\mu(x^\mu) = \sum_{\alpha=1}^{n} c_\alpha^\mu G(x^\mu - t_\alpha^\mu) \ .$$

Therefore another advantage of this technique is that the *additive components are now independent*, each of them being a one-dimensional Radial Basis Functions.

We can now use the same argument from section (1.3) to introduce a linear transformation of the inputs $\mathbf{x} \rightarrow \mathbf{W}\mathbf{x}$, where $\mathbf{W}$ is a $d' \times d$ matrix. Calling $\mathbf{w}_\mu$ the μ-th column of W, and performing the substitution $\mathbf{x} \rightarrow \mathbf{W}\mathbf{x}$ in eq. (17), we obtain

$$f(\mathbf{x}) = \sum_{\alpha=1}^{n} \sum_{\mu=1}^{d'} c_\alpha^\mu G(\mathbf{w}_\mu \cdot \mathbf{x} - t_\alpha^\mu) \ . \tag{18}$$

We now define the following one-dimensional function:

$$h_\mu(y) = \sum_{\alpha=1}^{n} c_\alpha^\mu G(y - t_\alpha^\mu)$$

and rewrite the approximation scheme of eq: (18) as

$$f(\mathbf{x}) = \sum_{i=1}^{d'} h_\mu(\mathbf{w}_\mu \cdot \mathbf{x}) \ . \tag{19}$$

Notice the similarity between eq. (19) and the Projection Pursuit Regression technique: in both schemes the unknown function is approximated by a linear superposition of one-dimensional variables, which are projections of the original variables on certain vectors that have been estimated. In Projection Pursuit Regression the choice of the functions $h_\mu(y)$ is left to the user. In our case the h_μ are one-dimensional Radial Basis Functions, for example cubic splines, or Gaussians. The choice depends, strictly speaking, on the specific prior, that is, on the specific smoothness assumptions made by the user. Interestingly, in many applications of Projection Pursuit Regression the functions h_μ have been indeed chosen to be cubic splines.

Let us briefly review the steps that bring us from the classical additive approximation scheme of eq. (8) to a Projection Pursuit Regression-like type of approximation:

1. the regularization parameters θ_μ of the classical approximation scheme (8) are considered as free parameters;
2. the number of centers is chosen to be smaller than the number of data points;
3. it is assumed that the true relevant variables are some unknown linear combination of the original variables;

We notice that in the special case in which each additive component has just one center ($n = 1$), the approximation scheme of eq. (18) becomes:

$$f(\mathbf{x}) = \sum_{\mu=1}^{d'} c^\mu G(\mathbf{w}_\mu \cdot \mathbf{x} - t^\mu) \ . \tag{20}$$

If the basis function G were a sigmoidal function this would be clearly a standard Multilayer Perceptron with one layer of hidden units. Although sigmoidal functions cannot be derived from regularization theory, not being symmetric functions, they are related to basis functions that can be derived from regularization, like the absolute value function (Girosi, Jones and Poggio, 1993).

1.4 Summary

A large number of approximation techniques can be written as multilayer networks with one hidden layer. Using results of a number of authors (Wahba, 1990; Hastie and Tibshirani, 1990; Girosi, Jones and Poggio, 1993) we have shown that it seems that there is now a theoretical framework that justifies a large spectrum of approximation schemes (networks) in terms of different smoothness constraints imposed within the same regularization functional to solve the ill-posed problem of function approximation from sparse data. The claim is that all the different networks and corresponding approximation schemes can be justified in terms of the variational principle

$$H[f] = \sum_{i=1}^{N} (f(\mathbf{x}_i) - y_i)^2 + \lambda\phi[f] \ . \tag{21}$$

They differ because of different choices of stabilizers ϕ, which correspond to different assumptions on the smoothness of the functions to be approximated.

2 Performance

In the previous part we have talked about different architectures, and their justifications, but we did not discuss their performances. It is clear that the final performance of a technique depends on the number of data points that are available, on the class of functions we want to approximate, on the approximation scheme we are using and on its number of free parameters. In this part of the paper we present some results about the rate of convergence to zero of the approximation error when the number of parameters tends to infinity, under the assumption of having infinite data. We also report two results (Barron, 1991, 1994; Niyogi and Girosi, 1993) that deal with the finiteness of the number of data. In the next section we review the problem of rates of convergence, together with some classical results. In section 2.2 we present a lemma, due to several authors (Maurey, 1981; Jones, 1992; Barron, 1991, 1993), that shows how to construct a sequence of functions f_n that approximate certain functions in a Hilbert space with a rate of convergence $O(\frac{1}{\sqrt{n}})$. In section 2.3 we will show an application of this lemma to a Radial Basis Functions technique, while in section 2.4 we will breifly review other similar results. In section 2.5 we will then draw some conclusions and sketch some open problems.

2.1 Degree of approximation

Let Φ be a normed space of functions and let A be a subset of Φ. The prototypical problem in approximation theory consists in approximating an element f of Φ by an element of A, that is looking for an element in A that has minimum distance from f. It is also natural to consider the *distance of f from A* as

$$\delta(f, A) \equiv \inf_{a \in A} \|f - a\| \tag{22}$$

and to study this quantity for different choices of A and $f \in \Phi$. In the classical theory of approximation the set A is usually a linear k-dimensional subspace $A_k \subset \Phi$ (Lorentz, 1986) (the algebraic or the trigonometric polynomials of given degree and the splines with fixed knots are typical examples of such subspaces), while in nonlinear approximation theory it is usually a k-dimensional manifold (DeVore, 1991). Usually one has a family of manifolds $\{A_k\}_{k=1}^{\infty}$ such that $\bigcup_k A_k$ is dense in Φ and

$$A_1 \subset A_2 \subset \ldots \subset A_n \subset \ldots$$

so that the quantity $\delta(f, A_k)$ is a monotone decreasing function of k converging to zero and the approximation in A_k gets arbitrarily close to f provided one takes k sufficiently large. It is clearly of interest to know the rate of convergence to zero of $\delta(f, A_k)$ as a function of k. This rate of convergence can be taken as a measure of the complexity of f with respect to the manifolds A_k, in the sense that "simple" functions should have a fast rate of convergence.

As an example, let us consider as space Φ the space $\Lambda^d_{s\alpha}$ of the functions whose partial derivatives of order s are bounded in the uniform norm on the

d-dimensional cube $I = [0,1]^d$ and satisfy a Lipschiz condition with exponent α (Lorentz, 1986, p. 50). On the space Φ we consider the uniform norm $\|f\| = \max_I |f(x)|$. Choosing as manifold A_k the set of polynomials of degree $n-1$ in each of the d variables, that is a linear space of dimension $k = n^d$, the following bound can be obtained (Lorentz, 1986):

$$\delta(f, A_k) \leq N d k^{-\frac{s+\alpha}{d}} \tag{23}$$

where N is a constant that depends on f and s.

From this example we see that the rate of convergence dramatically slows down when the dimension d increases, revealing the discouraging phenomenon known under the name of "curse of dimensionality" (Bellman, 1961). However, for every fixed number of dimensions, arbitrary inverse-power rates of convergence can be obtained if the smoothness index s is chosen big enough (although the bound 23 becomes meaningless when both d and s are very large). This result is typical in linear approximation theory since the computation of the n-width (Lorentz, 1986; Pinkus, 1986) of the space $\Lambda^d_{s\alpha}$ shows that the best linear technique cannot improve the rate of convergence $O(k^{-\frac{s+\alpha}{d}})$ (Lorentz 1986, p. 135).

Similar results hold even if nonlinear techniques are taken in account (DeVore, Howard and Micchelli, 1986; DeVore, 1991), and for other spaces of functions, in which smoothness is measured in a different way. We are therefore led to argue that in practical situations we can only approximate classes of functions that become more and more constrained when the dimension increases.

It is therefore interesting to fix a rate of convergence and a particular approximation technique, and to see what kind of functions we can approximate at that rate. In the case in which the rate of convergence is $O(\frac{1}{\sqrt{n}})$ some results have been obtained by a number of authors (Jones, 1992; Barron, 1991, 1993; Breiman, 1992; Girosi and Anzellotti, 1992, 1993; Girosi, 1993; Mhaskar, 1993). Most of these results are based on a simple lemma on iterative approximation in Hilbert spaces, that will be presented in the next section.

2.2 The Maurey-Jones-Barron Lemma

The results we present are based on a lemma by Jones (1992) on the convergence rate of an iterative approximation scheme in Hilbert spaces. A formally similar lemma, brought to our attention by R. Dudley (Dudley, 1991), is due to Maurey, and was published by Pisier in 1981. However Jones' lemma is constructive while Maurey's is not. Here we report a version of the lemma due to Barron (Barron, 1991; 1993) that contains a slight refinement of Jones' result:

Lemma 2.1 (Maurey-Jones-Barron) *If f is in the closure of the convex hull of a set $\mathcal{G}$ in a Hilbert space H with $\|g\| \leq b$ for each $g \in \mathcal{G}$, then for* *every $n \geq 1$ and for $c > b^2 - \|f\|^2$ there is a f_n in the convex hull of n points in $\mathcal{G}$ such that*

$$\|f - f_n\|^2 \leq \frac{c}{n}.$$

In order to exploit this result we need to define suitable classes of functions which are the closure of the convex hull of some subset $\mathcal{G}$ of a Hilbert space H. One way to approach the problem consists in utilizing the ***integral representation*** of functions. Suppose that the functions in a Hilbert space H can be represented by the integral

$$f(\mathbf{x}) = \int_{\mathcal{M}} G_{\mathbf{t}}(\mathbf{x}) d\alpha(\mathbf{t}) \tag{24}$$

where $d\alpha$ is some measure on the parameter set $\mathcal{M}$, and $G_{\mathbf{t}}(\mathbf{x})$ is a function of H parametrized by the parameter $\mathbf{t}$, whose norm $\|G_{\mathbf{t}}(\mathbf{x})\|$ is bounded by the same number for any value of $\mathbf{t}$. If $d\alpha$ is a finite measure, the integral (24) can be seen as an infinite convex combination, and therefore, applying lemma (2.1) one should be able to prove that there exists n coefficients c_i and n parameter vectors $\mathbf{t}_i$ such that

$$\|f - \sum_{i=1}^{n} c_i G_{\mathbf{t}_i}(\mathbf{x})\| \leq O(\frac{1}{\sqrt{n}})$$

In (Girosi and Anzellotti, 1993) we considered the case in which the functions $G_{\mathbf{t}}(\mathbf{x})$ are the translates $G(\mathbf{x}-\mathbf{t})$ of a fixed function G. In the next section we report a result (Girosi, 1993), that can be proved using the same technique of (Girosi and Anzellotti, 1993), in which we consider translates and dilates of the Gaussian function.

2.3 Translates and dilates of the Gaussian function

Let $G_m(\mathbf{x})$ be the Bessel-Macdonald kernel, that is the function whose Fourier Transform is

$$\tilde{G}_m(\mathbf{s}) = \frac{1}{(1 + \|\mathbf{s}\|^2)^{\frac{m}{2}}} \qquad m > 0,$$

and let L_{G_m} the set of functions f that can be written as $f = G_m * \lambda$, where λ is any signed Radon measure whose total variation $|\lambda|_{R^d} \equiv \|\lambda\|$ is finite and the symbol $*$ stands for the convolution operation. In (Girosi and Anzellotti, 1992, 1993) we have shown that, if m is larger than d, elements of the space L_{G_m}, and in particular of the Sobolev space $H^{m,1}$ with m even, are continuous functions that can be approximated with a superposition of n translates of the Bessel-Macdonald kernel with a rate of convergence $O(\frac{1}{\sqrt{n}})$

in the L_∞ norm. However, this result is not particularly useful, because an analytical expression for $G_m(\mathbf{x})$ is not available, and moreover the shape of basis function G_m changes with the dimension (since m has to be larger than d). Here we consider the case in which instead of the Bessel-Macdonald kernel a Gaussian function is used, and we allow not only for translates but also for dilates of the Gaussian function, a technique that has been extensively used in the neural network community (Moody and Darken, 1989).

Our result follows form the observation that the Bessel-Macdonald kernel has the following integral representation (Stein, 1970, p. 132):

$$G_m(\mathbf{x}) = \int_0^\infty H_\sigma(\mathbf{x}) d\mu_{m,d}(\sigma) \tag{25}$$

where we have defined the measure $d\mu_{m,d}(\sigma)$ as

$$d\mu_{m,d}(\sigma) = \frac{\pi^{-m}\, 2^{-(m+\frac{d}{4})}}{\Gamma(\frac{m}{2})} e^{-\frac{\sigma}{4\pi}} \sigma^{\frac{2m-d}{4}-1}\, d\sigma \tag{26}$$

and where $H_\sigma(\mathbf{x})$ is the Gaussian function:

$$H_\sigma(\mathbf{x}) = \left(\frac{2}{\sigma}\right)^{\frac{d}{4}} e^{-\pi\frac{\|\mathbf{x}\|^2}{\sigma}} .$$

Notice that, since we have made the assumption $m > d$, the measure $\mu_{m,d}$ is finite, with total variation $|\mu_{m,d}|$. Let now f be a function that belongs to L_{G_m}. Then we have that $f = G_m * \lambda$, where λ is a signed Radon measure of total variation $\|\lambda\|$. Using the integral representation (25) and applying Fubini's theorem we obtain the following integral representation for f:

$$f(\mathbf{x}) = \int H_\sigma(\mathbf{x}-\mathbf{t}) d\mu_{m,d}(\sigma) d\lambda(\mathbf{t}) . \tag{27}$$

The meaning of this expression is that a function belonging to L_{G_m} is an "infinite" convex combination of translates and dilates of the Gaussian function, and therefore it is not surprising that we can prove the following (Girosi, 1993):

Theorem 2.1 *Let f be a function such that $f = G_m * \lambda$, where λ is a signed Radon measure of bounded total variation $\|\lambda\|$. Then, for every $c > \|\lambda\|^2|\mu_{m,d}|^2 - \|f\|^2$ there exist n numbers c_α and σ_α, with $\sigma_\alpha > 0$, and n vectors $\mathbf{t}_\alpha$ such that*

$$\left\| f(\mathbf{x}) - \sum_{\alpha=1}^{n} c_\alpha e^{-\pi\frac{\|\mathbf{x}-\mathbf{t}_\alpha\|^2}{\sigma_\alpha}} \right\|_{L_2}^2 < \frac{c}{n}$$

Notice that, by the same argument used in (Girosi and Anzellotti, 1992, 1993), the same result holds in the sup norm, and in particular for functions belonging to the Sobolev space $H^{m,1}$ with $m > d$, m even.

Function space	Norm	Approximation scheme
$\int_{R^d} ds\, \lvert\tilde{f}(\mathbf{s})\rvert < +\infty$ (Jones, 1992)	$L_2(\Omega)$	$f(\mathbf{x}) = \sum_{i=1}^{n} c_i \sin(\mathbf{x}\cdot\mathbf{w}_i + \theta_i)$
$\int_{R^d} ds\, \lVert\mathbf{s}\rVert\lvert\tilde{f}(\mathbf{s})\rvert < +\infty$ (Barron, 1991)	$L_2(\Omega)$	$f(\mathbf{x}) = \sum_{i=1}^{n} c_i\sigma(\mathbf{x}\cdot\mathbf{w}_i + \theta_i)$
$\int_{R^d} ds\, \lVert\mathbf{s}\rVert^2\lvert\tilde{f}(\mathbf{s})\rvert < +\infty$ (Breiman, 1992)	$L_2(\Omega)$	$f(\mathbf{x}) = \sum_{i=1}^{n} c_i\lvert\mathbf{x}\cdot\mathbf{w}_i + \theta_i\rvert_+ + \mathbf{x}\cdot\mathbf{a} + b$
$e^{-\lVert\mathbf{x}\rVert^2} * \lambda \;,\lambda \in L_1(R^d)$ (Girosi and Anzellotti, 1992)	$L_\infty(R^2)$	$f(\mathbf{x}) = \sum_{\alpha=1}^{n} c_\alpha e^{-\lVert\mathbf{x}-\mathbf{t}_\alpha\rVert^2}$
$H^{2m,1}(R^d)$, $2m > d$ (Girosi and Anzellotti, 1992)	$L_\infty(R^2)$	$f(\mathbf{x}) = \sum_{\alpha=1}^{n} c_\alpha G_m(\lVert\mathbf{x}-\mathbf{t}_\alpha\rVert^2)$
$H^{2m,1}(R^d)$, $2m > d$ (Girosi, 1993)	$L_2(R^2)$	$f(\mathbf{x}) = \sum_{\alpha=1}^{n} c_\alpha e^{-\frac{\lVert\mathbf{x}-\mathbf{t}_\alpha\rVert^2}{\sigma_\alpha^2}}$

Table 1: Approximation schemes and corresponding functions spaces with the same rate of convergence $O(n^{\frac{1}{2}})$. See text for explanation.

2.4 Other approximation schemes

Lemma (2.1) has been applied to other approximation schemes and function spaces, and table 1 shows a summary of some of these results. Notice that the first 3 examples concern approximation by ridge functions, of the type commonly used in neural networks. The most used approximation scheme is probably the second one (Barron, 1991, 1993), where σ is a sigmoid function, that corresponds to the standard multilayer perceptron with one layer of hidden sigmoidal units. The third one (Breiman, 1992) is also known as "hinge function" approximation, since it represents a linear superposition of "hinging" hyperplanes.

2.5 Summary

We have seen in this part few results about rates of convergences "independent of the dimension". The results presented in this work may be deepened and generalized in several directions, some of which will be described below:

- when lemma (2.1) is applied to Radial Basis Functions techniques, the condition that the basis function has to belong to an Hilbert space, say L_2, is too restrictive, and does not allow us to deal with cases in which G is a function that grows to infinity. Many of the "interesting" Radial Basis Functions are of this type, and it would be interesting to apply lemma (2.1) to these basis functions as well.

- It is still not clear whether the spaces function considered in sections 2.3 and 2.4 are sufficiently large to include functions that could be encountered in practical cases. Moreover the relationship between these different spaces are not well understood, and it would be important to be able to say, given a function, or a set of data, which technique is more appropriate for that particular task.

- These results do not take in account the fact that, in practice, we only have a finite set of data, and can only minimize the mean square error. The joint effect of finite number of parameters and finite number of data can be taken in account and it has been considered by a number of authors (Barron, 1991, 1994; Niyogi and Girosi, 1993). Barron (1991, 1994) considers the function space and the approximation scheme shown in the second entry in table 1, and shows that the mean integrated squared error between the estimated network and the target function is bounded by

  $$O\left(\frac{1}{n}\right) + O\left(\frac{nd}{N}\log N\right) .$$

  For the function space and the approximation scheme shown in the fourth entry in table 1, Niyogi and Girosi (1993) show that the mean integrated squared error between the estimated network and the target function is bounded, with probability greater than $1-\delta$, by

  $$O\left(\frac{1}{n}\right) + O\left[\left(\frac{nd\ln(n) + \ln(1/\delta)}{N}\right)^{1/3}\right] .$$

Acknowledgements

I would like to thank M. Jones and T. Poggio, with whom part of the work presented in this paper has been done.

References

[1] N. Aronszajn. Theory of reproducing kernels. *Trans. Amer. Math. Soc.*, 686:337–404, 1950.

[2] A.R. Barron. Universal approximation bounds for superpositions of a sigmoidal function. Technical Report 58, Department of Statistics, University of Illinois at Urbana-Champaign, Champaign, IL, March 1991.

[3] A.R. Barron. Approximation and estimation bounds for artificial neural networks. Technical Report 59, Department of Statistics, University of Illinois at Urbana-Champaign, Champaign, IL, March 1991a.

[4] A.R. Barron. Universal approximation bounds for superpositions of a sigmoidal function. *IEEE Trans. Info. Theory*, 39(3):930–945, May 1993.

[5] A.R. Barron. Approximation and estimation bounds for artificial neural networks. *Machine Learning*, 14:115–133, 1994. (to appear).

[6] R.E. Bellman. *Adaptive Control Processes.* Princeton University Press, Princeton, NJ, 1961.

[7] M. Bertero. Regularization methods for linear inverse problems. In C. G. Talenti, editor, *Inverse Problems.* Springer-Verlag, Berlin, 1986.

[8] L. Breiman. Hinging hyperplanes for regression, classification, and function approximation. 1992. (submitted for publication).

[9] D.S. Broomhead and D. Lowe. Multivariable functional interpolation and adaptive networks. *Complex Systems*, 2:321–355, 1988.

[10] A. Buja, T. Hastie, and R. Tibshirani. Linear smoothers and additive models. *Annals of Statistics*, 17:453–555, 1989.

[11] R. DeVore, R. Howard, and C. Micchelli. Optimal nonlinear approximation. *Manuskripta Mathematika*, 1989.

[12] R.A. DeVore. Degree of nonlinear approximation. In C.K. Chui, L.L. Schumaker, and D.J. Ward, editors, *Approximation Theory, VI*, pages 175–201. Academic Press, New York, 1991.

[13] D.L. Donohue and I.M. Johnstone. Projection-based approximation and a duality with kernel methods. *Annals of Statistics*, 17(1):58–106, 1989.

[14] J. Duchon. Spline minimizing rotation-invariant semi-norms in Sobolev spaces. In W. Schempp and K. Zeller, editors, *Constructive theory of functions os several variables, Lecture Notes in Mathematics, 571.* Springer-Verlag, Berlin, 1977.

[15] R.M. Dudley. Comments on two preprints: Barron (1991), Jones (1991). Personal communication, March 1991.

[16] N. Dyn. Interpolation of scattered data by radial functions. In C.K. Chui, L.L. Schumaker, and F.I. Utreras, editors, *Topics in multivariate approximation.* Academic Press, New York, 1987.

[17] N. Dyn. Interpolation and approximation by radial and related functions. In C.K. Chui, L.L. Schumaker, and D.J. Ward, editors, *Approximation Theory, VI*, pages 211–234. Academic Press, New York, 1991.

[18] R. Franke. Scattered data interpolation: tests of some method. *Math. Comp.*, 38(5):181–200, 1982.

[19] R. Franke. Recent advances in the approximation of surfaces from scattered data. In C.K. Chui, L.L. Schumaker, and F.I. Utreras, editors, *Topics in multivariate approximation*. Academic Press, New York, 1987.
[20] J.H. Friedman and W. Stuetzle. Projection pursuit regression. *Journal of the American Statistical Association*, 76(376):817–823, 1981.
[21] F. Girosi. On some extensions of radial basis functions and their applications in artificial intelligence. *Computers Math. Applic.*, 24(12):61–80, 1992.
[22] F. Girosi. Rates of convergence of approximation by translates and dilates of a given function. 1993a. (in preparation).
[23] F. Girosi and G. Anzellotti. Rates of convergence of approximation by translates. A.I. Memo 1288, Artificial Intelligence Laboratory, Massachusetts Institute of Technology, 1992.
[24] F. Girosi and G. Anzellotti. Rates of convergence for radial basis functions and neural networks. In *Artificial Neural Networks with Applications in Speech and Vision*, London, 1993. Chapman & Hall.
[25] F. Girosi, M. Jones, and T. Poggio. Priors, stabilizers and basis functions: From regularization to radial, tensor and additive splines. A.I. Memo No. 1430, Artificial Intelligence Laboratory, Massachusetts Institute of Technology, 1993.
[26] R.L. Harder and R.M. Desmarais. Interpolation using surface splines. *J. Aircraft*, 9:189–191, 1972.
[27] R.L. Hardy. Theory and applications of the multiquadric-biharmonic method. *Computers Math. Applic.*, 19(8/9):163–208, 1990.
[28] T. Hastie and R. Tibshirani. Generalized additive models. *Statistical Science*, 1:297–318, 1986.
[29] T. Hastie and R. Tibshirani. Generalized additive models: some applications. *J. Amer. Statistical Assoc.*, 82:371–386, 1987.
[30] T. Hastie and R. Tibshirani. *Generalized Additive Models*, volume 43 of *Monographs on Statistics and Applied Probability*. Chapman and Hall, London, 1990.
[31] P.J. Huber. Projection pursuit. *Annals of Statistics*, 13(2):435–475, 1985.
[32] L.K. Jones. A simple lemma on greedy approximation in Hilbert space and convergence rates for Projection Pursuit Regression and neural network training. *Annals of Statistics*, 20(1):608–613, March 1992.
[33] E.J. Kansa. Multiquadrics – a scattered data approximation scheme with applications to computational fluid dynamics – . *Computers Math. Applic.*, 19(8/9), 1990.
[34] G. G. Lorentz. *Approximation of Functions*. Chelsea Publishing Co., New York, 1986.
[35] W.R. Madych and S.A. Nelson. Multivariate interpolation and conditionally positive definite functions. II. *Mathematics of Computation*, 54(189): 211–230, January 1990.

[36] B. Maurey. In: "Remarques sur un resultat non publiè de B. Maurey" by G. Pisier. In Centre de Mathematique, editor, *Seminarie d'analyse fonctionelle 1980–1981*, Palaiseau, 1981.
[37] J. Meinguet. Multivariate interpolation at arbitrary points made simple. *J. Appl. Math. Phys.*, 30:292–304, 1979.
[38] C. A. Micchelli. Interpolation of scattered data: distance matrices and conditionally positive definite functions. *Constr. Approx.*, 2:11–22, 1986.
[39] C. A. Micchelli. Interpolation of scattered data: distance matrices and conditionally positive definite functions. *Constr. Approx.*, 2:11–22, 1986.
[40] J. Moody and C. Darken. Fast learning in networks of locally-tuned processing units. *Neural Computation*, 1(2):281–294, 1989.
[41] V.A. Morozov. *Methods for solving incorrectly posed problems.* Springer-Verlag, Berlin, 1984.
[42] A. Pinkus. *N-widths in Approximation Theory.* Springer-Verlag, New York, 1986.
[43] T. Poggio and F. Girosi. A theory of networks for approximation and learning. A.I. Memo No. 1140, Artificial Intelligence Laboratory, Massachusetts Institute of Technology, 1989.
[44] T. Poggio and F. Girosi. Networks for approximation and learning. *Proceedings of the IEEE*, 78(9), September 1990.
[45] T. Poggio and F. Girosi. Regularization algorithms for learning that are equivalent to multilayer networks. *Science*, 247:978–982, 1990.
[46] M. J. D. Powell. Radial basis functions for multivariable interpolation: a review. In J. C. Mason and M. G. Cox, editors, *Algorithms for Approximation.* Clarendon Press, Oxford, 1987.
[47] M.J.D. Powell. The theory of radial basis functions approximation in 1990. Technical Report NA11, Department of Applied Mathematics and Theoretical Physics, Cambridge, England, December 1990.
[48] N. Sivakumar and J.D. Ward. On the best least square fit by radial functions to multidimensional scattered data. Technical Report 251, Center for Approximation Theory, Texas A & M University, June 1991.
[49] E.M. Stein. *Singular integrals and differentiability properties of functions.* Princeton, N.J., Princeton University Press, 1970.
[50] A. N. Tikhonov. Solution of incorrectly formulated problems and the regularization method. *Soviet Math. Dokl.*, 4:1035–1038, 1963.
[51] A. N. Tikhonov and V. Y. Arsenin. *Solutions of Ill-posed Problems.* W. H. Winston, Washington, D.C., 1977.
[52] V. N. Vapnik. *Estimation of Dependences Based on Empirical Data.* Springer-Verlag, Berlin, 1982.
[53] G. Wahba. Practical approximate solutions to linear operator equations when the data are noisy. *SIAM J. Numer. Anal.*, 14, 1977.
[54] G. Wahba. *Splines Models for Observational Data.* Series in Applied Mathematics, Vol. 59, SIAM, Philadelphia, 1990.

Self-Organizing Networks for Nonparametric Regression

Vladimir Cherkassky and Filip Mulier

Department of Electrical Engineering
University of Minnesota
Minneapolis, Minnesota 55455, U.S.A.
cherkass@ee.umn.edu

Abstract. Widely known statistical and artificial neural network methods for regression are based on function approximation, i.e. representing an unknown (high-dimensional) function as a decomposition/superposition of simpler (low-dimensional) basis functions. Such methods naturally follow the supervised learning paradigm. In this paper we discuss a different approach to nonparametric regression that is based on unsupervised learning. Unsupervised learning methods are commonly used for modeling an (unknown) density distribution and for Vector Quantization. However, it can be also used for adaptive positioning of units ("knots") along the regression surface, thereby providing discrete approximation of the unknown function. A method for adaptive positioning of knots called Constrained Topological Mapping(CTM) is discussed in detail. CTM is a modification of the biologically inspired method known as Kohonen's Self-Organizing Maps (SOM) suitable for regression. SOM and CTM methods effectively combine iterative (flow through) computation and local regularization to achieve robust performance and modeling flexibility. This paper describes SOM/CTM methods in the general framework of adaptive methods for regression. We also suggest several statistically motivated improvements of these methods.

1 Neural Network and Statistical Methods for Regression

In the last decade, neural networks have given rise to high expectations for model-free statistical estimation from a finite number of samples(examples). However, several recent studies clearly point out that Artificial Neural Networks(ANNs) represent inherently statistical techniques subject to well-known statistical limitations [Barron et al, 1988; Geman et al, 1992; White, 1989; Ripley, 1993]. Moreover, many neural learning (adaptation) procedures can be readily recognized as a special case of stochastic approximation techniques proposed in the early 50's. Whereas many early neural network application studies have been mostly empirical, more recent research successfully applies statistical notions (such as overfitting, resampling, bias-variance dilemma, the curse of dimensionality etc.) to improve neural network performance. Statisticians can also gain a lot from analyzing neural network models as a new tool for data analysis. It may be interesting to note that many recently proposed statistical methods have their neural network counterparts. For example, there is a close similarity between MARS[Friedman, 1991] and a tree-structured network proposed by Sanger[1991]; the popular backpropagation networks use the same functional representation as Projection Pursuit Regression[Friedman and Stuetzle, 1981]; and Breiman's PI-method[1991] is related to sigma-pi networks [Rumelhart and McClelland, 1986] as both seek to represent an output (function) in the sum-of-products form.

Here we consider regression problems. Using mathematical notation, we seek to estimate a function f of $N-1$ predictor variables (denoted by vector $\mathbf{x}$) from a given set of n training data points, or measurements, $\mathbf{z}_i = (\mathbf{x}_i, y_i)$ $(i = 1, \ldots, n)$ in N-dimensional sample space:

$$y = f(\mathbf{x}) + \text{error} \tag{1}$$

where error is unknown (but zero mean) and its distribution may depend on $\mathbf{x}$. The distribution of training data in $\mathbf{x}$ is also unknown and can be arbitrary.

Nonparametric methods make no or very few general assumptions about the unknown function $f(\mathbf{x})$. Nonparametric regression is hard due to:

(1) the finite number of training samples implies that any estimate of an unknown function is always inaccurate (biased), i.e., the problem itself is ill-posed. In particular, meaningful predictions are possible only for sufficiently smooth functions [Poggio and Girosi, 1990]. We emphasize that the function smoothness is measured with respect to sampling density of the training data.

(2) the curse or complexity of dimensionality, or inherent sparseness of finite training data in high-dimensional settings (see Friedman's paper in this volume).

(3) the problem in distinguishing between the variations due to (unknown) additive noise and true function variations, given finite training sample. This is known as bias-variance dilemma in statistics[Geman et al, 1992].

Many ANN application studies successfully tackle the problems with tens and hundreds variables, in spite of the fact that nonparametric methods face the problem of sparse data in high dimensions. The reasons for this disagreement between statistical theory and practical applications of ANNs are not very clear [Cybenko, 1990]. A possible explanation is that application studies employ clever preprocessing or data encoding techniques, so that the network has to learn simple functions or decision surfaces[Cherkassky and Lari-Najafi, 1992]. Another possibility is that in high-dimensional applications many input variables are interdependent, so that the *effective* problem dimensionality is small. Yet another plausible explanation is that high-dimensional real data typically has a very non-uniform distribution (i.e. appears in clusters) - this may explain the success of *local* methods, such as Radial Basis Functions and Fuzzy Inference Systems.

Most statistical methods utilize the whole training set (batch mode), whereas ANN methods typically use iterative processing (one sample at a time) known as flow-through computation in Statistics. It appears that gradient-descent style training procedures are used in ANN methods mainly for historical reasons, since most studies report off-line training where the whole training set is available.

Hence, according to Ripley[1994], general unconstrained minimization methods (i.e. quasi-Newton and conjugate gradient descent) usually work better than empirically chosen variants of gradient descent (backpropagation). However, Finnoff[1994] argues that a common variant of backpropagation is less likely to get stuck in local minima than the batch training process. Whereas batch methods are usually much faster than gradient-descent style iterative methods, there are several advantages to iterative ANN methods. They tend to be very simple computationally, albeit at the expense of recycling (multiple presentations) of the training data. Another advantage is that models can be generated in real time as the data becomes available.

It may be interesting to note that batch mode processing fits naturally into the framework provided by *global* error minimization and *global* complexity penalization formulations common in statistical and ANN methods (see papers by Friedman and Girosi in this volume). Here global refers to the error (cost) function and the penalization terms defined over the entire domain of $\mathbf{x}$ (predictor variables). Availability of the complete training set (batch mode) naturally enables analytic treatment using minimization of global error on the training data with an added global penalization term. However, such global penalization formulation usually allows analytic treatment under the assumption that an estimated function is *uniformly smooth* over the entire domain of $\mathbf{x}$. In many practical applications, an unknown function may have different smoothness properties in various parts of $\mathbf{x}$. Hence, it seems reasonable to penalize more in one part of the domain of $\mathbf{x}$, and less in another. Local regularization is difficult to implement *analytically*, since the function itself is unknown. However, flow through methods that process one training sample at a time, can potentially achieve local regularization by allowing "unequal" treatment of different data points, depending on the current local estimate of the function.

Computational methods for regression fall into three major groups [Friedman, 1991]:

- *Global parametric methods*, which assume that an unknown function in (1) has a fixed (parametric) form, or can be represented as a combination of (predetermined, fixed) basis functions globally defined in $\mathbf{x}$. Examples include Linear and Polynomial Regression.
- *Piecewise parametric or locally parametric methods* try to approximate an unknown function by several simple parametric functions each defined over a different subregion of domain of independent variables. These methods are also equivalent (at least in low dimensions) to local or kernel smoothers [Friedman et al, 1989]. In these methods the training data enters explicitly into a parametric model. Examples are piecewise-linear regression, splines[de Boor, 1978] and statistical kernel methods.
- *Adaptive computation methods* which dynamically adjust their strategy to the training data, in order to take into account the behavior of the unknown function.

The motivation for adaptive methods is due to the fact that for high-dimensional problems locally parametric techniques fail to estimate the underlying function faithfully because there is usually not enough data points in the training set. Since global parametric methods inevitably introduce bias and local parametric methods are applicable only to low-dimensional problems (given a limited-size training set), *adaptive* methods are the only practical alternative in high-dimensions.

We further distinguish several types of adaptive methods:
- *Global Adaptive Methods* that seek regression estimate within a rich class of functions defined globally in the domain of predictor variables $\mathbf{x}$. Global adaptive methods are based on the existence theorems from Function Approximation stating that any "reasonable" function can be represented as superposition of simpler functions of lower dimensionality[Barron et al, 1988; Breiman, 1991]. Frequently, such a superposition of parametric and/or nonparametric functions(components) can be regarded as a network of components. In ANN research, these methods are known as *adaptive* networks, where the network topology (i.e. the number of hidden units) is not fixed in advance. Examples include: Projection Pursuit[Friedman and Stuetzle, 1981]; feedforward networks, polynomial networks[Barron et al, 1988] etc.;
- *Local Adaptive Methods* seek an unknown function as a sum of local functions, i.e. functions that are large only in a small region in $\mathbf{x}$-space and small (or zero) elsewhere. Coefficients in the linear combination ("weights") and parameters associated with each basis function (that determine a region where the function is large) are determined from the training data. Examples of local adaptive methods include adaptable-span kernel methods, radial basis function (RBF) networks, regularization networks, networks with locally tuned units etc. [Broomhead et al, 1988; Moody et al, 1989; Poggio et al, 1990; Specht, 1991];
-*Partitioning Methods* seek to partition domain of $\mathbf{x}$ into several regions, so that each region is using its own (simple) parametric function to model the response. Partitioning methods differ on both the choice of the partitioning strategy and the choice of parametric functions. However, the partitioning strategy is usually more important, so we can further classify partitioning methods as:
- Recursive Partitioning methods that employ recursive (greedy) partitioning strategy to minimize lack-of-fit (squared residual) error. Examples include CART and MARS[Breiman et al, 1984; Friedman, 1991] ;
- Non-recursive Partitioning or Adaptive Function Quantization Methods that provide discrete approximation of the regression surface using (non-recursive) partitioning methods borrowed from Pattern Recognition and ANN research[Cherkassky and Lari-najafi, 1991; Cherkassky, 1992]. The goal is to provide piecewise-constant approximation of the unknown function by specifying $(\mathbf{x}, y)$ locations of the finite set of "knots" or "network units". The domain of independent variables is partitioned into many (unequal) subregions, assuming constant response value for each subregion. The center of each subregion corresponds to the knot location, and thus the problem of knot location is equivalent to piecewise-constant quantization of the regression surface into many subregions:

$$\text{if } \mathbf{x} \in R_m, \text{ then } f(\mathbf{x}) = c_m \qquad (2)$$

where disjoint subregions R_m and c_m are unknown response values for each subregion are determined by an adaptive algorithm. Thus adaptive function quantization can be viewed as adaptive placement of "knots" along an (unknown) regression surface, as discussed next.

2 Adaptive Knot Location and Self-Organization

This section discusses the connection between the problem of knot placement frequently encountered in statistical methods for regression, and a neural network model of self-organization. Notice that in this paper the term "knots" is used generically to describe a grid of points (units) representing regression surface. This should not be confused with a specific notion of knots usually associated with spline methods in statistics. For example, in the methods described in this paper the units (knots) *can not* be viewed as free parameters as in many applications of spline methods.

2.1 Motivation: the Problem of Knot Location

One of the challenging problems in implementation of adaptive methods for multivariate regression is adaptive positioning of knots along the regression surface. Usually, the method of interpolation between the knots is fixed (i.e. by the order of the spline in spline methods) and the only way the method can adapt to the target function is through knot placement. We consider the simplest type of interpolation between the knots (piecewise constant), in order to focus attention on the problem of the knot location. In fact, for high-dimensional problems the most important part of an adaptive method is its knot placement (partitioning) strategy, and not the interpolation method used. For example, results produced by MARS do not depend significantly on the type of splines used. The problem of knot placement is often discussed under different names in various adaptive methods, i.e. partitioning strategy in recursive partitioning methods, learning center locations in Radial Basis Function methods, etc.

The common approach to knot positioning is to choose first $\mathbf{x}$-coordinates, and then determine y-values for the knots. Typically, knot positions in the domain of $\mathbf{x}$ are chosen as a subset of the training data set, or knots are uniformly distributed in $\mathbf{x}$. Once $\mathbf{x}$-locations are fixed, commonly used data-driven methods can be applied to determine the number of knots [Friedman and Silverman, 1989], and the y-values can be found from the training data (usually by the standard least squares techniques). Unfortunately, optimal positioning of knots in $\mathbf{x}$-space depends on y-values. For example, de Boor[1978] showed that a polynomial spline with unequally spaced knots can approximate an arbitrary function much better than a spline with equally spaced knots. Unfortunately, the minimization problem involved in determination of the optimal placement of knots is highly nonlinear and the solution space is not convex[Friedman and Silverman, 1989]. Hence, the performance of many recent algorithms that include adaptive knot placement (e.g. MARS) is difficult to evaluate analytically. There are several factors which contribute to the complexity of the knot positioning problem:
High-dimensional problems. For a single-variable function, it can be shown that the optimal local knot density is (roughly) proportional to the squared second derivative of the function and the local density of the training data, and inversely proportional to the local noise variance [Brockmann et al, 1993]. No analytic results are available for higher dimensions or data-dependent noise, but similar results probably hold true.

Estimating the second derivative of a true function is necessary for optimal knot placement. Yet, the function itself is unknown and its estimation depends on the good placement of knots. This may suggest the need for some iterative procedure that alternates between function estimation(smoothing) and knot positioning steps.
Finite-sample variance. Given a (sparse) training sample, it may not be a good strategy to place knots at a subset of data set, as done in many statistical methods. A sparse sample may be a poor approximation of an underlying distribution. Hence, knot location can be determined better by applying some smoothing to the scatterplot of $\mathbf{x}$-coordinates of the training data, in order to find a more accurate estimate of the unknown distribution.
Assumed class of the basis functions. Even though all major methods for regression for a one-variable case(kernel methods, smoothing splines, nearest neighbor etc.) are quite similar, at least for uniform data points, this is not true in high dimensions. For multivariate problems, the good strategy for knot placement strongly depends on the class of basis functions used to approximate the regression surface. For example, Friedman's MARS uses partitioning approach to knot selection that fits naturally into his regression splines of the tensor product type. Alternatively, a network for function estimation proposed by Poggio and Girosi[1990] effectively implements regression with Radial Basis Functions (RBF) or thin plate splines. In the thin plate spline case the strategy for choosing "knots" (or RBF centers) is different from MARS partitioning approach. In both cases knot selection is a nontrivial part of each method, as noted by Gu and Wahba in their discussion section in [Friedman, 1991].

2.2 Self-Organizing Maps for Adaptive Knot Location

In the spirit of self-organizing networks, we may attempt to approximate an unknown regression surface (or distribution) using a fixed number of "units" (or local "prototypes"). This corresponds to piecewise constant approximation between the knots in statistical formulation. In statistical spline methods knot locations are typically viewed as free parameters of the model, and hence the number of knots directly controls the model complexity. Alternatively, one can introduce topological ordering between the knots, and then impose *local regularization* constraints on adjacent knot locations, so that neighboring knots cannot move independently (this requires the notion of "neighborhood"). Such an approach is effectively implemented in the model of self-organization known as Kohonen's Self-Organizing Maps (SOM) [Kohonen, 1984]. This model uses a set of units ("knots") with a neighborhood relation between units defined according to a fixed topological structure (typically 1D or 2D grid). An M-dimensional map consists of units arranged in M-dimensional grid topology. The neighborhood relation between the units i and j on the map is specified as the *topological distance* between these units, i.e. the number of hops in the shortest path from i to j. The goal of the SOM model is to approximate an unknown statistical distribution (given by a finite training set) by a topological map of low dimensionality (typically, 1D or 2D). This is achieved by repeated presentations of the training data to the network (map). During training or self-organization, data points are presented to the map iteratively, one at a time, and the unit closest to the data moves towards it, also pulling along its topological neighbors. This can be summarized as a two-step process [Kohonen, 1984]:

1. Given a data sample, find the unit with value nearest the data using some distance measure in the input (data) space. This unit is then designated the "winner".
2. Move the "winner" along with its neighborhood towards the data. The amount of motion for each unit depends on its topological distance from the winner in the model space.

Decrease the learning rate and the neighborhood.

Commonly, the Euclidean distance in the sample space is used as the measure in the first step. Step 2, the unit update, can be written as:

$$\mathbf{w}_j(k) = \mathbf{w}_j(k-1) + \beta(k)C_j(i(k),k)\left[\mathbf{z}(k) - \mathbf{w}_j(k-1)\right] \tag{3}$$

Where $\mathbf{w}_j(k)$ is the vector denoting the location of unit j at iteration k ($k = 1, 2, \ldots, kmax$), $\mathbf{z}(k)$ is the sample vector presented at time k, β is the learning rate that decreases with k, C is the neighborhood function dependent on unit indices j and $i(k)$ -the winning unit index at time k. C is often taken to be a Gaussian function of the index j with mean at $i(k)$ and standard deviation decreasing with k. Many empirical rules for choosing the learning rate and the neighborhood schedule exist. A common choice is the exponentially decreasing learning rate and neighborhood function [Ritter, Martinetz and Schulten, 1991]:

$$\beta(k) = \beta_0 \left(\frac{\beta_f}{\beta_0}\right)^{\frac{k}{kmax}} \quad (4) \qquad C_j(i,k) = exp\left(\frac{-\|i-j\|^2}{(\beta(k)S_0)^2}\right) \quad (5)$$

In the above equations $kmax$ is the total number of iterations and S_0 is the number of units per dimension in the map.

Empirical results given by Kohonen and many other researchers show that following many presentations the SOM approximates faithfully an unknown distribution. In other words, following training, the input space is divided into a number of regions (given by to the number of units in the map), and each unit's coordinates serve as a prototype vector for the its region. Notice that an N-dimensional probabilistic distribution is effectively approximated using an M-dimensional map (usually $M < N$).

The goals of the original SOM algorithm are:

- adaptive vector quantization or density estimation using discrete number of prototypes (map units);
- dimensionality reduction, when a high-dimensional distribution is approximated using a low-dimensional map. This can be also interpreted as finding a nonlinear low-dimensional projection of the distribution.

2.3 CTM Algorithm for Regression

Cherkassky and Lari-Najafi [1990, 1991] proposed to interpret the units of a topological map as the dynamically movable knots for regression problems. Correspondingly, the problem of finding a regression estimate can be stated as the problem of forming an M-dimensional topological map using a set of samples from N-dimensional sample space (where $M \leq N-1$). Regression fitting is achieved by training a map to approximate training samples $\mathbf{z}_i = (\mathbf{x}_i, y_i)$ in N-dimensional input space. Unfortunately, straightforward application of the SOM algorithm to regression problem does not work well. The reason is that the original Kohonen's algorithm is intended for density estimation and it does not preserve the functionality of the regression surface. In particular, the presence of noise (in y-dimension) in the training data can fool the algorithm to produce a map that is a multiple-valued function of the predictor variables in formulation (1). This problem is overcome in the Constrained Topological Mapping (CTM) algorithm, where the best-matching unit is found *in the space of predictor variables*, rather than in the input (sample) space [Cherkassky and Lari-Najafi, 1991]. An approach of using SOM for time series prediction very similar to CTM was proposed independently by Walter, Ritter and Schulten [1990].

Following training, CTM with piecewise-constant interpolation between the units effectively partitions domain of predictor variables $\mathbf{x}$ into many (unequal) subregions, so that there is a constant response value for each subregion. Locations of the trained CTM units specify subregions and the function response for each subregion. The goals of regression are smoothing in y-dimension and, possibly, extracting *effective dimensionality* for high-dimensional data sets with *dependent/correlated* predictor variables. The number of regions may be larger than the number of training samples (i.e., in high-dimensional problems), so there is usually no goal of data compression.

We present next a concise description of the CTM algorithm. Using formulation (1) for regression, the training data are N-dimensional vectors $\mathbf{z}_i = (\mathbf{x}_i, y_i)$, where y_i is a noisy observation of an unknown function of $N-1$ predictor variables given by vector $\mathbf{x}_i$ (of dimension $N-1$). Also assume deterministic or probabilistic dependencies given by K *unknown constraints* on predictor variables (the *number of constraints*, K, is known). Then the number of independent variables, or *effective problem dimensionality*, is $M = N-1-K$. Frequently $M = N-1$ (i.e. all predictor variables are independent, as in most low-dimensional problems). The CTM algorithm constructs an M-dimensional map in N-dimensional sample space as follows:

0. Initialize the M-dimensional topological map in N-dimensional sample space. For example, $\mathbf{x}$-coordinates of units can be initialized uniformly over the range of predictor variables, with y-coordinates set to small random values or zero.
1. Given an input training data vector $\mathbf{z}(k) = (\mathbf{x}(k), y(k))$ in N-dimensional sample space at time k, find the closest (best matching) unit i in the $\mathbf{x}$-space (of predictor variables). Closeness is usually measured using Euclidean distance as a metric.

2. Adjust the weights of the units in the full space $(\mathbf{x}, y)$ exactly as in the Kohonen SOM algorithm - see equation (3).
3. Decrease the learning rate and the neighborhood.

Note that both the learning rate and the neighborhood are gradually reduced as the training continues. Original CTM specifies exponentially decreasing learning rate and neighborhood schedule according to equations (4, 5). Gradual decrease in the learning rate is typical for neural network training viewed as a special case of stochastic approximation [White, 1989]. However, decrease of the neighborhood function does not have an obvious statistical interpretation/explanation.

3 Relationship Between SOM/CTM and Other Methods

Based on empirical comparisons[Cherkassky and Lari-Najafi, 1991; Cherkassky, Lee and Lari-Najafi, 1991], CTM algorithm appears competitive against other methods for low-to-medium-dimensional problems. Unfortunately, theoretical properties of the CTM algorithm are difficult to derive. In this section we provide some qualitative insights into the properties of CTM and its relationship to other methods. CTM algorithm interpretation can be greatly simplified by considering training (self-organization) process in $\mathbf{x}$-space of predictor variables *separately* from y-dimension (response variable). It can be readily seen, that $\mathbf{x}$-coordinates of CTM units during training follow the standard Kohonen SOM algorithm. Therefore, trained CTM units approximately follow the distribution of the training data in the space of predictor variables. This capability is related to other methods, such as Sammon's method for low-dimensional projections[Sammon, 1969] and Principal Curves/Manifolds[Hastie and Stuetzle, 1989]. On the other hand, in y-dimension CTM method is similar to the flow-through version of kernel methods known as the Method of Potential Functions[Mendel and Fu, 1970]. The main distinct feature of CTM appears to be the concept of the topological neighborhood, that can be interpreted as a *local regularization* constraint imposed on the (topologically) adjacent map units. Detailed comparisons of SOM/CTM with other methods for density modeling and regression are discussed below.

3.1 Kohonen Maps, Principal Surfaces and Dimensionality Reduction

As mentioned above, movement of CTM units in $\mathbf{x}$-space is independent of y-values of the training data, and amounts to vector quantization and dimensionality reduction in $\mathbf{x}$-space. Such dimensionality reduction is often possible because of correlation or dependency among variables in real data sets. Sammon's method[1969] also achieves dimensionality reduction. The main advantage of Kohonen's maps over Sammon's method seems to be the concept of the *topological neighborhood*, which provides for better robustness, generalization and interpretability of the model[Kraaijveld et al, 1992].

In statistics, the notion of principal curves(or manifolds) has been introduced by Hastie and Stuetzle[1989] to approximate a scatterplot of points from an unknown probability distribution. They argue that principal component analysis technique summarize the data with a straight line, and hence may produce a poor fit when the linearity assumption does not hold. Hence, they use a smooth non-linear curve called a principal curve, to approximate the joint behavior of the two variables. Obviously, the objectives of the Kohonen method are similar to the goal of finding principal curves, even though Hastie and Stuetzle, evidently, were not familiar with Kohonen's work. Surprisingly, there is a lot of similarity between Hastie and Stuetzle's algorithm for finding principal curves, and Kohonen's algorithm for adaptive positioning of units(knots) of a one-dimensional map. To make a meaningful comparison, consider the batch-mode version of SOM [Kohonen, 1993], since the Principle Curve approach uses batch processing. The H&S algorithm for finding principal curves consists of two steps:

1. *The Projection Step* of finding for each sample point its projection (or the closest point) on the curve. This is similar to finding the best matching unit step in Kohonen's algorithm. The principal curve algorithm uses line segments to approximate the principle curve between the projected data points, while the SOM algorithm uses a piecewise constant approximation given by the units of the one-dimensional map.
2. *The Conditional-Expectation Step*, implemented via scatterplot smoothing. Scatterplot smoothing is applied to the projected values along the length of the principal curve, which is parameterized according to arc length. H&S suggest the following "most successful" empirical strategy for choosing span selection: "initially use a large span, and then decrease it gradually". This is similar to neighborhood reduction in SOM. In particular, in the batch-mode version of SOM, unit updating can be formulated as a kernel scatterplot smoothing applied to the units in the topological space with a decreasing span. The effect of the smoothing is different in each algorithm, due to the differences in parameterization of the principle curve vs. the topological map. Since the principle curve is parameterized according to arc length, the smoothing span is defined in terms of a distance in the sample space. The parameterization of the SOM map is according to the map topology, which is fixed and not related to the distance between the units in the sample space. This causes qualitative differences in the structure of the principle curve compared to the batch-mode self-organizing map, especially in the initial stages of operation for each algorithm. At the start of self-organization, when the neighborhood width is large, nearly each unit is updated by every data sample so the map units form a tight cluster around the centroid of the data distribution. At this point there is a high degree of smoothness in the model (topological) space since topologically near units have very similar values. On the other hand, the Principle Curve algorithm tends to approximate the first principle component line during the initial iterations (when a high degree of smoothing is applied) since smoothness is defined directly in the sample space.

In summary, Kohonen's method can be viewed as a computational procedure for finding discrete approximation of principal curves(or surfaces) by means of a topological map of units (knots)[Ritter, Martinetz and Schulten, 1991]. This connection between Kohonen's maps and Principal Surfaces also suggests the types of problems for which CTM may be particularly useful:

- errors-in-variables regression, i.e. when there is randomness in the predictor variables;
- highly correlated or dependent predictor variables.
- reducing variance due to finite sample size, achieved by CTM algorithm smoothing effect (due to the concept of neighborhood). Hence, adaptive knot positioning by CTM is superior to the usual strategy of placing knots at **x**-locations of a (small) training sample.

3.2 Local Regularization and CTM Neighborhood

Regularization/penalization methods are commonly used in Statistical and ANN methods. In spite of their theoretic appeal, their practical use is limited by the use of *global* complexity terms. This is equivalent to an assumption that a function is uniformly smooth over the entire domain of **x**. In many practical applications, an unknown function may have different smoothness properties in various parts of **x**. Hence, it seems reasonable to penalize more in one part of the domain of **x**, and less in another. Local regularization may be accomplished using an iterative computational approach, such as CTM. In CTM algorithm, the map of units can be viewed as the model that adaptively adjusts itself to the training data. During the adaptation process given by CTM algorithm, the neighborhood effectively introduces *local regularization* effect into the algorithm. For example, increasing the number of units(knots) does not result in overfitting, as in many statistical methods. It is shown empirically that the quality of CTM smoothing of pure noise does not depend on the number of knots used[Cherkassky and Lari-najafi, 1991]. However, this effect is difficult to describe analytically, since the neighborhood itself is reduced during training.

3.3 CTM, Method of Potential Functions and Kernel Smoothers

The CTM algorithm is closely related to the method of potential functions (MPF) [Mendel and Fu, 1970]. The Potential Function is essentially a kernel function, and the MPF method seeks a regression estimate iteratively, with every training sample presentation:

$$f_{k+1}(x) = f_k(x) + \beta(k)h(x - x_k)\big(y_k - f_k(x)\big) \tag{6}$$

where k is the discrete time step, h is a kernel (potential) function with its center locations given by the training data points. Learning rate $\beta(k) = 1/k$ is given according to standard conditions prescribed by stochastic approximation. The method of potential functions recursively updates an estimate of the unknown function with every new observation (noisy data point). Thus MPF method can be viewed as a flow-through implementation of a kernel smoother. Recursive estimation (6) has some similarity with CTM unit update in y-space using equation (3). However, an important difference is that in CTM the map space is distinctly different from the sample space. Traditional kernel smoothers seek regression estimates in the original sample space, whereas CTM transforms the *model* of the data, represented by a map. Hence, the number of units and the dimensionality of

CTM can be set different from the number of training points and the number of predictor variables, respectively. For example, a two-dimensional map can be used to model intrinsically two-dimensional problems, even with large number of predictor variables (see examples in section 3.4 below). In summary, the CTM neighborhood can be interpreted as a kernel in the model (map) space, and training is analogous to kernel smoothing in the map space.

3.4 CTM Comparisons

Maechler et al[1990] compare prediction performance of a backpropagation network vs. Projection Pursuit(PP) for several 2-variable regression problems of various complexity, i.e. simple interaction, radial, harmonic, additive and complicated interaction functions. They conclude that both methods achieve similar prediction accuracy, but that PP is computationally much faster(by two orders of magnitude). Later, Cherkassky, Lee and Lari-Najafi[1991] applied CTM method to the same data set, and achieved overall improvement in the prediction accuracy. These results are particularly encouraging, since CTM results are degraded by the quantization error peculiar to the current CTM implementation (piecewise-constant regression). Friedman [personal communication, 1991] applied MARS to the same data, and obtained further improvement over CTM for all functions, except the harmonic function, where CTM still performed best. Results of the latter comparison are not surprising, since CTM is similar to kernel methods which are known to work best for harmonic functions.

We show next comparison of different methods on regression problems with collinear variables, using artificial data sets in Table 1. For example, in the case of function 1, the variable y is dependent on only two variables a and b, however, the data set consists of three predictor variables x_1, x_2 and x_3. It is important that the nonparametric modeling method be able to take advantage of the implicit constraints in order to reduce the effective problem dimensionality. The training and test sets each consisted of 100 samples with normally distributed noise (with standard deviation σ given in Table 1). The normalized RMS error for the test set was used as a performance index. Four methods were compared: k-nearest neighbors, CTM, MARS, and GMBL [Atkeson, 1990]. Generalized memory-based learning (GMBL) is an advanced version of locally weighted regression [Cleveland et al, 1988], i.e., it applies weighted nearest-neighbor or locally weighted linear interpolation with parameters selected by cross-validation. For each method, the smoothing parameters were varied over a large range to achieve the best results.

Table 1. Functions used to create the artificial data sets.

number	function	noise
1	$x_1 = a^2,\ x_2 = b^2,\ x_3 = cos(a^2 + b^2),\ y = a + b$	σ=.1
2	$x_1 = a,\ x_2 = sin(a),\ y = cos(a)$	σ=.05
3	$x_1 = a,\ x_2 = cos(a),\ x_3 = a,\ x_4 = a^2,\ x_5 = a^3,$ $y = sin(a)$	σ=.05
4	$x_1 = a,\ x_2 = b,\ x_3 = a^2,\ x_4 = ab,\ x_5 = b^2,$ $y = sin(2\pi a)cos(2\pi b)$	σ=.05

Table 2. Best normalized RMS error of the test set.

number	k NN	GMBL	MARS	CTM
1	.29	.28	.28	.26
2	.40	.36	.34	.35
3	.12	.11	.11	.11
4	.63	.44	1.0	.67

Naturally, problems with an intrinsic dimensionality of two (functions 1,4), tend to be more difficult for every method to handle than those with intrinsic dimensionality of one (functions 2,3). The most difficult problem, based on normalized RMS error, (function 4), also has more variation in the quality of the models. The results also show that the modeling difficulty is not related to the number of predictor variables. This can be seen by comparing functions 2 and 3. Both of these functions have a intrinsic dimensionality of one and have similar sinusoidal dependence, but function 3 has 5 predictor variables while function 2 has 2. The modeling results for function 3 are much better than those of function 2. A possible explanation for this is that some of the predictor variables of function 3 are powers of a which are the terms in the Taylor approximation for the sinusoid. The variable y depends on some of the predictor variables linearly, so this is in fact a simple modeling task. This example shows that it is misleading to judge the difficulty of a problem based solely on the dimensionality of the data set. The above results show that CTM can be successfully applied to regression problems with collinear variables. In particular, the best results using CTM method were achieved with the map dimensionality equal to the intrinsic dimensionality of a problem.

The data used for the following comparison is the result of a designed experiment on a 3M drying process. There are three input variables and seven output variables in the data set. The set was divided so that 50 samples were used for training and 25 samples used for testing. The first step taken in the analysis was to look at the linear correlation coefficients between the predictor and response variables (Table 3).

Table 3. Correlation coefficients between the variables.

	y1	y2	y3	y4	y5	y6	y7
x1	-0.93	-0.92	-0.04	-0.87	-0.85	0.27	0.27
x2	0.98	0.98	0.04	0.91	0.90	-0.36	-0.38
x3	0.58	0.60	0.11	0.45	0.46	-0.34	-0.39

Among the output variables, y1, y2, y4, y5 have a high linear correlation with the independent variables. Variables y3, y6, and y7 have low linear correlation with the independent variables. This indicates that either the independent variables have no effect on these dependent variables or that the effect is non-linear, making them difficult variables to model. A number of modeling methods were applied to the training data and the normalized RMS error for predicting the test set was determined. For each method the smoothing parameters were varied in order to achieve the best results for the test set. Only the best result for each method is shown in Table 4.

Table 4. Normalized RMS error for the test set.

	k-NN	GMBL	MARS	backprop	CTM
y1	.28	.35	.30	.30	.22
y2	.31	.34	.33	.33	.26
y3	.97	1.14	1.00	.85	.78
y4	.42	.33	.34	.26	.32
y5	.52	.75	.48	.46	.43
y6	.80	.64	.90	.69	.76
y7	.62	.60	.83	.67	.58

Modeling y1 and y2 should have been an easy task due to the high linear correlation with the independent variables. MARS and backpropagation performed as well as linear regression with first order terms and GMBL performed worse. The CTM map which performed the best was one dimensional for both y1 and y2. This may indicate that some constraints exist between the predictor variables. Variables y4 and y5 were of medium modeling difficulty. In this case backpropagation and CTM gave the best results. Variables y3, y6, and y7 had the lowest linear correlation with the input variables. In all three cases, the best models turned out to be CTM with a map dimensionality of two.

4 Extensions and Improvements of SOM/CTM Methods

In this section we discuss several recent extensions and improvements of self-organizing networks for density estimation (SOM) and regression (CTM) from finite training samples. Specific improvements discussed next are not intended to present an exhaustive survey of recent developments on SOMs.

4.1 Dynamic Map Topology

Topological maps discussed in this paper have fixed structure or static topology, i.e. 2D grid topology. Such maps can adapt well to continuous unstructured (convex) distributions. However, many real-life data sets have structured (non-convex) distribution and disjoint clusters. Moreover, it is likely that a high-dimensional data set may have low intrinsic dimensionality that varies in different parts of the input space. Fixed topology networks may have difficulty in modeling such structured/clustered/variable-intrinsic-dimension distributions. This inability is usually manifested in the existence of unused/underutilized units of the trained map and large quantization (approximation) error. Notice, that in spite of such a mismatch between fixed topology and structured distributions, a fixed 2D map is frequently used *to visualize* metric-topological relationships of high-dimensional data [Kohonen, 1984; Varfis and Versino, 1992].

Recent proposals for flexible map topologies that enable modeling arbitrary distributions fall into two major groups:

(1) *Constructive* methods that provide incremental growth of the map (during training) by adding more units as required by training data. For example, Blackmore and Mikkulainen [1993] propose a method for incremental growth of the 2-D topology to model arbitrary (high-dimensional) distributions. This approach is very appealing because the 2-D structure of the map can greatly assist in interpretation of the input data. Another approach called Growing Cell Structures was recently proposed by Fritzke [1993]. This method automatically finds a suitable network structure and size through a controlled network growth process (which also includes occasional removal of units).
(2) *Dynamic Topology* methods use the same (fixed) number of units and the training follows standard SOM two-step procedure outlined in section 2.2. However, the topological relationships between the units (may) *change* dynamically *during each iteration* (sample presentation), as dictated by the training data. Examples include dynamic Minimum Spanning Tree (MST) topology by Kangas et al (1989) and the Neural Gas network by Martinetz et al (1993). In the dynamic MST method, the map units are connected according to the minimum spanning tree topology (defined in the sample space) during each training iteration. Then the topological distance from the winning unit is defined in this MST topology, i.e. as the number of hops in MST. The neighborhood is reduced as the training proceeds, as in the original SOM method. This method is especially suitable for modeling (connected) structured but intrinsically low-dimensional distributions, since it always produces a tree topology. On the other hand, the Neural Gas network provides a more flexible approach, and it can be used to model arbitrary distributions. In the Neural Gas model, the topological relationship between map units is determined (at each iteration) according to linear (1-D) ordering of units based on their distance (closeness) to the winning unit (in the sample space). This approach appears to be especially suitable for modeling clustered and variable intrinsic dimensionality distributions. Empirical comparisons [Martinetz et al, 1993] demonstrate superiority of the Neural Gas method over standard Kohonen SOM, K-means and Maximum-entropy algorithms for modeling clustered data. However, their comparison results are based on using empirically chosen (exponentially decreasing) learning rate and neighborhood schedules. In fact, such a choice may result in suboptimal results, as discussed in the next section.

4.2 Statistical Analysis of SOM Learning Rate Schedules

The major weakness of many flow-through artificial neural network (ANN) methods is a heuristic choice of the learning rate schedules. Flow-through methods process training data one point at a time, and the training set is usually repeatedly presented to the network (or recycled) many times. Hence, the final model of the trained network may be sensitive to the order of presentation of the training data. In some cases, the theory of stochastic approximation can be used to develop good learning rate schedules and asymptotic performance bounds. For example, feed-forward ANN models can use standard learning rate schedules prescribed by stochastic approximation for parameter (weight) updates[White, 1989]. The learning rates should satisfy standard conditions from stochastic approximation theory [Ljung, 1977]:

$$\sum_{k=0}^{\infty}\beta(k)=\infty,\quad \sum_{k=0}^{\infty}\beta^2(k)<\infty \tag{7}$$

Even though classical theory of stochastic approximation assumes an infinite sequence of training samples, the same conditions on learning rate generally hold true for finite samples with recycling, commonly used in ANNs [White, 1991].

Let us consider the choice of the learning rate schedule for Kohonen's Self-Organizing Maps (SOM). The original SOM model [Kohonen, 1984] does not provide specific form of the learning rate and the neighborhood function schedules, so many heuristic schedules have been used [Kohonen, 1990; Ritter, Martinetz, and Schulten, 1991]. Straightforward generalization over the classical rates given by stochastic approximation does not seem an easy task, because of the complexity introduced by the concept of neighborhood. Mulier and Cherkassky[1993] propose statistical kernel interpretation of self-organization. For a given empirical learning rate schedule, this interpretation makes it possible to analyze (computationally) the contribution of a given training data point on the final location of the trained map units. Such analysis indicates potential pitfalls of the commonly used exponentially decreasing learning rate [Kohonen, 1990; Ritter, Martinetz, and Schulten, 1991; Cherkassky and Lari-najafi, 1991]. Furthermore, statistical kernel interpretation of SOM enables derivation of improved learning rates that represent a suitable generalization of the standard rates given by stochastic approximation theory for a self-organizing map of units.

4.2.1 Kernel Interpretation of Self-Organization

During Kohonen training or self-organization, units of a map move in the input space in response to repeated presentations of the training samples. Following notation in section 2.2, Kohonen SOM training or self-organization is described by the iterative unit (weight) update equation (3), which can be rewritten as:

$$\mathbf{w}_j(k)=\left[1-a_j(i(k),k)\right]\mathbf{w}_j(k-1)+a_j(i(k),k)\mathbf{z}_j(k)$$
$$\text{given } \mathbf{w}_j(0) \text{ as an initial condition} \tag{8}$$

where

$$a_j(i(k),k)=\beta(k)C_j(i(k),k) \qquad 0\le a_j\le 1$$

Unfolding recurrent update equations (8) results in explicit expression for the unit locations at time k as a weighted sum of the initial position of the units and every data point presented to the algorithm:

$$\mathbf{w}_j(k)=d_j(k)\mathbf{w}_j(0)+\sum_{n=1}^{k}d_j(k,n)\mathbf{z}_j(n) \tag{9}$$

The weights of the weighted sum then quantify the contribution of the initial conditions and of each presentation of the data on the position of the map at a later stage of self-organization. The coefficient $d_j(k)$ describes the contribution of the initial position of unit j on the position of unit j at time k. The coefficients $d_j(k,n)$ describe the contribution of the presentation at time n on the position of unit j at the time k. Since these coefficients depend on knowing the winning unit at each presentation step, the equations are evaluated numerically as the self-organization proceeds.

Evaluating (9) for particular data sets gives some insight into the self-organization process and can be used to answer two questions. First, how does the value of a training sample affect its contribution to the final location of each unit? Second, how does the order of presentation affect a training sample's contribution to the final location of each unit? The results depend on the specific learning rate and neighborhood function used during self-organization. Our analysis concentrates on the use of the exponentially decreasing learning rate and the Gaussian neighborhood function given in equations 4 and 5. The initial and final learning rates in all experiments are $\beta_0 = 1.0$, $\beta_f = 0.05$.

Several experiments using uniform 1D distribution of training data result in the following conclusions [Mulier and Cherkassky, 1993]:

(a) Contribution of the initial unit position on its final location is negligibly small, i.e. initial conditions do not affect the final results of self-organization.

(b) Each unit of the trained map is affected only by the training data near that unit. For example, Fig. 1a shows distribution of contributions of training samples on the 10 units of a one-dimensional map. Note that the contribution of the training samples on the unit location have *kernel-shaped* distribution.

(c) Generally, the contribution of training data (on a unit location) is larger in the area of low density samples than in the area of high-density samples (see Fig. 1b). Further experiments have shown that the width of the contribution kernel also depends on local data density.

(d) Contributions of the training samples (within each kernel) on the final position of a unit vary wildly, especially when the number of training samples is large (relative to the number of units). This is shown in Fig. 2.

The last observation suggests that *unequal* contribution of training samples with nearly the same value on the final unit locations may be due to their order of presentation during training. In particular, it can be shown that exponential learning rate schedule results in unequal contribution of the training samples on the final unit locations, so that typically only the last portion of the training data presented to the map have a significant affect on the results of self-organization (final position of the map units). This effect can be clearly seen by plotting the contribution of training data on the final unit locations as a function of the samples' ordering in the training set. See Fig 3. In this experiment, the training data was presented to the algorithm several times (recycled) in the same order. The same effect can be observed if the presentations are randomly selected from the training set with replacement, so that the ordering of the training set has no effect on the order of presentation. In this case only the last presentations of training data significantly affect the unit locations[Mulier and Cherkassky, 1993]. The under-utilization of training data can be a problem, especially in situations where there are a large number of samples with high noise. In these cases, the accuracy of the estimation method depends on its ability to smooth out the effects of the errors using all the samples. Data under-utilization increases the variance of the estimates. If self-organization using a poorly chosen learning rate is repeated a number of times for the same (randomly presented) training data, the sequence of maps generated will have a high variability, since each will be based on a different small portion of the training data.

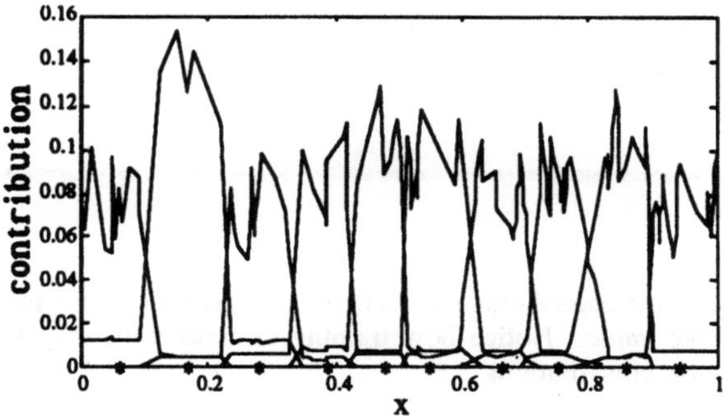

(1a)

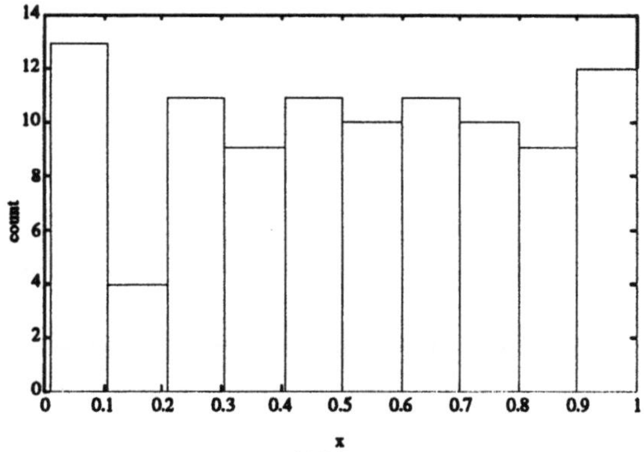

(1b)

Figure 1 Plots showing the contribution of the data on the final unit location and the histogram of the data. Notice that in the area where there is a lower concentration of data each data point has a larger contribution. (1a) Plot of $d_j(kmax, n)$ vs. $x(n)$ for $j = 1, \ldots, 10$. The 10 functions (one for each unit) showing the contribution of the data samples on the final unit location. (1b) The histogram of the data.

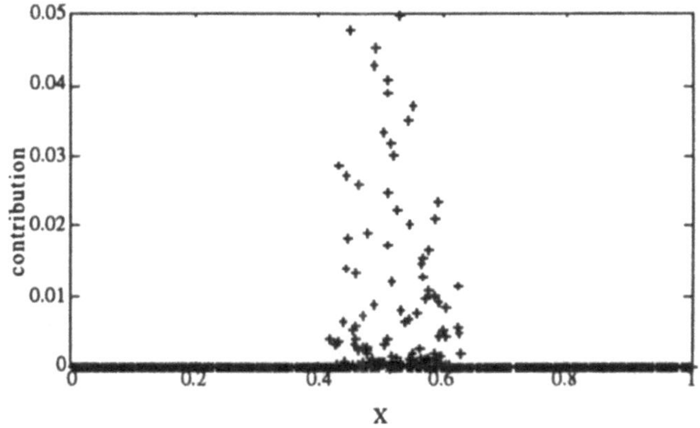

Figure 2 A plot of the contributions of data on a single unit of a 5 unit map with 1-D topology vs. sample value. Notice how training samples with very similar x values have wildly varying contributions.

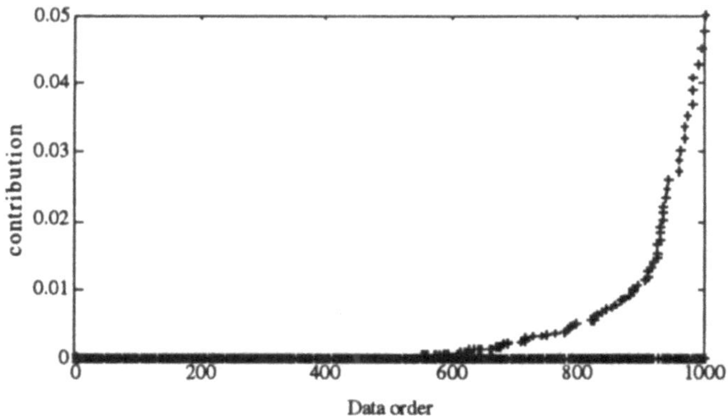

Figure 3 Plot of the contributions of data on a single unit of a 5 unit map with 1-D topology vs. presentation index. In this case only 20% of the presentations contribute significantly.

Past work on CTM [Cherkassky and Lari-Najafi, 1991; Cherkassky and Mulier, 1992] and on SOM [Kohonen, 1990; Ritter, Martinetz, and Schulten, 1991] using the exponential learning rate schedule have not been able to identify these effects because they only manifest themselves in certain situations. If there exists a statistical difference between, say, the first half of the training data and the last half in terms of ordering, the final map unit locations will more closely model the last half of the data. In most past experiments there was no statistical difference between the first half of the data and the last half, so a model based on only the last half would apply just as well to the rest of the data. In this case it would be hard to determine if the model was based on the whole data set or just the last half, looking just at the final unit locations. However, the problems caused by the underutilization of training data (i.e., high model variance) still occur undetected. Problems of underutilization of data can occur even if random sampling of the training set is done (as in most studies of the SOM). The solution to this problem is in the careful choice of learning rate schedule. A major difficulty in determining this schedule analytically is the interaction of the neighborhood function and the complexity of updating multiple units. Mulier and Cherkassky [1993] develop a learning rate schedule for SOM based on the results of an algorithmic search. The schedule is optimal in the sense that each presentation contributes equally to the final position of all the map units. This condition was devised so that the choice of neighborhood did not affect the analysis, although the results of self-organization will depend greatly on the choice of neighborhood and its decrease rate. Notice also that the condition is overly strict in that it enforces equal contribution for *each presentation* rather than equal contribution for *every sample* in the training set. This stricter condition may not be optimal in terms of the results of self-organization. The schedule based on this condition is

$$\beta(k) = \frac{1}{m(k-1)+1} \qquad m = \frac{1-\dfrac{P}{kmax}}{P-\dfrac{P}{kmax}}. \tag{10}$$

where P is the total number of units and $kmax$ is the total number of presentations. In the case of a single unit ($P = 1$), the equation becomes $\beta(k) = 1/k$ which is the running average schedule and conforms to the well-known conditions on learning rates used in stochastic approximation methods (7). Also, when $kmax$ is large, the rate becomes:

$$\beta(k) = \frac{1}{P^{-1}(k-1)+1} \tag{11}$$

which is similar to the schedule used by the k-means algorithm [MacQueen, 1967]. Note that k-means can be seen as a specific case of self-organization where the neighborhood consists of only one unit and each unit has its own independent learning rate which is decreased when that unit is updated. The self-organization algorithm has a global learning rate because several units are updated with each iteration. If one assumes that each unit is updated equiprobably during self-organization, then the two learning rates are comparable.

4.3 CTM Knot Placement Based on Estimated Second Derivative of a Function

Existing CTM method does not place more knots where the underlying function changes rapidly. By estimating and employing the second derivative of the function, the modified CTM algorithm can be made more flexible around regions with large second derivative.

The problem with estimating second derivative is that the function itself is unknown. This suggests using an iterative strategy for building a model, i.e., start with a crude model, estimate the second derivative based on this crude model, use the estimated second derivative to refine the model, etc. This strategy can be easily incorporated into the CTM algorithm due to its iterative nature. Specifically, in CTM method the map of knots(i.e., the model) becomes closer and closer to the final regression model as the training proceeds. Therefore, at each iteration, the modified algorithm estimates the second derivative at the best matching unit (closest to the presented data point in $\mathbf{x}$-space), and allows additional movement of units (towards the training sample) proportional to this estimate. Estimating the second derivative from the map (instead of using the training data) makes sense due to smoothing properties of CTM. The improved strategy for CTM knot placement in $\mathbf{x}$-space takes into account estimated second derivative of a function was proposed by Najafi and Cherkassky [1994] as described next:

1. Present training sample $\mathbf{z}(k)=(\mathbf{x}(k), y(k))$ to the map and find the closest (best matching) unit i in the space of predictor variables. (same as in the original CTM)
2. Move the map (i.e., the best matching unit and all its neighbors) toward the presented data point (same as in the original CTM)
3. Estimate average second derivative of the function at the best matching unit based on the current positions of the map units.
4. Normalize this average second derivative to an interval of [0,1].
5. Move the map toward the presented data point at a rate proportional to the estimated normalized average second derivative and iterate.

For multivariate functions only gradients along directions given by the topological structure of the map can be estimated in step 3. For example, given a 2-dimensional mesh that approximates function $f(x_1, x_2)$, every unit of the map (except the border units for which there will be only one neighbor) has two neighboring units along each topological dimension. These neighboring units can be used to approximate the function's gradients along the corresponding topological dimension of the map. These values along each dimension can then be averaged to provide a local gradient estimate at a given knot. In step 4, estimated average second derivative f'' is normalized to [0,1] range using $\psi_i = 1 - exp(|f''| / tan(\tau))$. This is done because the value of the second derivative is used as the learning rate. In step 5, the map is modified according to the following equation:

$$\mathbf{w}_j(k) = \mathbf{w}_j(k-1) + (1-\beta(k))\psi_i(k)C_j(i(k),k)[\mathbf{z}(k) - \mathbf{w}_j(k-1)] \quad (12)$$

It is this second movement of the map that allows for more flexibility around the region of the map where the second derivative is large. The process described by equation 12 is equivalent to pulling all units towards the data, with the learning rate proportional to estimated second derivative at the best matched unit. Note that the influence of the second derivative is gradually increased during the process of self-organization by the factor $(1-\beta(k))$. This accounts for the fact that the map becomes closer and closer to the underlying function during self-organization; hence, providing a more reliable estimate of second derivative.

An experiment was done in which training samples $(\mathbf{x}_i, y_i)$ were generated according to (1), with $\mathbf{x}_i$ randomly drawn from a uniform distribution in the closed interval [-1,1], and the *error* drawn from the normal distribution $N(0,(0.1)^2)$. Resulting knot locations produced by the original CTM and the improved CTM algorithm are shown in Figs. 4 and 5 for two example functions. Visual comparison of results shows that the increase in local knot density (around the regions with large second derivative) introduces more flexibility into the model and makes the model less biased around these regions. However, this additional flexibility of the modified CTM algorithm does not result in overfitting.

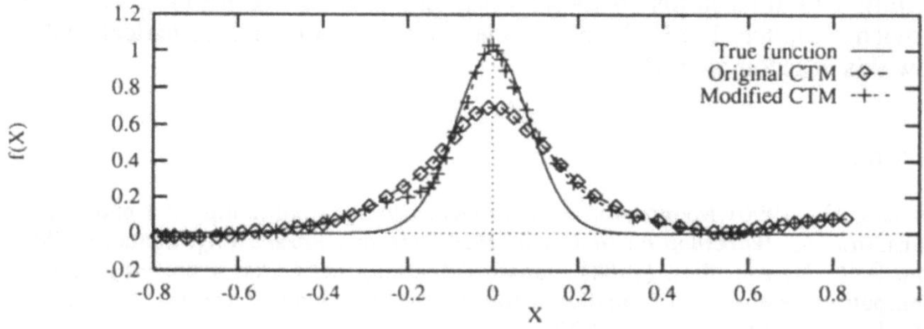

Figure 4 A 50 unit map formed by the original and modified algorithm for the Gaussian function

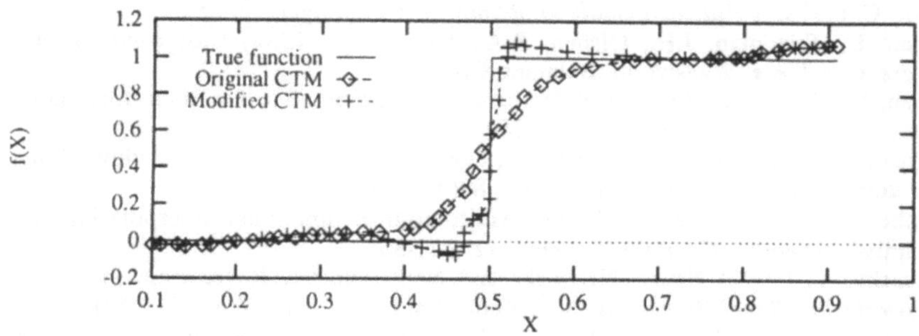

Figure 5 A 50 unit map formed by the original and modified algorithm for the step function

5 Conclusions

We discussed application of self-organizing networks for nonparametric regression. Training (self-organization) can be interpreted as the process of adaptive positioning of knots (units) along the regression surface. CTM method is shown to be a practical alternative to other popular methods for regression, at least for problems of low- to-medium dimensionality. CTM can be viewed as a flow-through local smoother, where smoothing is performed in the map (model) space rather than in the sample space.

Future progress in ANN modeling would require more rigorous analysis of heuristic ANN methods and establishing connections with similar methods in other (more mature) fields. With this in mind, we discussed similarities (and differences) between SOM/CTM and several statistical methods, such as Sammon's Projections, Principal Curves, kernel smoothers and Method of Potential Functions. Furthermore, it is demonstrated how statistically motivated considerations can be used to improve SOM/CTM methods.

Future work on application of self-organizing networks for regression may be concerned with analysis of the decreasing neighborhood. Whereas it is widely believed that the decreasing neighborhood schedule achieves the effect of simulated annealing and thus helps to avoid local minima during training[Martinetz, Berkovich, Schulten, 1993], there is no clear understanding/ mathematical analysis of how this is accomplished.

References

Atkeson, C.G. (1990) Memory-based approaches to approximating continuous functions, in *Proc. Workshop on Nonlinear Modelling and Forecasting*, Santa Fe NM

Barron, A.R., Barron, R.L. (1988) Statistical learning networks: a unifying view, in Computing Science and Statistics, *Proc. of the 20th Symp. Interface*, E. Wegman, ed., American Stat. Assn., 192-203,

Blackmore, J., Mikkulainen, R. (1993) Incremental grid growing: encoding high-dimensional structure into a two-dimensional feature map, *Proc. Int'l Conf. on Neural Networks*, IEEE Press, 450-455

de Boor, C. (1978) *A Practical Guide to Splines*, N.Y., Springer Verlag

Breiman, L., Friedman, J.H., Olshen, R.A., Stone, C.J. (1984) *Classification and Regression Trees*, Wadsworth, Belmont, CA

Breiman, L. (1991) The PI method for estimating multivariate functions from noisy data, *Technometrics*, v.3, no.2, 125-160

Brockmann, M., Gasser, T., Herrmann, E., (1993) Locally adaptive bandwidth choice for kernel regression estimators, *JASA*, 88(424), 1302-1309

Broomhead, D.S. , Lowe, D. (1988) Multivariable functional interpolation and adaptive networks, *Complex Systems*, v2, 321-355

Cherkassky, V. (1992) Neural Networks and Nonparametric Regression, in *Neural Networks for Signal Processing*, S.Y. Kung et al (Eds.), IEEE Press, 511-521

Cherkassky, V., Lari-Najafi, H. (1990) Self-organizing neural network for non-parametric regression analysis, *Proc. INNC*, Paris, France, 370-374

Cherkassky, V., Lari-Najafi, H. (1991) Constrained topological Mapping for Nonparametric Regression Analysis, *Neural Networks*, Pergamon, v.4, 27-40

Cherkassky, V., Lari-Najafi, H. (1992) Data representation for diagnostic neural nets, *IEEE Expert*, 7, 5, 43-53

Cherkassky, V., Lee, Y., Lari-Najafi, H. (1991) Self-organizing network for regression: efficient implementation and comparative evaluation, *Proc. IJCNN*, v.1, 79-84

Cherkassky, V., Mulier, F. (1992) Conventional and neural network approaches to regression, *Proc. SPIE Conf. on Applic of Artificial Neural Networks.*, SPIE vol. 1709, 840-848

Cleveland, W.S., Delvin, S.J. (1988) Locally weighted regression: an approach to regression analysis by local fitting, *JASA*, 83(403), 596-610

Cybenko, G. (1990) Complexity theory of neural networks and classification problems, *Proc. Eurasip Workshop on Neural Networks*, L. B. Almeida and C. J. Wellekens (Eds.), Springer Verlag, 26-44

Finnoff, W. (1994) Diffusion approximations for the constant learning rate backpropagation algorithm and resistance to local minima, *Neural Computation* 6, 285-295

Friedman, J.H. (1991) Multivariate adaptive regression splines (with discussion), *Annals of Statistics* 19, 1-141

Friedman, J.H.(1991) Personal communication

Friedman, J.H., Silverman, B. W. (1989) Flexible Parsimonious Smoothing and Additive Modeling, *Technometrics*, v.31, 1, 3-21

Friedman, J.H., Stuetzle, W. (1981) Projection Pursuit Regression, *JASA*, v.76, 817-823

Fritzke, B. (1993) Growing Cell Structures - a self-organizing network for unsupervised and supervised learning, *Int'l Computer Science Institute*, TR-93-026, Berkeley

Geman, S., Bienenstock, E., Doursat, R. (1992) Neural Networks and the Bias/Variance dilemma, *Neural Computation*, 4, 1-58

Hastie, T., Stuetzle, W. (1989) Principal Curves, *JASA*, v.84, no.406, 502-516

Kangas, J. et al (1989) Variants of self-organizing maps, *Proc. IJCNN*, IEEE Press, v.2, 517-522

Kraaijveld, M., Mao, J., Jain, A.K. (1992) A Non-linear projection method based on Kohonen's topology preserving maps, *Proc. 11th IAPR Conf. on Pattern Recognition*, 41-45

Kohonen, T. (1984) *Self-organization and Associative Memory*, Berlin: Springer-Verlag

Kohonen, T. (1990) The self-organizing map, *Proc. of the IEEE*, 78, 9, 1464-1479

Kohonen, T. (1993) Things you haven't heard about the self-organizing map, *Proc. IEEE Int. Joint Conf. on Neural Networks*, San Francisco, 1147-1156

Ljung, L. (1977) Analysis of recursive stochastic algorithms, *IEEE Trans. Automat. Contr.*, AC-22, 551-575

MacQueen, J. (1967) Some methods for classification and analysis of multivariate observations, *Proc. 5th Berkeley Symp. Math. Stat. Prob.* 1, 281-298

Maechler, M., Martin, D., Schimert, J., Csoppensky, M., Hwang, J. N. (1990) Projection Pursuit learning networks for regression, *Proc. Int'l Conf. on Tools for AI*, IEEE Press, 350-358

Martinetz, T., Berkovich, S., Schulten, K. (1993) "Neural -gas" network for vector quantization and its application to time series prediction, *IEEE Trans. on Neural Networks*, 4, 558-569

Mendel, J.M., Fu, K.S. (1970) Eds., *Adaptive Learning and Pattern Recognition Systems: Theory and Applications*, Academic Press, NY

Moody, J., Darken, C.J. (1989) Fast learning in networks of locally tuned processing units, *Neural Computation* 1, 281

Mulier, F., Cherkassky, V. (1993) Statistical analysis of self-organization, *Neural Networks* (under review)

Najafi, H.L., Cherkassky, V. (1994) Adaptive knot placement for nonparametric regression, to appear in *Advances in Neural Information Processing Systems* 6, J.D. Cowan et al (eds.), Morgan Kaufman, San Mateo, CA

Poggio, T., Girosi, F. (1990) Networks for approximation and learning, *Proc. of the IEEE*, v.78, no.9, 1481-1497

Ripley, B.D. (1993) Neural networks and flexible regression and discrimination, in *Statistics and Images*, ed. K. V. Mardia, Advances in Applied Statistics, Abingdon: Carfax

Ripley, B.D. (1994) Neural networks and related methods for classification (with discussion), *J. Roy. Statist. Soc. B* 56

Ritter, H, Martinetz, T., Schulten, K. (1991) *Neural Computation and Self-Organizing Maps*, Addison-Wesley

Rumelhart, D.E., McClelland, J.L., PDP Research group (1986) (Eds.), *Parallel Distributed Processing*, MIT Press

Sammon, J.W. (1969) A non-linear mapping for data structure analysis, *IEEE Trans. Comp.*, C-18, 401-409

Sanger, T.D. (1991) A Tree-structured additive network for function approximation in high-dimensional spaces, *IEEE Trans. on Neural Networks*, v.2, no.2, 285-293

Specht, D.F. (1991) A General regression neural network, *IEEE Trans. Neural Networks*, 2,6, 568-576

Varfis, A., Versino, C. (1992) Clustering of socio-economic data with Kohonen Maps, *Neural Network World*, 2, 6, 813-834

Walter, J., Ritter, H., Schulten, K. (1990) Nonlinear prediction with self-organizing maps, *Proc. IJCNN*, v.3, San Diego, CA, 589-594

White, H. (1989) Learning in Artificial Neural Networks: a statistical perspective, *Neural Computation*, 1, 425-464

White, H. (1991) Parametric statistical estimation with artificial neural networks, TR, Dept. of Economics, UC San Diego

Neural Preprocessing Methods

Luís B. Almeida

INESC/IST, R. Alves Redol, 1000 Lisboa, Portugal
lba@inesc.pt

Abstract. When using data, real or artificial, it is often convenient to perform on them some form of preprocessing. This preprocessing is often aimed at extracting the most important features of the data, thus performing dimensionality reduction, or at changing the data to a more convenient format (e.g. decorrelating the components of the data vectors). This paper presents an overview of unsupervised, neural-style preprocessing algorithms. It starts by analyzing criteria for unsupervised feature extraction, and then proceeds to describe some of the most important feature extraction algorithms. Here, the emphasis is placed on linear algorithms that extract principal components or their linear combinations.

Subsequently, a simple decorrelation algorithm is analyzed, and an application is described, to the acceleration of training of supervised networks.

Keywords: Preprocessing, dimensionality reduction, feature extraction, principal components, decorrelation, orthogonalization, fast training.

1. Introduction

In pattern recognition situations, as well as in other forms of data processing, one often needs to perform some kind of unsupervised preprocessing of the input data. This preprocessing can have two main aims, namely the reduction of the dimensionality of the data and the transformation of the data into a more suitable format for further processing. Dimensionality reduction is also often called *feature extraction*. We should stress that here we are interested only in the unsupervised forms of feature extraction, i.e. those which do not use information on the further processing that is to be applied to the data. Among the examples of transformations of the data format, we will mention decorrelation, which will be of most interest to us here.

This paper presents an overview of the main neural-style algorithms for performing these two kinds of operations, which have a strong inter-relationship with each other. We first review the most important criteria for unsupervised feature extraction, and then present an overview of some of the most important algorithms for both feature extraction and decorrelation. Finally, we center ourselves with greater detail on a simple decorrelation and normalization algorithm, and study both its properties and one of its applications. In this paper we will not present formal proofs about the algorithms. These proofs can be found in the referenced literature.

2. Criteria for feature extraction

Assume that we have a finite or infinite set of random data vectors $\boldsymbol{x}$, of dimension n, with a certain probability distribution $p(\boldsymbol{x})$ (which is normally unknown). There are several possible criteria for extracting the most significant features from these data. We will call these features $y_i = f_i(\boldsymbol{x}), \quad i = 1,\ldots,m$ with $m < n$.

2.1. Minimum variance

A simple criterion for feature selection is to choose the m first principal components of the distribution $p(\boldsymbol{x})$. These are the linear features that minimize the "remaining variance", i.e. the average variance of $\boldsymbol{x}$ given $\boldsymbol{y}$. They are uncorrelated, i.e. $E(y_i y_j) = 0$ if $i \neq j$ (we will also refer do uncorrelated features as *orthogonal* ones, taking the expected value $E(y_i y_j)$ as the inner product between the components y_i and y_j).

Principal components are well known from the theory of statistics, and their determination can be done by algebraic methods. Here, however, we are interested in their determination by parallel distributed methods, with connectionist flavor. It is worth noting that, for some distributions, linear principal components are not adequate, and we would like to have some kind of *nonlinear principal components* (Fig. 1).

2.2. Optimal reconstruction

A criterion which is more elaborate than minimum variance, and which allows the extraction of nonlinear features, is to select the features y such that a reconstruction of the form $\hat{x}_i = g_i(\boldsymbol{y})$ (with unconstrained g_i) would minimize the expected value of some cost functional $C(\boldsymbol{x},\hat{\boldsymbol{x}})$. Often, the quadratic error, $C(\boldsymbol{x},\hat{\boldsymbol{x}}) = \|\boldsymbol{x} - \hat{\boldsymbol{x}}\|^2$, is chosen as cost functional, but other functionals can be more adequate in certain circumstances.

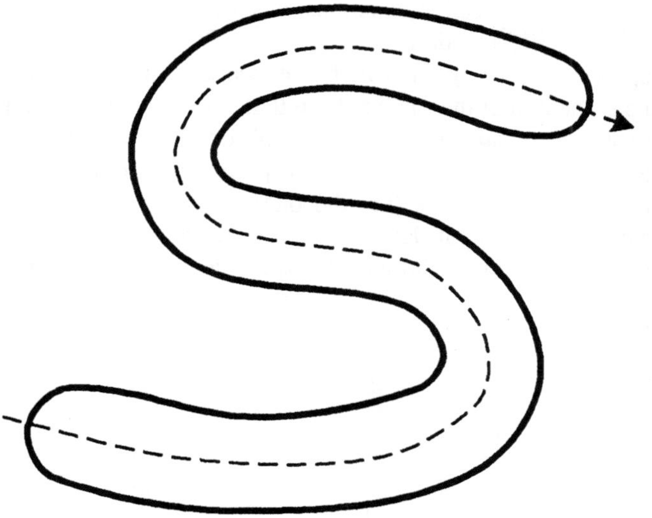

Fig. 1 - Need for nonlinear principal components. The thick line depicts the outline of the data distribution. The desirable nonlinear component would be measured along the dashed line.

2.3. Maximum information preservation (Infomax)

Another reasonable criterion for selecting the features is to minimize the average information-theoretic uncertainty about x given y, i.e. $H(x|y)$, which measures the amount of information lost in the feature extraction process. Minimizing $H(x|y)$ can easily be shown to be equivalent to maximizing the mutual information between x and y, given by $H(x) - H(x|y)$, or equivalently by $H(y) - H(y|x)$, which is the information about x contained in y. For this reason, this criterion, which was introduced by Linsker [1], is called *infomax*. Like the optimal reconstruction criterion, infomax is also able to extract nonlinear features.

3. Algorithms for unsupervised preprocessing

3.1. Nonlinear methods

Using the Infomax principle with some additional constraints, Linsker has been able to exemplify the self-organization of topological maps, and the emergence of feature detectors similar to those that occur in the visual system [1,2]. However, the Infomax principle is normally hard to apply and to analyze, giving rise to complex, or even intractable equations, when one wishes to derive optimization formulas for specific situations.

Self-supervised learning (in which a network with a bottleneck is trained to reproduce at the output the same pattern that is presented at the input, see Fig. 2) can be viewed as an implementation of optimal reconstruction, extracting nonlinear features from the input data [3]. During training, the network has to jointly optimize the features (i.e. the outputs of the bottleneck units) and the reconstruction of the input data. Often, for this purpose, multilayer perceptrons are used, with training through backpropagation [4]. Of course, such an

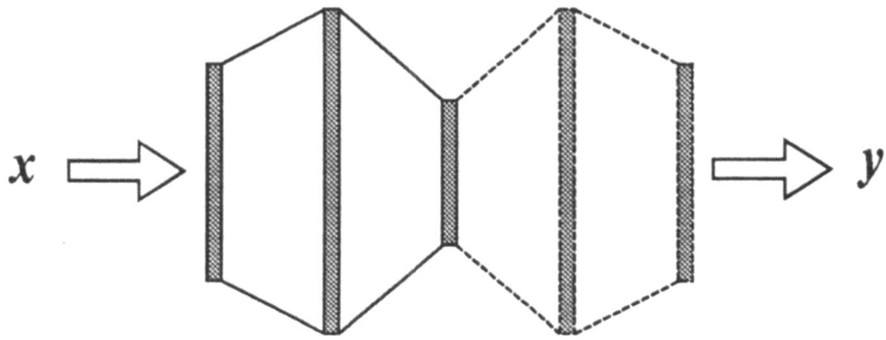

Fig. 2 - Self-supervised learning. Each rectangle represents a layer of units. The outputs of the units of the bottleneck layer become nonlinear features of the input data. After training, the dashed part can be discarded.

implementation of the optimal reconstruction criterion is subject to the limitations of the network architecture and training algorithm in use. For example, the optimum may not be reached due to the existence of local minima of the error surface. Backpropagation is normally employed, with the quadratic cost functional, for optimization. We should stress, however, that nothing prevents the use of other cost functionals with the backpropagation algorithm, as long as they are differentiable relative to the network outputs.

In the special case that the network is linear and the cost function is the quadratic error, it can be shown that self-supervised learning simply extracts a *principal subspace* (i.e. a linear combination of the first principal components) [5]. Note that, as will happen with several other methods to be described below, the solution found by self-supervised linear networks is not unique, since there is an infinite number of different linear combinations of the first principal components.

Another well known method for nonlinear feature extraction is the use of topological maps of patterns [6]. When a pattern is presented to a well trained map, the coordinate(s) of the winning unit, on the topology specified for the map, are discrete nonlinear features of the input pattern. If continuous features are desired, the discrete values that are obtained can be interpolated, on the basis of the distances from the input vector to the winning unit and to its neighbors.

3.2. Linear methods

There is a large class of methods for unsupervised preprocessing that are based on linear networks. One of these was already mentioned above: self-supervised learning with a linear network.

Most of the other linear methods are based on the fact, shown by Oja [7] that if a linear unit, with output $y = \boldsymbol{w} \cdot \boldsymbol{x}$, is trained with a Hebbian rule of the form $\Delta w_i = \alpha x_i y$, with a normalization $\|w\| = 1$, its output will converge to the first principal component of the input distribution. The specific weight update equation proposed by Oja was

$$\Delta w_{ij} = \alpha(x_j y_i - w_{ij} y_i^2),$$

where the second term within the parentheses is a normalization term.

This basic method would only allow the extraction of the first principal component, but several authors have then expanded it in different ways. Oja and Williams, independently developed a technique known as the *subspace algorithm*, or *error-correction learning*, which extracts a principal subspace [8,9]. In this method, as in many of the ones to follow, a linear single-layer feedforward network is used. For each pattern that is presented, one starts by computing the output vector of the network,

$$\boldsymbol{y} = \boldsymbol{W}\boldsymbol{x}$$

Then, the outputs are propagated back to the input, using the same weights:

$$\boldsymbol{z} = \boldsymbol{W}^T \boldsymbol{y}$$

where the superscript T denotes transposition. The error between the reconstructed input z and the actual input is given by

$$\boldsymbol{e} = \boldsymbol{x} - \boldsymbol{z}$$

and is used for updating the weights, through

$$\Delta \boldsymbol{W} = \alpha\, \boldsymbol{y}\, \boldsymbol{e}^T$$

It was shown in [9] that, under mild conditions, the principal subspace is an attractor of this algorithm, and that the weight vectors of the output units (i.e. the lines of W) become orthogonal to one another and normalized. However, the outputs normally don't become the principal components themselves.

Oja then proceeded to develop the subspace algorithm further, into the *weighted subspace algorithm*, which can extract the principal components themselves [8]. In the original subspace algorithm, the update equation for each weight could be written as

$$\Delta w_{ij} = \alpha\, y_i (x_j - z_j).$$

The modification introduced by Oja consisted of the introduction of *symmetry-breaking factors* θ_i on the reconstructed input, resulting in

$$\Delta w_{ij} = \alpha\, y_i (x_j - \theta_i z_j).$$

These factors, which are assumed to obey $0 < \theta_1 < \theta_2 < \cdots < 1$, lead the units to align themselves with the principal components, y_1 being the first, y_2 the second, etc. The weight vectors do not become normalized to unity, but instead, upon convergence, $\|w_i\| = 1 / \sqrt{\theta_i}$.

Sanger [10] developed an architecture, called *generalized Hebbian learning*, for the extraction of any number of principal components, by using a technique that is reminiscent of Gram-Schmidt orthogonalization, combined with Hebbian learning. The first unit is trained using simple Hebbian learning. The second unit is trained with Hebbian learning, but the component already detected by the first unit is first subtracted from the input. For the third unit, the components detected by the first two units are subtracted, and so on. The weight update formula is

$$\Delta w_{ij} = \alpha\, y_i (x_j - \sum_{k \le i} w_{kj} y_k),$$

where the term $k = i$, in the sum, corresponds to Oja's normalization term, and the terms $k < i$ correspond to the components already extracted by previous units. This algorithm extracts the principal components, in order of decreasing importance.

Several authors, including Földiak [11], Leen [12], Rubner and Schulten [13] and Kung and Diamantaras [14], have exploited different ways of using anti-Hebbian terms, in conjunction with Hebbian ones, for obtaining orthogonal outputs that span the principal subspace. In some of these cases, the networks extract the principal components themselves, while in other ones they simply extract a principal subspace. Of these, we will only briefly describe the APEX algorithm, of Kung and Diamantaras, which is one of the simplest which allow the extraction of the principal components. The network architecture corresponding to this algorithm is depicted in Fig. 3. Each unit receives contributions both from the network inputs (with weights w_{ij}) and from the units above it (with weights a_{ij}). Note that, though there are connections running from right to left in the figure, the network is not recurrent, since these connections do not form loops.

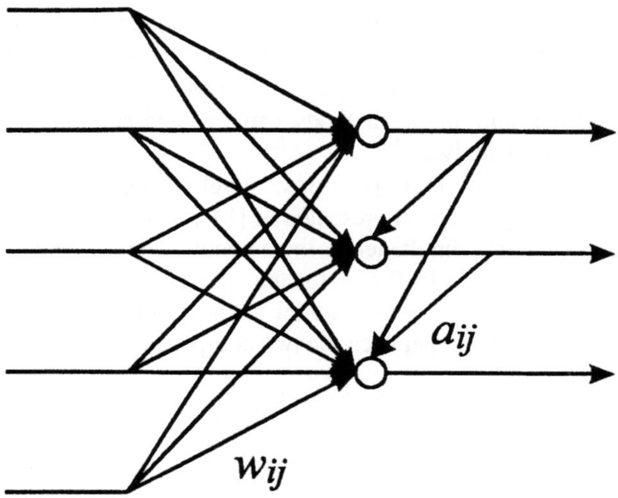

Fig. 3 - Network used in the APEX algorithm.

The unit outputs are given by

$$y = Wx + Ay$$

where A is lower triangular, with a null diagonal, which ensures that there is no recurrence. The weight update rules are

$$\Delta w_{ij} = \beta\,(y_i\,x_j - y_i^2\,w_{ij})$$

$$\Delta a_{ij} = -\gamma\,(y_i\,y_j + y_i^2\,a_{ij}) \qquad \text{for } i > j$$

The term in $y_i\,x_j$, in the first equation, is the usual Hebbian term, that tends to align the unit's weight vector with the main principal component. The term in $y_i\,y_j$, in the second equation, is an anti-Hebbian term, due to its negative sign. It tends to make each unit's output orthogonal to those of the preceding units. These two terms lead each unit to align itself with the main principal component that is orthogonal to those extracted by the units above it. Therefore, the units will extract the principal components in order of decreasing importance, from top to bottom.

4. A simple decorrelation algorithm

4.1. The algorithm

Orthogonalization and principal component extraction have one very important point in common, namely that principal components are orthogonal to one another. Therefore, if we need to preform orthogonalization, we can always use a principal component extraction algorithm. However, if orthogonalization is all we need, simpler and faster methods can be devised, than those suited for principal component analysis.

A simple algorithm that performs simultaneous orthogonalization and normalization, which has been presented in [14], is based on the idea of applying what could be called "simultaneous incremental Gram-Schmidt orthogonalization", which is illustrated in Fig. 4 for the case of two components: From each component, we subtract a vector parallel to the other component, whose length depends on the correlation between the two components.

The batch form of the weight update rule is given by

$$\Delta w_{ij} = \alpha(w_{ij} - \sum_k w_{kj} r_{ik}), \qquad (1)$$

where $r_{ik} = E(y_i y_k)$ is the correlation between outputs, computed over the whole training set. To better understand this rule, we can transform it:

$$\Delta w_{ij} = -\alpha \sum_{k \neq i} w_{kj} r_{ik} + \alpha w_{ij} (1 - r_{ij}).$$

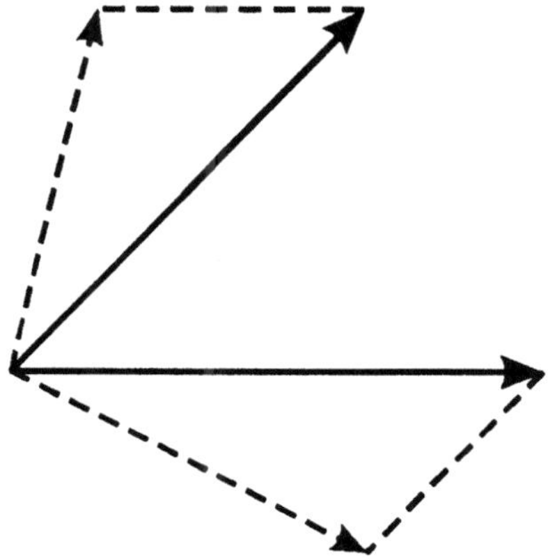

Fig. 4 - Simultaneous orthogonalization of two components. Solid vectors: before the orthogonalization. Dashed vectors: after one orthogonalization iteration.

The first term in the right-hand side corresponds to the above mentioned subtraction of vectors parallel to other components, with a length dependent upon the correlation with the component being updated. The second term normalizes the component being updated, so that its RMS value goes to 1.

The stochastic version of the weight update rule is

$$\Delta w_{ij} = \alpha(w_{ij} - y_i \sum_k w_{kj}\, y_k)$$

where the cross-correlation r_{ik} has been replaced by its instantaneous estimate, $y_i\, y_k$.

It can be shown that the batch algorithm converges if the following conditions are met: (1) the weight matrix is initialized with the identity, i.e. $w_{ij} = \delta_{ij}$, (2) $\alpha < 0.5$, and (3) $\alpha < 1/(\lambda_{max} - 1)$, where λ_{max} is the largest eigenvalue of the input autocorrelation matrix.

Only a sketch of the proof will be given here. From the update equation (1) one can derive a recursive equation for the output correlation matrix $\boldsymbol{R} = [r_{ij}]$:

$$\begin{aligned} \boldsymbol{R}_{n+1} &= (i+\alpha)^2 \boldsymbol{R}_n - 2\alpha(1+\alpha)\boldsymbol{R}_n^2 + \alpha^2 \boldsymbol{R}_n^3 \\ &= P(\boldsymbol{R}_n) \end{aligned}$$

where $P(\cdot)$ denotes the polynomial that is given in full in the first line. If we make an eigenvalue decomposition

$$\boldsymbol{R}_n = \boldsymbol{V}_n\, \Lambda_n\, \boldsymbol{V}_n^T$$

it is easy to see that

$$\boldsymbol{R}_n^k = \boldsymbol{V}_n\, \Lambda_n^k\, \boldsymbol{V}_n^T$$

and that, therefore,

$$\Lambda_{n+1} = P(\Lambda_n)$$

However, since Λ is diagonal, the same recursion still applies to each of the eigenvalues individually. If λ is a generic eigenvalue,

$$\lambda_{n+1} = P(\lambda_n).$$

From Fig. 5, which sketches $P(\lambda)$, one sees that the recursion has three fixed points, of which only $\lambda = 1$ can be stable. For it to be stable, it suffices that $\alpha < 0.5$. For the recursion to converge to this point, it is sufficient that it be started below the local minimum, i.e. that $\lambda_0 < 1 + 1/\alpha$, where λ_0 is the initial value of λ. If we initialize the weight matrix with the identity, the initial output autocorrelation is the same as the input autocorrelation. If $\alpha < 0.5$ and $\alpha < 1/(\lambda_{max} - 1)$, then all eigenvalues will converge to 1, and the output autocorrelation will converge to the identity matrix, which means that all outputs will be decorrelated and normalized.

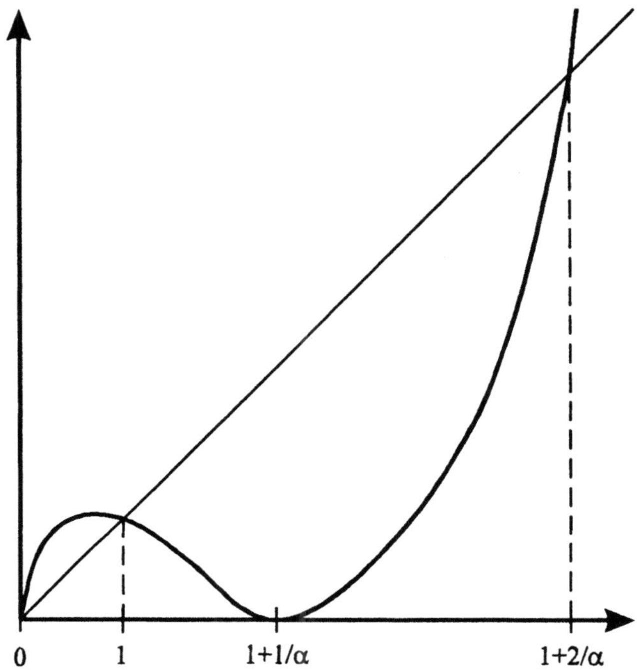

Fig. 5 - Sketch of $P(\lambda)$.

For the stochastic case, we must vary the step size α with n, and conditions (2) and (3) above are replaced by the usual Robins-Monro conditions: (2') $\Sigma\alpha^2(n) < \infty$ and (3') $\Sigma\alpha(n) = \infty$. Experimental tests have confirmed the convergence of the two forms of the algorithm [15].

4.2. An application

It is well known from adaptive filter theory that the convergence of the training of a single linear unit is fastest if its inputs are uncorrelated and normalized. It has been conjectured that the same would happen, in general, with sigmoidal units, even if they were embedded into a network. This has led to the proposal of an architecture [16] in which unsupervised, decorrelating layers alternate with normal, supervised ones (Fig. 6)[1]. The unsupervised layers provide uncorrelated, normalized inputs to the supervised units. During training, the unsupervised layers are trained with the algorithm presented above, and the supervised ones are trained with backpropagation (the backpropagation of errors has to be performed also through the unsupervised units, though it is not used to update their weights). Note that the inputs to the first layer can be orthonormalized off-line, once and for all, using any standard algorithm (e.g. Gram-Schmidt, plus straightforward normalization), since their statistics don't change with the training. Only the inputs to subsequent layers need to be adaptively orthonormalized during training, since their statistics change, due to the training of previous layers.

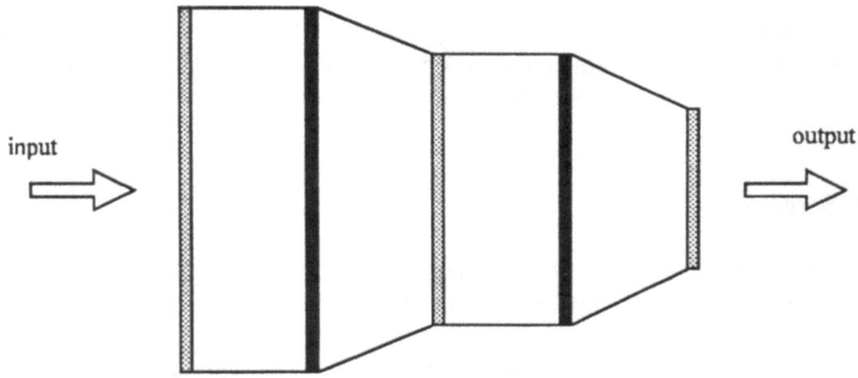

Fig. 6 - Fast learning architecture. Gray rectangles represent normal, supervised layers, trained by backpropagation. Black rectangles represent unsupervised, orthonormalizing layers, adapted by the algorithm described in section 4.1. The input to the first layer can be orthonormalized off-line.

Experimental tests have confirmed that this kind of architecture learns significantly faster than the usual, purely supervised one. The actual speed gains that are obtained depend on the topology of the network that is to be implemented, but for the architectures that have been tested, they typically were of a factor of 5 or more, in terms of CPU time, in comparison with an accelerated backpropagation algorithm [16].

---

[1] A related architecture has been proposed in [17].

5. Conclusion

There are a variety of algorithms for unsupervised, neural-style preprocessing of data. They can have two main purposes: extraction of features from the data, or changing the data format to a more convenient one.

For feature extraction, three main criteria exist: minimum variance, optimal reconstruction and maximum information preservation. Algorithms such as topological maps, or self-supervised training of networks with a bottleneck, implement an approximation to the extraction of nonlinear features by optimal reconstruction. Minimum variance leads to the extraction of linear principal components. For this purpose, several different algorithms exist, which employ linear feedforward or recurrent networks, and which extract the principal components themselves, or just a principal subspace.

For a special case of data formatting (orthogonalization) the principal component extraction algorithms can be employed, but they exceed that purpose quite a bit. A simpler orthonormalization algorithm has been presented in this paper, together with its application to fast training of supervised networks.

References

[1] R. Linsker, "How to generate ordered maps by maximizing the mutual information between input and output signals", *Neural Computation*, vol. 1, 1989.

[2] R. Linsker, "An application of the principle of maximum information preservation to linear systems", *Advances in Neural Information Processing Systems 1*, Morgan Kaufman, 1989.

[3] J. Elman and D. Zipser, "Learning the hidden structure of speech", *ICS Report 8701*, Institute of Cognitive Science, UCSD, 1987.

[4] D. Rumelhart, G. Hinton and R. Williams, "Learning internal representations by error propagation", in *Parallel Distributed Processing. Exploration of the Microstructure of Cognition*, vol. 1, D. Rumelhart, J. McClelland et al. (eds.), MIT Press, 1986.

[5] H. Bourlard and Y. Kamp, "Auto-association by multilayer perceptrons and singular value decomposition", *Biological Cybernetics*, vol. 59, 1988.

[6] T. Kohonen, "Clustering, taxonomy and topological maps of patterns", *Proc. Int. Conf. Pat. Recognition*, 1982.

[7] E. Oja, "A simplified neuron as a principal components analyser", *J. Math. Biol.*, vol. 15, 1982.

[8] E. Oja, H. Ogawa and J. Wangviwattana, "PCA in fully parallel neural networks", *Artificial Neural Networks 2*, Elsevier Science Publishers, 1992.

[9] R. Williams, "Feature discovery through error correction learning", *ICS Report 8501*, Institute of Cognitive Science, UCSD, 1985.

[10] T. Sanger, "Optimal unsupervised learning in a single-layer linear feedforward network", *Neural Networks*, vol. 2, 1989.

[11] P. Földiak, "Adaptive network for optimal linear feature extraction", *Proc. Int. Conf. Neural Networks*, June 1989.

[12] T. Leen, "Dynamics of learning in recurrent feature-discovery neural networks", *Advances in Neural Information Processing Systems 1*, Morgan Kaufman, 1991.

[13] J. Rubner and K. Schulten, "Development of feature detectors by self-organization. A network model", *Biol. Cybern.*, vol. 62, 1990.

[14] S. Kung and K. Diamantaras, "A neural network algorithm for adaptive principal component extraction (APEX)", *Proc. IEEE Int. Conf. Acoust., Speech, Sig. Proc.*, 1990.

[15] F. Silva and L. Almeida, "A distributed solution for data orthonormalization", in T. Kohonen (ed.), *Artificial Neural networks*, Elsevier Science Publishers, 1991.

[16] F. Silva and L. B. Almeida, "Speeding-up backpropagation by data orthonormalization", in T. Kohonen (ed.), *Artificial Neural networks*, Elsevier Science Publishers, 1991.

[17] S. Orfanidis, "Gram-Schmidt Neural Networks", *Neural Computation*, vol. 1, no. 4, 1990.

Improved Hidden Markov Models for Speech Recognition Through Neural Network Learning

Chris J. Wellekens
Institut EURECOM - 06904 Sophia Antipolis France

Abstract. Multilayer perceptrons generate a posteriori probabilities related to emission probabilities of Hidden Markov Models through Bayes rule. This property is used to improve the discrimination of *HMM*. Moreover, it gives rise to many statistical interpretations which can be cast in neural architectures for nonlinear prediction and triphone probability estimation.

Keywords. Multilayer perceptrons, Hidden Markov Models, Speech Recognition, Discrimination.

1 Introduction

Mathematical formalization is definitely the intellectually most satisfactory approach to solve technical issues. It offers a continuous and clear insight into the problem since any intermediate step in the computing process can be observed and has a mastered physical meaning. Unfortunately, some problems get so intricate that the number of equations or their nature prevent any reasonable mathematical treatment e.g. the model of sophisticated robot arm with multiple degrees of freedom and nonlinearities which should be real time operated. Other problems involve unexplained behavior of industrial plants or human beings e.g. the auditory or visual human apparatus. In both cases, the unability to formalize forces to alternative methodologies. In microphysics, the huge number of particles prevents any traditional use of the laws of mechanics and a combined use of statistics and mechanics gave rise to one of the most impressive discipline. In that case, hypotheses on the hidden phenomena help the scientist formalize the statistical behavior. If no reasonable hypotheses can be made, the sole approach relies on observations which are used for model training.

This is the case in speech recognition where the phonatory process is quite versatile depending on speaker's identity, stress status, cultural history and even inconsistency. Best results in speech recognition have been obtained by using statistical models the parameters of which are estimated in a training phase on speech databases. Hypotheses were made on statistics which restrict to some extent the power of this approach. Weaker and weaker hypotheses are accepted leading to improved models. However, the number of parameters grows up with the generality of the models and any significant training requires huger and huger data bases. Neural networks provide an elegant method to estimate statistics with few hypotheses and few parameters. The joint use of neural networks and statistical models lead to speech recognizers the performances of which compare favorably with the best known techniques and require less a priori knowledge on the speech production process. Also less parameters are necessary to describe the underlaying statistics and as a consequence, less training material. However, the training process of neural networks is known to be so CPU time greedy that research work is impaired by the unacceptable delays between research tests and the expected results! Dedicated machines have been built which partly circumvent the problem. While training is part of the design phase and consumes such expensive computing resources, recognition can be achieved very fast using custom devices.

For all the reasons above, speech recognition has been identified as a particularly *representative research field for neural networks and statistics.*

Speech recognition relies on comparisons between an utterance and a cascade of speech unit models. Since the pertinent information for recognition is hidden and mixed with other features (like phase lags and prosody) in the waveform, a preprocessing is required. Section 2 gives a quick summary of this representation problem.

In the early years of automatic speech recognition (ASR), word models were plain utterances of words. Speaker's variability was not easily taken into account: the only manner was to use several models per word at the price of a prohibitive computation time in the recognition phase and of storage needs. Recognition was based on the time alignment between reference and test signals: this alignment results in a distorted path in the matrix of local distances between acoustic vectors of speech frame pairs from the reference and the test signal. This distortion is known as *time warping* [17]. The resulting distortion score is used as a classification criterion.

Statistical models (Hidden Markov Models (HMM)) have been introduced by Jelinek [1] and proved to be very efficient to create robust and even speaker independent models. From that time, the idea of learning was included as a major issue in ASR. Very soon, embedded training was proposed: the speech data base consisting in sentences of connected words is "matched" by Viterbi training on a global model formed by concatenating word models in the same order as they appear in the sentence. The most commonly used training criterion is the likelihood that an utterance be associated with a given model but it does not yield the best recognition rates due to an inherent lack of discrimination. Indeed, a word model is tuned to be highly probable for the corresponding word but no care is brought to make it as less probable as possible for the other words. Section 3 will describe in more detail this statistical approach which will be combined later with a neural network approach in a hybrid recognizer.

Neural networks are known for their learning capabilities. Interesting results in speech recognition were obtained with Time-Delay-Neural Networks ($TDNN$) i.e. multilayer perceptrons endowed with memory at each layer [2]. Memory adds on contextual representation to the static signal but $TDNN$'s hardly take time warping into account. Most interesting results were obtained for phoneme and isolated word recognition without any use of HMM.

Section 4 will be devoted to the use of Multilayer Perceptrons (MLP) in ASR. It will be showed that outputs of MLP's used for classification can be interpreted as a posteriori probabilities [3-5] of observing a given class when a signal is observed. These probabilities are related by Bayes rule to the emission (local) probabilities of HMM's. These MLP-derived probabilities are more robust than Gaussian parametric densities traditionally used in HMM because they are obtained from discriminant training with neither assumption on the shape of probability density functions (pdf's) nor quantization errors as observed in a quantized representation space. MLP architecture eases incorporation of contextual information by extension of the input field to right and left informations [4]. Nonlinearities of neural nets extend the capabilities of class partitioning [6].

Hybrid models using MLP-derived probabilities in conjunction with HMM's combine the advantages of both techniques: time warping is taken into account and discrimination is significantly improved by MLP classifier training. Recent results show that scores obtained with hybrid HMM/MLP's compare favorably with those obtained with carefully designed traditional triphone HMM's [7].

Thanks to the statistical meaning of MLP classifier outputs, most of standard laws of statistics can be cast into connectionist architectures. For instance, the difficult problem of triphone (phoneme in left and right contexts) model training can be simplified [8-9].

The emission probabilities in HMM can be extended to the probability of observing an acoustic vector on a state given the previous vector: the prediction error can then be used as a local distance between a state and an acoustic vector [10]. To alleviate the restriction of linear prediction, neural architectures have been proposed [11] to train nonlinear predictors.

2 Speech representation

2.1 Waveform preprocessing

Since speech waveforms contain information under different forms not all essential for the recognition, a preprocessing is required to provide an efficient representation in term of what is called *acoustic vectors*. Speech is by nature a nonstationary process. However due to the mechanical inertia of the phonatory apparatus, it may be considered stationary on short time intervals of a centisecond duration called *time frames*. Spectral analysis can be performed on overlapping intervals defined by a window spanning two or more centisecond time frames. The results of this analysis are stored in a vector called ***acoustic vector***. Its content could be either some linearly or nonlinearly (MEL Scale) frequency spaced values of the smoothed spectrum or LPC (linear prediction coefficients) or cepstral coefficients or any other description of the speech signal over the window (PLP or Rasta-PLP coefficients)[20-21]. Analysis windows are shifted by one centisecond so that there is one acoustic vector ($\in R^d$) associated with each time frame. Some representation parameters suit better for some applications (speaker dependent or not, recognition over the phone, robust to noise recognizers). A multiresolution analysis could probably improve recognition rates.

Spectral analysis based on an FFT roughly applied to the waveform samples in an analysis window, results in a spectrum exhibiting formant peaks but also, in case of voiced speech, a fine structure due to the fundmental frequency of the glottal excitation (*pitch* is in the range of 100 to 200 Hz according to speaker's sex). Since pitch information is commonly admitted not to be pertinent for speech recognition (mainly because it is related to high level analysis like semantics and hard to deal with at the front end analysis layer!), only spectral envelope will be kept by smoothing and decimation (data compression).

Another way to get rid of pitch information is to apply homomorphic filtering [18-19]. Since the speech spectrum is the product of the vocal tract transfer function modulus and the Fourier transform of the pitch, application of a log operator transforms it into a sum. Taking the FFT of that sum generates the cepstrum which is a function of a new variable denoted quefrency that has dimension of time. By removing the high quefrency components of the cepstrum (quefrency has the dimension of time and forms with frequency the Fourier variable pair in the log domain), pitch information is liftered (i.e. filtering in the quefrency domain) out. This operation amounts to spectral smoothing. Moreover cepstral coefficients are independent of the acquisition channel gain except c_0 which is thus frequently discarded. Both spectral and cepstral approaches obviously overlook phase information since only moduli are considered.

Linear prediction is a parametric representation since it assumes an underlaying speech production model (i.e. source coding). Only information on the vocal tract model is retained i.e. the LP coefficients or any other equivalent representation set such as Parcor's or log-area ratios [17-19]. Cepstral coefficients can also be derived from the prediction coefficients but they differ from those obtained through homomorphic analysis since contrary to the latter ones, they assume an underlaying source model.

Speech representation is denoted *continuous* in opposition with the *discrete* one obtained when acoustic vectors are replaced the nearest vector taken out of a codebook. Codebook clusters are computed with vector quantization algorithms such as K-Means or LBG [22] applied on a large amount of the acoustic vectors of the preprocessed speech data base.

2.2 Lexicon representation

Speech recognition relies on comparisons between a preprocessed utterance and a cascade of speech unit models. If the number of words in the lexicon is small (less than 50), word models are used. For larger lexicons, sub-units like phonemes or triphones (phonemes in right an left contexts) are mandatory: indeed any lexicon regardless to its size can be represented in terms of a limited number of sub-units (about 40 phonemes or 2500 triphones). The addition of a new word in a lexicon amounts then to give its transcription in terms of sub-units. A transcription may be read in a dictionary but also could be automatically generated by a grapheme to phoneme algorithm as used in the front end of a text-to-speech system. Mostly, word models are merged into a lexical tree resulting in a saving of computation and storage.

Grammars used to constraint word sequences and so to reduce the search space may be either a priori described or stochastically trained. Discussions of these aspects fall beyond the scope of this paper.

3 Hidden Markov Models

Speech variability causes most of the difficulties in recognition: indeed, pronunciation of words depends of course on the speaker but even the same speaker articulates words unconsistently. To take the variability of speech into account, it is useful to create a statistical model for each speech unit: *Hidden Markov Models* [1] are perfectly suited. An utterance of a speech unit (a time sequence of acoustic vectors) is viewed as being generated by a state machine. Each time a state is visited, an acoustic vector is emitted according to a probability density function (pdf) associated with the current state. Usually due to the time progressive nature of speech, only left to right models are considered i.e. states are ordered and transitions are allowed from left to right only. No other loops but self-loops on states are accepted (fig. 1).Self loops and jumps over states allow duration control of the utterance. Two kinds of probabilities appear in an HMM: emission pdf's and transition probabilities. Emission probabilities are either computed from a parametric pdf's (Gaussian, Gaussian mixture or Laplace densities) or read from a look-up table if the representation space is vector quantized. In the latter case, no assumption on the pdf is made but a distance definition between acoustic vectors and clusters is assumed. Transition probabilities are estimated by plain frequencies. The parameters of the models are determined by training.

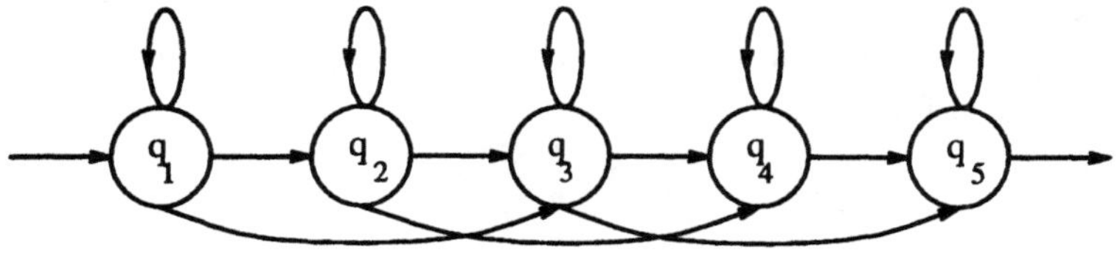

Figure 1: A left-to-right Hidden Markov Model

3.1 Training

Two main criteria are used for training. The first one is the maximum likelihood criterion where the probability that several utterances of the word corresponding to the model is maximized by iterative reestimation of the parameters (Estimate-Maximize algorithm). This probability is the sum of the probabilities associated with all possible paths through the model from the input state to the output one. Probabilities of all paths are considered in the *forward backward* algorithm proposed by Baum and Welch [19].

In the sequel, we will focus on a second criterion known as *Viterbi's criterion*, which is a simplified version of the maximum likelihood where only the best path is considered. So, HMM training amounts in aligning a large amount (N) of utterances of the corresponding sub-unit W on the model. The best match is measured by the accumulated probability of the optimal (most probable) path computed with the Viterbi algorithm (Bellman's dynamic programming) in the matrix of the local emission probabilities:

$$\max \prod_{j=1}^{N} P(X_j|W) \tag{1}$$

where $X_j = \{x_{j,1}, x_{j,2}, \ldots, x_{j,m_j}\}$ stands for an utterance of word W consisting in a sequence of m_j acoustic vectors ($\in R^d$).

Bellman's principle consists in solving a sequence of subproblems. In our case, the best scores computed from the first acoustic vector of the test utterance to any subsequent one. They represents the probability that this part of the utterance can be matched with the model. Frame by frame, it is then possible to recurrently compute the score up to the last frame. During this forward process, one keeps track of the optimal local decisions and eventually the optimal path is obtained by backtracking. It should be pointed out that the path is globally optimal: no hypotheses have been discarded during the forward process.

In practice, probabilities are commonly replaced by the opposite of their logarithms and can be viewed as local distances. Pdf's parameters are estimated by collecting all vectors emitted on a given state and transition probabilities by plain counting during the backtracking process. For instance, for Gaussian pdf's associated with a given state, the mean vector μ is estimated by the classical formula:

$$\mu = \frac{1}{n}\sum_i x_i \tag{2}$$

where n denotes the number of vectors x_i emitted on that state along the optimal path.

In case of discrete models, pdf's are the observation probabilities of cluster prototypes on the current state (look-up table). The probability of emitting cluster ξ on a given state q is estimated by:

$$\hat{p}(\xi|q) = \frac{n_\xi}{n} \tag{3}$$

where n_ξ and n are respectively the number of emissions of cluster ξ and the number of vectors emitted on state q.

Isolated utterances of speech units (as words for instance) are not mandatory for training. *Embedded training* makes use of word labeled but unsegmented (detection of boundaries between words) sentences. Optimal alignment results in a path in the matrix of local emission probabilities. This path generates the segmentation of the training material as a by-product. It is interesting to notice that this process can be extended to the training of subunits such as phonemes if the training sentence can be labeled in subunits: the tedious and unaccurate segmentation process by experts is avoided.

Using short subunits such as phonemes leads to less accurate results but requires less models and less training material. An additional advantage is the possibility to add a new word to the lexicon by just giving its phonetic spelling. A word model is then built by concatenating phoneme models. The recognition degradation comes from the *coarticulation effects*: the utterance of a phoneme is indeed strongly affected by its left (due to the continuity of the motion of the articulatory apparatus) and right (due to anticipation in the speech production process) neighbors. Occurrences of a speech-unit in various contexts are merged into a single signal model and reduces coarticulation to some extent but a definite improvement is obtained by replacing phonemes by triphones i.e. phonemes in right and left contexts. Triphone training sets up new problems: a larger training data base should be available and the frequencies of triphones span over a wide range. Significance of the estimators is questionable if no special interpolation techniques are used. However, using short subunits is the only way to tackle the large vocabulary recognition task.

An important improvement was observed when taking spectral (or cepstral) contextual effects into account. The easiest way was to increase the size of the representation space by concatenating two neighboring acoustic vectors or one vector and the difference with its neighbor [12]. Even second order differences are commonly used. The increased space dimension slows down the recognition process since the local probability computation consumes more

CPU time. Another technique is to define local probability given a previous vector: it has been shown that the logarithm of this local probability is closely related to a linear prediction of acoustic vectors [10]. Both techniques require larger training data bases.

Equation (1) shows the criterion used for training word W model. So, no correlation between word models is taken into account during the training process which does not enforce discrimination; indeed, the objective is to maximize the global probability produced by an HMM when it matches a corresponding utterance but a very close probability might be observed when it is matched a wrong word. Several attempts to modify the criterion have been proposed such as Minimum Mutual Information Estimator ($MMIE$) or corrective training. Unfortunately, no convergence proofs can be given if such approaches are used: these techniques should be considered as heuristics.

Training capability is not restricted to HMM. In particular, studies in discriminant classification put into evidence the role of the perceptrons [13]. Unfortunately, perceptrons can be trained only on linearly separable data sets for two reasons: first, the criterion used is looking for an exact solution and does not use an LMS approach and second, the monolayer structure is not rich enough to describe non convex or non connected partitions. Multilayer perceptrons trained along a LMS criterion remove these severe restrictions[6].

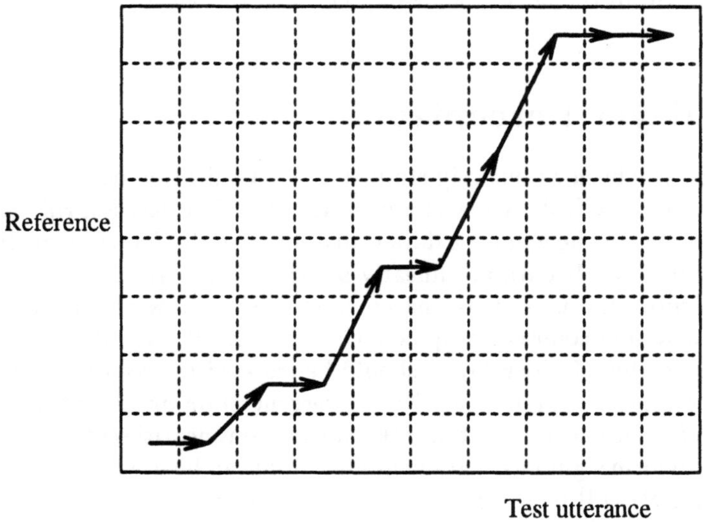

Figure 2: Viterbi alignment

3.2 Recognition

Isolated word recognition is based on the comparison of the test utterance with all word models. The highest score identifies the recognized word. Scores are nothing but the probabilities computed using either a Baum Welch algorithm or a Viterbi alignment. So recognition uses the same algorithm as for training except backtracking. This is no longer the case for connected word recognition.

Concatenated word recognition amounts to find an optimal path aligning the test utterance with a sequence of word models. The best alignment is obtained by a generalization of Viterbi's algorithm which allows discontinuities (cfr figure 3) of the optimal path; they correspond to jumps between the end of a word and the beginning of the next one. Possible starting points are the grey-colored entries while ending points are in black-colored entries. Here the absolute value of the score does not matter but the optimal path is crucial since it yields the word sequence and boundaries simultaneously. Since determination of the best path is crucial to segment and label the test sentence, Viterbi algorithm is traditionally used [23-24].

The process can also be applied to *phonemic segmentation* but results in low recognition scores due to the intrinsic fragility of phonemic models. Word models can be built as phoneme concatenations: this word description can be viewed as a syntactical constraint on the phonemes and allows description of a full lexicon from the small phonemic set: it is the mostly used lexicon description.

4 Multilayer Perceptrons

The perceptron has been extensively studied as a classification device having an abrupt decision law [13]. A major advantage of such a decision rule is in its squashing property: how much a data is distant from the *linear* separation surface does not care. If data are linearly separable, a convergent training algorithm assigning the perceptron parameters exists. However, by trivial non linearly separable counterexamples such as the XOR, algorithm failure is easily demonstrated. Hidden layers should be inserted between the output (decision) field and the input one. No convergent training algorithm has been proposed for such structures but if the abrupt nonlinearities of nodes are smoothed out to form sigmoids, a gradient algorithm can be used (Error Back Propagation *EBP*) [14] to compute the optimal values of the connections. *EBP* is nothing else but a clever use of Newton's formula for derivating functions of functions to get gradient corrections.

Supervised training offers a powerful manner to learn mappings between input/output pairs of data. Unfortunately *EBP* is extremely time consuming. When used in the classification mode i.e. with all outputs equal to zero but one which corresponds to the class the input data belong, they produce a

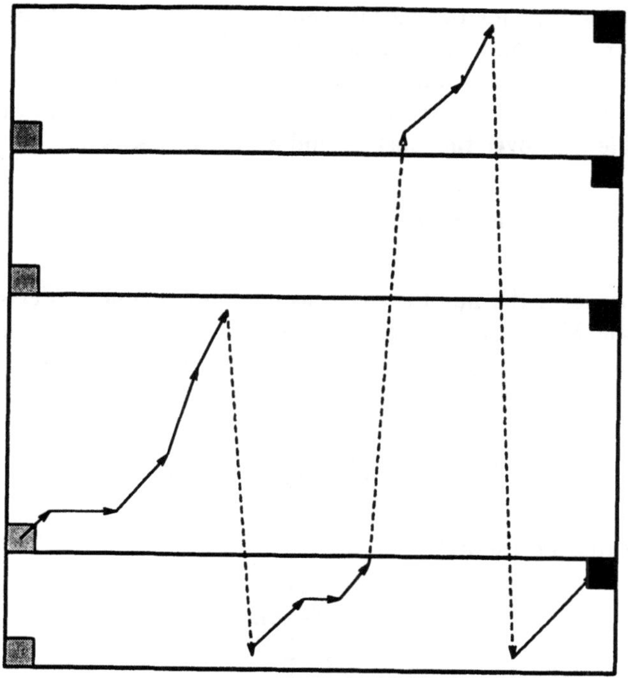

Figure 3: One-level method for connected word recognition

posteriori probabilities $p(C_j|x)$ after training. Here C_j denotes classes and x is an input vector. Application of this result to speech recognition has been proposed in [4] with vector quantized inputs. While justification for continuous inputs has been published by Lippmann [5], we focus in this paper on the discrete approach for the sake of simplicity [25].

Let us thus assume the acoustic vectors of the training database have been replaced by their nearest clusters and I denotes the number of different clusters. The sequence of vectors becomes a sequence of indices i_n where $n \in [1, N]$ and $i_n \in [1, I]$. Each acoustic vector is also known to belong to a given class C_k where $k \in [1, K]$. An MLP with I inputs and K output is trained to map a sequence of N input index vectors y_n (all entries equal to zero but the one corresponding to the input cluster index) to a sequence of output index vectors (all entries equal to zero but the one corresponding the current class). The same cluster vector can show up in different classes depending on its time of occurrence in the sequence (class overlapping). The objective LMS function is thus:

$$E = \sum_{n=1}^{N} \sum_{k=1}^{K} [g_k(i_n) - d_k(i_n)]^2$$

where $g_k(i_n)$ stands for the output value of the k-th output given the i_n-th input is turned on and $d_k(i_n)$ is a target equal to one or zero according to the current input is associated with class C_k. If we partition the terms of () to form groups corresponding to the same input cluster, sum over n is split into a double sum over the clusters and over the classes:

$$E = \sum_{i=1}^{I}\sum_{k=1}^{K}\sum_{\ell=1}^{K} n_{ik}[g_\ell(i) - d_\ell(i)]^2$$

where n_{ik} denotes the number of occurrences of cluster i in class C_k. Thus, whatever the MLP topology may be i.e. number of layers and number of units per layer, the optimal output values $g_\ell^{opt}(i)$ are obtained by canceling the partial derivatives of E with respect to the $g_\ell(i)$:

$$\frac{\partial E}{\partial g_\ell(i)} = 2\sum_{k=1}^{K} n_{ik}[g_\ell(i) - d_\ell(i)] = 0$$

So, the optimal values are:

$$g_\ell^{opt}(i) = \frac{\sum_{k=1}^{K} n_{ik} d_\ell(i)}{\sum_{k=1}^{K} n_{ik}}$$

or by using the definition of $d_\ell(i)$:

$$g_\ell^{opt}(i) = \frac{n_{i\ell}}{\sum_{k=1}^{K} n_{ik}}.$$

This expression can be interpreted as the *a posteriori* probability:

$$g_\ell^{opt}(i) = P(C_\ell|y_i).$$

This is the key result leading to hybrid HMM's: indeed, MLP's generate at their outputs a posteriori probabilities which are related to the emission probabilities of HMM by Bayes rule. The emission probabilities obtained from a MLP's generated a posteriori probabilities are more discriminant since discrimination between classes was taken into account by forcing outputs to be index vectors during the training phase.

4.1 Hybrid HMM/MLP's

By assuming for the sake of simplification that a state in a HMM corresponds to a class, we observe the local emission probabilities defined in the previous section $P(x|q)$ do not correspond to the a posteriori probabilities $P(q|x)$ but are related to them through Bayes rule:

$$P(x|q) = \frac{P(q|x)P(x)}{P(q)}. \tag{4}$$

Since in the alignment process, $P(x)$ is constant in each time frame, this factor can be discarded and $P(x|q)$ can be replaced by $P(q|x)/P(q)$. In place of using parametric pdf's or non discriminant probability look-up tables, MLP outputs divided by the a priori probability of state visits can be used in HMM : this approach is usually known as hybrid HMM/MLP. A major advantage lays in the discriminant training of $P(q|x)$ as explained above: this probability will be high or low according to the fact x belongs to state q or not.

Taking account of spectral or cepstral contexts is quite easy with hybrid HMM/MLP's. MLP's input is split into several fields: the central one contains the current vector while left anf right fields contain neighboring vectors (fig. 2). Inputs are fully connected to all hidden units, regardless to the field they belong.

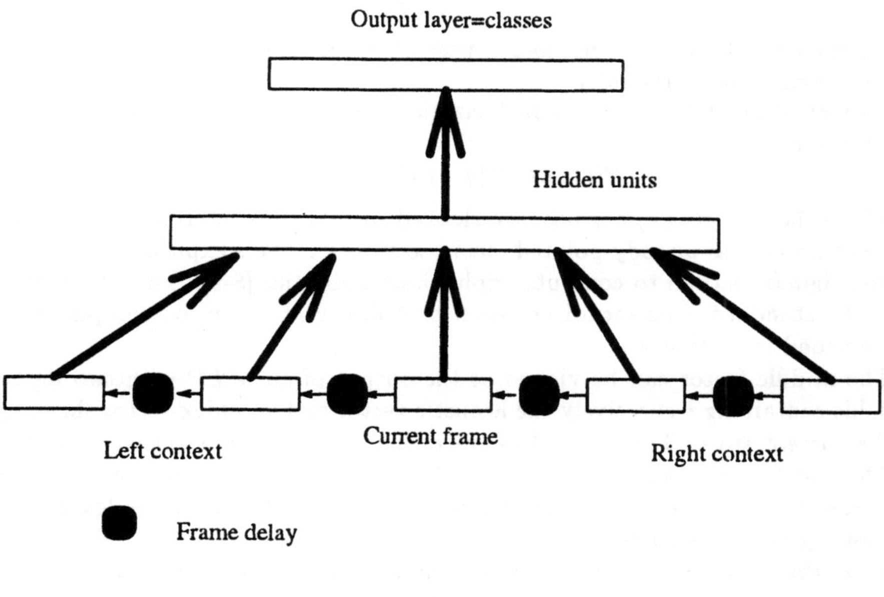

Figure 4: Context-dependent multilayer perceptron classifier

An obvious objection could be: "How do you segment your data in state intervals as it is required in a supervised training?". Actually, embedded training also applies for hybrid HMM/MLP [15]: an initial guess segmentation is defined and EBP training is applied. Then a Viterbi alignment is performed using the probabilities generated by the trained MLP resulting in a new segmentation in state intervals. The process is iterated. Since EBP is also an iterative process, the training program contains a double iteration loop: but using crossvalidation data subset to control both loops, the training process duration can be kept within reasonable limits. However for ambitious

ASR tasks like speaker independent 1000 word vocabulary continuous speech recognition (or more), dedicated boards are required [16]. The restriction of having one state per phoneme is removed since no segmentation is required. Segmentation even in states if necessary may result from embedded training.

4.2 Triphone emission probabilities

In the previous section, triphones have been shown an efficient but expensive way to cope with coarticulation effects. The local probability of a state taking left and right contexts into account can be written $P(x|q, c^{\ell}, c^{r})$ where c^{ℓ} and c^{r} respectively denote left and right phonemes. where c^{ℓ} and c^{r} respectively denote left and right phonemes.It factorizes according standard probability rules:

$$P(x|q, c^{\ell}, c^{r}) = \frac{P(q, c^{\ell}, c^{r}|x).P(x)}{P(q, c^{\ell}, c^{r})}$$

Let us denote by L the number of possible contexts (regardless they appear on the right or on the left).

Using standard probability factorization properties, numerator of (4) can be written:

$$P(q|x).P(c^{r}|q, x).P(c^{\ell}|q, x, c^{r}). \tag{5}$$

where the factor $P(x)$ has been overlooked since it plays no role in the alignment process as already pointed out in section 4.1. This expression suggests an original method to compute triphone probabilities [8-9]. The first factor is the standard a posteriori emission probability and may be computed as described in section 4.1.

The middle factor can be viewed as the output of an MLP with two input fields containing respectively the acoustic vector and an index vector showing the current state. This MLP has one output per possible right context (L). The last factor has also L outputs but three input fields: one contains the acoustic vector, the second the current state and the third is an index vector showing the right context.

Thus three MLP's can be used to compute the factors leading to the numerator of the triphone emission probability. The last two ones are shown in figure 5.

Some restrictions on the MLP architecture simplifies the amount of computations f.i. of $P(c^{\ell}|q, x, c^{r})$ [8-9]. Slight assumptions allow to merge these three MLP's resulting in a substantial weight saving when compared with the single MLP which could produce the triphone probability without going to the factorization formula. Weight saving implies training data saving.

The denominator is also factorized in a similar way:

$$P(q).P(c^{r}|q).P(c^{\ell}|q, c^{r}). \tag{6}$$

These factors depend on the lexicon only, are easily estimated by counting once for ever and stored in a look-up table.

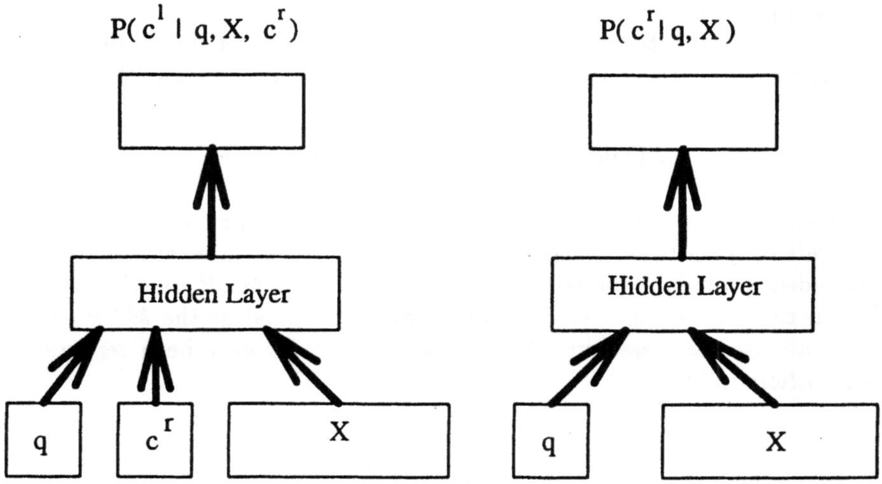

Figure 5: Triphone emission probabilities estimation by MLP's

4.3 Nonlinear predictors

In [10], Wellekens showed that taking context into account in a Gaussian emission probability amounts to use the error of a acoustic vector prediction based on this context as a representation of the signal. This vectorial prediction error is then equivalent to a distance in log-presentation ($-logP$ equivalent to a distance) of the algorithm. Levin [11] got rid of the Gaussian assumption and the linear predictor and suggested to extend the concept to nonlinear prediction by using an MLP to generate the predictor of any acoustic vector. The principle is illustrated in figure 6. Theoretically, ther should be one such predictor per state, but in practice an additional input field (not shown on the figure) controls the state dependency. The prediction error $x(t) - \hat{x}(t)$ is then used as a local distance. The corresponding emission probability is then:

$$P(x_t|q, X_{t-p}^{t-1}) \tag{7}$$

where X_{t-p}^{t-1} stands for $\{x_{t-1}, x_{t-2}, \ldots, x_{t-p}\}$. Training is easy since the target is to minimize the LMS prediction error on a large database. In that case, the predicted value is generated as an output. No interpretation in terms of probability is possible. Prediction error is directly used as a local distance. Unfortunately, results with nonlinear predictors have never reached the recognition scores obtained with the MLP used as classifiers. This is probably because the discriminant properties are no longer enforced in the training process.

It is interesting to observe that application of Bayes rule leads another method to compute context dependent probabilities [8-9]. Indeed,

$$P(x_t|q, X_{t-p}^{t-1}) = \frac{P(x_t|X_{t-p}^{t-1}).P(q|X_{t-p}^{t})}{P(q|X_{t-p}^{t-1})}$$

The first factor in the denominator is irrelevant for time alignment since it depends only on the the signal itself and not on the states and the context dependent probability is estimated as the ratio of two *MLP* classifier outputs. In this case, discriminative constraints can be enforced on the *MLP*'s which are both used as classifiers. No comparative results have been reported by the authors [8-9].

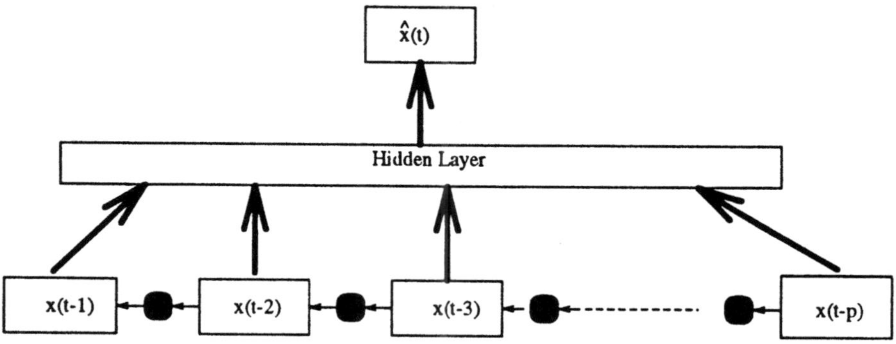

Figure 6: Nonlinear prediction using *MLP*'s

5 Conclusions

In the long history of *ASR*, a major step was the introduction of statistical techniques. But since the underlaying statistical rules completely escape to our knowledge and also for the sake of simplification, standard parametric pdf's have been hypothesized for the description of the speech production process. Even when discrete pdf's were considered, the clustering process was constraining the generality of the statistical behavior through distance definition.

The relationship between Least Mean Square minimization and statistics has been known for several decades. The idea to interpret outputs of *MLP* classifiers as probabilities is thus not new. However, relationship through the Bayes rule with the emission probabilities and discriminant properties inherited from the training process lead very soon to significant scores comparing favorably with very sophisticated recognizers affected by the above constraints. The price to pay was a CPU time greedy training algorithm but the regular structure of the MLP architectures allows design of modular dedicated boards and integrated chips for fast training.

Statistical interpretation of *MLP* outputs shows the way to cast standard results of statistics into new architectures. Building on statistics and neural networks, researchers may still expect significant progresses in *ASR* and more generally in most of applications where complexity forbids any explicit formulation and forces to accept training on examples as the only reasonable approach.

References

[1] F.Jelinek, Continuous Recognition by Statistical Methods, Proceedings IEEE, vol. 64 no 4, pp.532-555, 1976.

[2] A.Waibel, T.Hanazawa, G.Hinton, K.Shikano, K.Lang, Phoneme Recognition : Neural Networks vs. Hidden Markov Models, Proc. Intl. Conf. on Acoustics, Speech and Signal Processing, New York, vol.1, pp107-110, 1988.

[3] H.Bourlard & C.J.Wellekens, Multilayer Perceptrons and Speech Recognition, IEEE Proc. of the First International Conf. on Neural Networks, vol IV, pp.407-416, San Diego, CA, 1987.

[4] H.Bourlard & C.J.Wellekens, Links between Markov Models and Multilayer Perceptrons, Computer, Speech and Language, vol.3,pp.1-19, 1989

[5] R.P.Lippmann, Neural Network Classifiers Estimate Bayesian a Posteriori Probabilities, Neural Computation, vol.3, no 4, pp. 461-484, 1991.

[6] R.P.Lippmann, An Introduction to Computing with Neural Nets, IEEE Acoustic, Speech, and Signal Processing Magazine, vol. 4, no 2, pp.4-22, 1987.

[7] M.Cohen, H.Franco, N.Morgan, D.E.Rumelhart & V.Abrash, Hybrid Neural Network/Hidden Markov Model Continuous Speech Recognition, Proc. Intl. Conf. on Spoken Language Processing, vol2, pp. 915-918, Banff, Canada, 1992.

[8] H. Bourlard, Continuous Speech Recognition: From Hidden Markov Models to Artificial Neural Networks, Doctoral Dissertation, Faculté Polytechnique de Mons, Belgium, Feb.1992.

[9] H.Bourlard, N.Morgan, Chuck Wooters & Steve Renals, CDNN: A Context Dependent Neural Network for Continuous Speech Recognition, IEEE Proc. Intl. Conf. on Acoustics, Speech and Signal Processing San Francisco, CA, vol.2 pp. 349-352, 1992.

[10] C.J.Wellekens, Explicit Time Correlation in Hidden Markov Models in Speech Recognition, Proc. IEEE Conference on Audio, Speech and Signal Processing, pp.384-387, April 1987.

[11] E.Levin, Speech Recognition Using Hidden Control Neural Network Architecture, IEEE Proc. Intl. Conf. on Acoustics, Speech, and Signal Processing, pp. 433-436, Albuquerque, NM, 1990.

[12] S.Furui, Speaker Independent Isolated Word Recognizer Using Dynamic Features of Speech Spectrum, IEEE Trans. on Acoustic, Speech, ans Signal Processing, vol.34, no 1, pp 52-59, 1986.

[13] M.Minsky & S.Papert, Perceptrons, Cambridge, MA : MIT Press, 1969.

[14] D.E. Rumelhart, G.E.Hinton & R.J.Williams, Parallel Distributed Processing. Exploration of the Microstructure of Cognition. vol.1: Foundations, Ed. D.E.Rumelhart & J.L.McClelland, MIT Press, 1986.

[15] N.Morgan & H.Bourlard, Continuous Speech Recognition Using Multilayer Perceptrons with Hidden Markov Models, IEEE Intl. Conf. on Audio, Speech and Signal Processing, pp. 413-416, Albuquerque, New Mexico, 1990.

[16] N.Morgan, J.Beck, P.Kohn, J.Bilmes, E.Allman & J. Beer, The Ring Array Processor (RAP): A multiprocessing peripheral for connectionist applications, Journal of Parallel and Distributed Computing, 1992.

[17] L.R.Rabiner, B.H.Juang, "Fundamentals of Speech Recognition", Prentice Hall, 1993.

[18] L.R.Rabiner, R.W.Schafer, "Digital Processing of Speech Signals", Prentice Hall, 1978.

[19] J.R.Deller, J.G.Proakis, J.H.L.Hansen,"Discrete-Time Processing of Speech Signals", Mc Millan, 1993.

[20] H.Hermansky, Perceptual Linear Predictive (PLP) Analysis of Speech, Jl of Acoustical Soc. of America, vol 87, no 4.

[21] H.Hermansky, J-C Junqua, Optimization of Perceptually-Based ASR Front-End, ICASSP 88, pp. 219-222.

[22] Y.Linde, A.Buzo, R.M.Gray, An Algorithm for Vector Quantizer Design, IEEE Trans. on Communications, vol 28, no 1, pp. 84-95, 1980.

[23] H.Ney, The Use of One-Stage Dynamic Programming Algorithm for Connected Word Recognition, IEEE Trans. on Acoustic, Speech and Signal Processing, pp 833-836. (1984)

[24] J.S.Bridle, M.D.Brown, R.M.Chamberlain, An Algorithm for Connected Word Recognition, ICASSP 1982, pp.899-902.

[25] H.Bourlard, C.J.Wellekens, Links between Markov Models and Multilayer Perceptrons, IEEE Trans. on Pattern Analysis and Machine Intelligence, vol 12, no 12, pp. 1167-1178.

Neural Network Architectures for Pattern Recognition

Françoise Fogelman Soulié
SLIGOS-CSIA/LRN, Tour Anjou, 33 quai de Dion Bouton- 92814 Puteaux cedex-France - fogelman@laforia.ibp.fr

Abstract
It is argued that maximal benefit is gained from complex Neural Network architectures. A formalism to train Multi Modular Architectures is given. Examples of such MMAs for various applications in image and speech processing, and time series prediction are shown, which illustrate the benefits of using MMAs.
Keywords
Neural Network, Multi-Modular Architecture, cooperative training. Optical Character Recognition. Speaker identification. Speech recognition. Scene analysis. Time series prediction.

1 Introduction

Are Neural Networks (NNs) a new class of statistical model? Are NNs something more than Statistics made simple (if not simplistic) for everybody's use? Is there anything brought by NNs, which could not have been by Statistics?
Well, those are the questions that any scientist interested in Statistics and NNs should address. I think that the answer to all three previous questions is yes, and in this paper I would like to give some arguments to support my belief (and at the time being, I do not think that there is ground for more than "educated" belief in one direction or the other).
The basic line of my argument goes as follows.
NNs are indeed a class of statistical models: they need the same care to gather data, prepare experiments, evaluate performances, interpret results. The NN community at large is not always aware enough of the existing literature and efforts in Statistics, but many have already pointed to the necessity of using NN with the usual "statistical" care.
In fact, plain simple NNs are probably not anything else but Statistics: by which I mean that there is a statistical model to which the NN is *equivalent* , i.e. performances are exactly the same (providing of course that the user is educated enough to be able to correctly manipulate the model he wants to use). Examples of such equivalences are Projection Pursuit -PP-, Principal Component Analysis -PCA- or Discriminant Analysis -DA. There is thus no reason whatsoever to use such a NN instead of the statistical model -or the opposite- except as a matter of taste or convenience. Most people, when they first start hearing about NNs, tend to believe that a NN is a MultiLayer Perceptron (MLP) with one (usually) hidden layer fully connected to the input and the output layers. This is the prototype of the plain sim-

ple, not so useful NN: the only thing one could expect from such a NN is just what a non-linear statistical technique could give or slightly more (usually not much more, although NNs can be easier to implement ?).
So "plain simple NNs" are, from a statistician point of view, useless. Let us then see what could be a non plain, non simple NN. There are two ingredients to a NN: its learning mechanism (which has of course its counterpart in any statistical model) and its architecture. Although some models in Statistics can be made to incorporate some "architecture", i.e. some particular form of the model adapted to the problem at hand, this is not very widespread in Statistics. In the Neural Network framework, the architecture question is right at the core: how many modules constitute the architecture ? how many neurons, layers? how are they interconnected? These architectural details are fully determining the final performances of the system.
Let me take the example of Optical Character Recognition -OCR-. A team at AT&T Bell labs has worked for years now on proposing various architectures for the OCR of hand-written digits (with a data base of digits coming from the US-Post Office). Some of their early results are worth mentionning [27] (fig. 1). They obviously show that a fully connected MLP performs basically as well (or as badly) as a linear classifier. But performances can be tremendously increased by working out an appropriate architecture: shared weights architectures or TDNNs [26] are useful in image and speech processing.

architecture connections	-- FC	-12- FC	-8x8-4x4- LC	-8x8x2-4x4- SW	-8x8x2- 4x4x4- SW
performanc on test set (%)	80	87	88.5	94	98.4

Figure 1: generalization performances of 5 network architectures. -m- is a MLP with input 16x16, 10 outputs and hidden layer(s) of size m. FC: fully connected, LC: locally connected, SW: shared weights

Now, how do we get these nice architectures? First way is by hand: available knowledge can be incorporated into the very structure of the NN. Local connections and shared weights for example come from similar ideas in image processing and are just a translation from that literature into the NN setting. Otherwise, the architecture can be obtained automatically (and this is more like in Statistics): there are various techniques to do so, which are more or less efficient. Some learning algorithms grow/prune architectures while learning [34]. The regularization framework allows to impose constraints on the architecture (e.g. on the a priori distribution of weights [35]); the Bayesian framework allows model selection [30], network pruning [37] and very efficient performances [31]! Multi-experts networks, with the EM algorithm [23], learn to specialize (become expert) on specific parts of the task; whereby the trained architecture has a structure adapted to that task.
In this latter approach, the architecture is a set of cooperating experts, which have learnt to decompose the task, and then have specialized each to an individual part of the task. The problem of task decomposition is hard to automatize. The only existing results still apply to small problems. So that, most often, in practice that decomposition has to be done by hand, before training. Anyway the resulting architecture

is not anymore a simple, fully connected NN; but more probably a set of various NNs. We thus have to handle multi-modular architectures if we want to get something really better from NNs.
After a brief discussion of modularity (section 2), I will present a formalism which allows to train multi-modular architectures (section 3) and will then illustrate, through real-size applications, the performances obtained by such architectures: in face recognition (section 4), speaker identification (section 5), OCR (section 6) and speech recognition (section 7).

2 Why Multi-Modular Architectures?

2.1 Modularity

Modularity is a technique largely used in Computer Science, intended to provide the following properties:
- mastering complexity: by decomposing a problem into modules, one expects to have each module be simpler than the overall task. This *divide and conquer* strategy does not kill-off complexity of course, but eases the task for the designer who can take successive, hopefully simple steps.
- insulating: each module can be developed independently from the others, e.g. by different programmers. One has to be careful enough in the specification of the modules and provide a clear separation between the inner part of each module and its interface to the rest of the system. Insulation also allows for easy replacement of individual modules.
- reusability: generic modules can be ported from one application to another.

One problem raised by such an approach is the optimality of the global system: each module can be assumed to be locally optimized, but for the system to be globally optimal, there must exist some interaction between the modules. Of course, this is in contradiction with the insulation requirement. Hence, some compromise must be found between total insulation and total interaction.
All the remarks above indeed apply to the design of applications involving Neural Networks. But those also call for additional desirable properties:
- robustness: one of the problems with Neural Networks is the necessity to come-up with the best architecture. This requires a lot of trial-and-error and fine-tuning; whereby model parameters are chosen by cross-validation. It would be extremely useful to have principled design methods leading to architectures with performances robust with slight variations in architecture details (i.e. performances do not vary very much when the number of hidden units changes). In the Bayesian framework [30], model selection is one level of the overall training process and is thus "automatic". However, there is of course nothing in this framework which calls for the above mentioned robustness property.
- combining good individual module properties: various Neural Networks will have different capabilities. Combining them into a global architecture might allow one to cope with the errors of another. One should not expect to have a unique Neural Network type be the universal solution to all possible problems.
- getting generic design principles: each time one has to solve a new application, one has to design a new architecture. It would be useful to have a method to build

an architecture, possibly not optimal, but as generic as possible vis à vis the application.
We do not have solutions which would guarantee all these desired features, but we will show in the following a few techniques which are heading this way. One should not expect to have any given algorithm be best in all possible cases. And of course, this also applies to NNs. However, we will show that our design methodology provides architectures which are always (sofar) better than simple NNs.
One of the major problems with NNs is their generalization ability: various results [38], [22] have shown that the NN complexity must be matched to the problem complexity and the number of available examples. Too complex a network will perfectly learn the training set (achieve low bias), while generalizing very poorly (high variance). Controlling the complexity of the NN is thus a necessity to ensure good generalization. There are many ways to do so. In *stopped training*, training is stopped as soon as the generalization error on a validation set starts increasing (during training, weights tend to increase; at initialization, small random values of weights produce basically linear transfer functions; with larger weights, increasing non-linearities appear, thus leading to increasing complexity [19]); in *shared weights* architectures, neurons are forced to share the same weights, thus decreasing the number of free parameters [26]; in *structural risk minimization* [39], an embedded sequence of networks is explored to optimize the *capacity* or complexity of the network. Finaly, techniques exist to directly simplify the weights distributions: either static techniques, where a network is trained, then its complexity reduced, e.g. by *pruning*; or dynamic, where the network capacity is progressively reduced during training (e.g. by *regularization*). Modularity is another way to control the complexity: by sub-dividing the architecture into sub-modules, we obtain more simple individual NNs. We should thus gain increased generalization ability, while requiring less examples.
We now describe a simple example which illustrates some of the previous remarks.

2.2 Waveforms

Let us consider the following classification problem, introduced by Breiman et al. [15]. We define three vectors H^1, H^2 and H^3 or *waveforms* (fig. 2) in a 21-dimension space $\Re^{21}$. Example x is a vector defined by:

$$x_i = u H_i^m + (1 - u) H_i^n + \varepsilon_i \qquad 0 \leq i \leq 20 \qquad (1)$$

where m, n $\in$ { 1, 2, 3 }, u and ε_i are random variables (u uniformly distributed in [0, 1] and ε_i gaussian with 0 mean and unit variance).

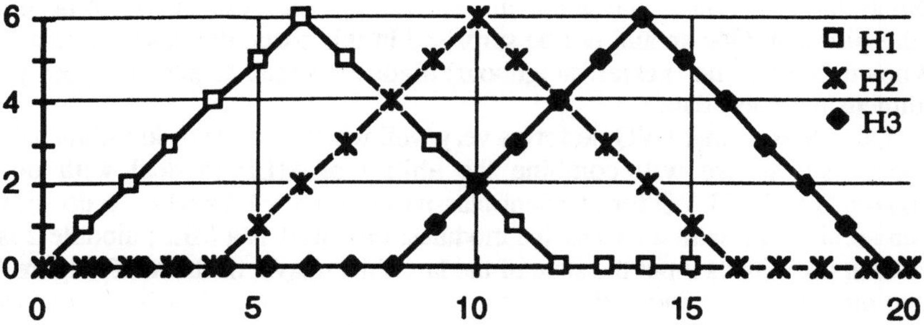

Figure 2: Waveforms H1, H2 and H3.

We can then define 3 classes of such vectors x, for the various pairs (m, n): class 1 for (1, 2), class 2 for (2, 3) and class 3 for (3, 1). In the H1-H2-H3 space the three classes are gaussian blurs of the 3 sides of a triangle, with vertices the H_i.
The learning set has 100, 85 and 115 points respectively for classes 1, 2 and 3 [15]. The test set has 5000 examples, with equal proportions for the 3 classes. We call this problem `problem1`.
We now define `problem2` as follows [4, 5, 6, 7]. Each vector is of dimension 40 and is defined by:

x_i = \F(u H^m \D\ba8 ()\S\do6(i) + (1 - u) H^n \D\ba8 ()\S\do6(i) ;5) + ε_i $0 \le i \le 20$ (2)

$x_i = \varepsilon_i \qquad 21 \le i \le 40$

Classes are defined as for `problem1`: `problem2` is thus a noisy version of `problem1`.
Various algorithms have been compared on `problem1`: conventional [15] and Neural Networks [4]. The optimal Bayes classifier can be computed analytically in `problem1` [15]. A MLP (Multi Layer Perceptron) and a LVQ (Learning Vector Quantization) have been evaluated for both `problem1` and `problem2` [7]. Generalization results are shown in figure 3 [7]. Error bars are computed at 95 % confidence level [2].

Method	Bayes	CART	k-means	LVQ	MLP	MLP+LVQ
Perf. (%)	86 ± 0.99	80 ±1.13	82 ±1.09	84.6 ±1.03	81.6 ±1.10	83.8 ±1.05
Perf. (%)			53.2 ±1.39	77 ±1.19	80.5 ±1.12	81.1 ±1.10

Figure 3: Generalization performances for various techniques on the waveforms `problem1`(top) and `problem2` (bottom).

The MLP is a fully connected-2 hidden layers network (21-15-9-3 for `problem1` and 40-30-20-3 for `problem2`). The LVQ network is trained with the LVQ1 algorithm and has 2 references per class. As can be seen in figure 2, the LVQ is better

than MLP in `problem1`, and worse in `problem2`: the best algorithm depends upon the problem. One should not be surprised in this particular case, since it is a well known fact that nn (nearest-neighbour) algorithms tend to perform poorly on high-dimension, noisy data.
Figure 3 also tells us that LVQ performs very well when data are of low-dimension, not too noisy: so we will combine the ability of MLP to deal with noise (`problem2`) and of LVQ for efficient classification (`problem1`). To do so, we build an architecture with 2 successive modules: module 1 is a MLP; module 2 is a LVQ which takes as its input the state of the last hidden layer of the MLP (figure 4). The two modules are trained one after the other: the MLP can thus be viewed as a pre-processor for the LVQ. After passing through the MLP module, data have reduced dimension and noise level, which makes the LVQ module more efficient.

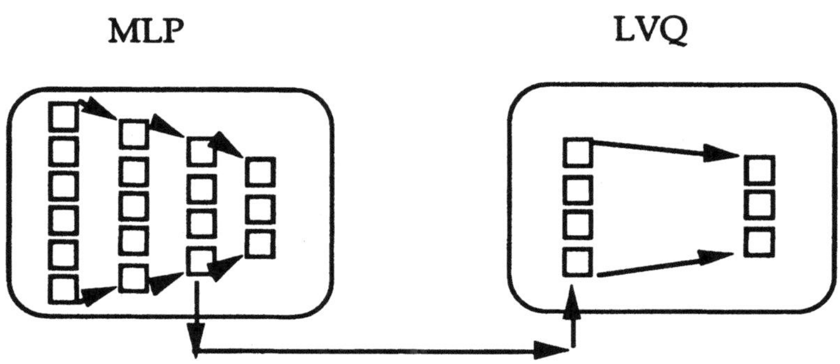

Figure 4: MLP reduces dimension and noise, LVQ is trained on examples pre-processed by MLP.

The results given in figure 3 in column MLP+LVQ show that this multi-module architecture is:
- always better than MLP alone
- as good as or better than LVQ alone.

This multi-module architecture is thus not so dependent upon the application as the individual modules were. Another interesting feature of this multi-modular architecture is that it is fast to train. The MLP architecture requires about 250 sweeps through the database for complete training. However, if one plugs the LVQ network after 20 sweeps only (fig. 5), the final results are better: the code extracted in the last hidden layer of the MLP must not be "too" optimal for the last classifying layer of the MLP. Hence, the multi-modular architecture is best trained by a few sweeps to initialize the MLP weights and then training of the LVQ (which is always very fast, about 20 sweeps). So this method allows to cut the training time of the MLP, while retaining its good properties for noise filtering and dimensionnality reduction. This property is somewhat similar to the *stopped training* idea or, more generaly to the *non-convergent* methods [19].

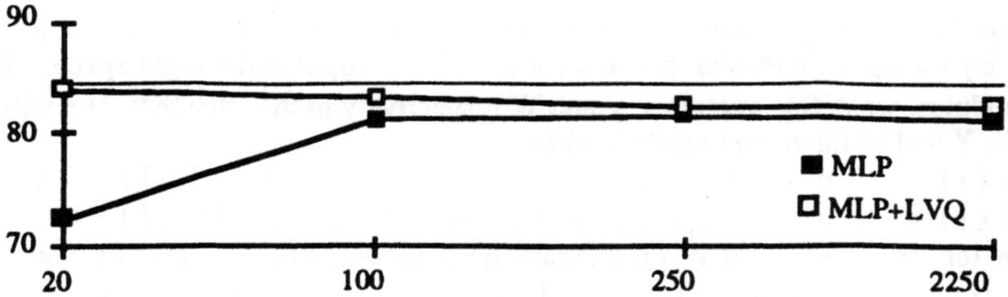

Figure 5: Final performances of the MLP and MLP+LVQ architectures as a function of the number of sweeps used for training the MLP.

2.3 Conclusion

We have shown in this simple example that it is possible to design an architecture made of two successive Neural Networks which has the following properties:
- the Multi-Modular Architecture (MMA) has better performances than the individual modules
- the MMA correctly deals with the two different problems.

In addition, the MMA is faster to train than just the MLP. In this setting, the 2 modules are trained one after the other (we call this *sequential training*): one can easily guess that the resulting architecture is only sub-optimal. The LVQ is optimized for the MLP, but the MLP has no way to take into account the requirements of the LVQ: some global mechanism is necessary to deal with such a problem. In the next section, we provide a general formalism, which allows to derive such a global mechanism, allowing us to achieve *cooperative training*.

3 A Formalism for Cooperative Training

3.1 Modular learning systems

Suppose that we have a Multi-Modular Architecture composed of a succession of modules $M_1, \ldots, M_N$ interconnected so that their connection graph has no cycle (fig. 6).

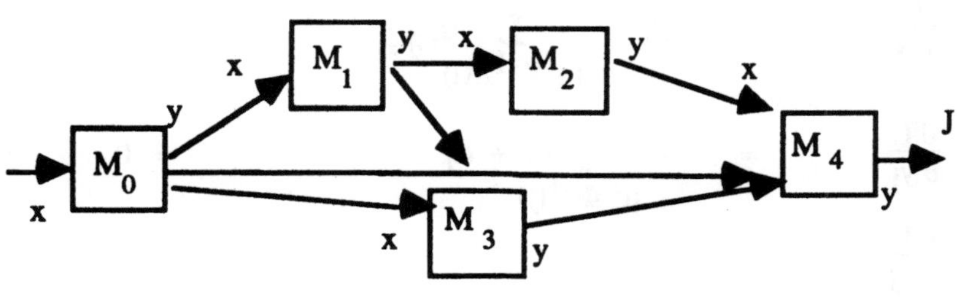

Figure 6: Multi Modular Architecture

Each module is characterized [8,9] by its input, output and weight (or parameter) vectors. By taking the cartesian products of the input, output and weight spaces of the N modules, we define vectors x, y and W respectively in $\Re^I$, $\Re^J$, $\Re^w$. We will denote X, Y and W the mappings defined by:

$$X(i) = n \quad \text{if } x_i \text{ is an input to module } M_n \qquad i \in \{1 \ldots I\} \tag{3}$$
$$Y(j) = n \quad \text{if } y_j \text{ is an output of module } M_n \qquad j \in \{1 \ldots J\}$$
$$W(\omega) = n \quad \text{if } W_\omega \text{ is a parameter of module } M_n \qquad \omega \in \{1 \ldots w\}$$

Thus $X^{-1}(n)$ (respectively $Y^{-1}(n)$, $W^{-1}(n)$) is the set of indices i (resp. j, ω) such that x_i (resp. y_j, W_ω) is an input to (resp. output, parameter of) module M_n. Inputs x to a module are outputs from other modules, as defined by the interconnection structure:

$$x_i = y_{\Phi(i)} \quad i \in \{1 \ldots I\} \tag{4}$$

Each module is characterized by its transfer function:

$$y_j = f_j\left[(x_i)_{i \in X^{-1}Y(j)}, (W_\omega)_{\omega \in W^{-1}Y(j)} \right] \quad j \in \{1 \ldots J\} \tag{5}$$

The first module M_0 just transfers the example χ to the MMA and the last module computes the global cost $C(\chi, x, W)$ of the system (a measure of how well the MMA performs for example χ): the last module M_N thus has a unique output y_J defined by:

$$y_J = C(\chi, x, W) = f_J\left[(x_i)_{i \in X^{-1}Y(J)}, (W_\omega)_{\omega \in W^{-1}Y(J)} \right] \tag{6}$$

The goal of learning is to minimize the cost $C(\chi, x, W)$, which is done using a Lagrangian formalism: let L be the Lagrangian of the system, defined by:

$$L(x, y, W) = C(\chi, x, W) + \sum_{i=1}^{I} \beta_i \left[x_i - y_{\Phi(i)} \right] + \sum_{j=1}^{J} \alpha_j \left(y_j - f_j\left[(x_i)_{i \in X^{-1}Y(j)}, (W_\omega)_{\omega \in W^{-1}Y(j)} \right] \right) \tag{7}$$

α_j and β_i are the Lagrange multipliers. Then the minimum of C under the constraints, expressed by (4) and (5) is obtained for:

$$\nabla L = 0$$

i.e. $$\frac{\partial L}{\partial x_i} = \frac{\partial L}{\partial y_j} = \frac{\partial L}{\partial W_\omega} = 0$$

($\frac{\partial L}{\partial \beta_i} = \frac{\partial L}{\partial \alpha_j} = 0$ just give back constraints (4) and (5)).

but: $$\frac{\partial L}{\partial x_i} = \beta_i - \sum_{j \in Y^{-1}X(i)} \alpha_j \frac{\partial f_j}{\partial x_i} = 0 \tag{8}$$

$$\frac{\partial L}{\partial y_j} = - \sum_{i \in \Phi^{-1}(j)} \beta_i + \alpha_j = 0 \qquad j \neq J$$

$$\frac{\partial L}{\partial y_J} = 1 - \alpha_J = 0$$

$$\frac{\partial L}{\partial W_\omega} = \frac{\partial C}{\partial W_\omega} - \sum_{j \in Y^{-1}W(\omega)} \alpha_j \frac{\partial f_j}{\partial W_\omega} = 0$$

which simplifies into:

$$\beta_i = \frac{\partial C}{\partial x_i} \quad \text{if } i \in X^{-1}(N) \tag{9}$$

$$\beta_i = \sum_{j \in Y^{-1}X(i)} \left[\sum_{k \in \Phi^{-1}(j)} \beta_k \right] \frac{\partial f_j}{\partial x_i} \quad \text{otherwise}$$

$$\frac{\partial C}{\partial W_\omega} = \sum_{j \in Y^{-1}W(\omega)} \left[\sum_{k \in \Phi^{-1}(j)} \beta_k \right] \frac{\partial f_j}{\partial W_\omega}$$

Weights are updated according to the usual stochastic gradient rule:

$$W_\omega^{t} = W_\omega^{t-1} - \varepsilon^{t} \frac{\partial C}{\partial W_\omega} (\chi^{t}, x, W) \tag{10}$$

This learning rule (9-10) thus allows to update weights W_ω and Lagrange multipliers β_i through forward and backwards computations, very similar to the Gradient Back Propagation algorithm.

Training a Multi Modular Architecture thus simply requires being able to define the interconnection structure of the modules, through a function Φ, and a cost function C; each module being characterized by its transfer function (5).

The formalism we have just presented is thus a generalization of Gradient Back Propagation to a "network" composed of modules instead of layers. In general, a global MMA will be too large to be efficiently trained by the above algorithm and we will use the following procedure:

phase 1- individually train each module, i.e. use sequential training

phase 2- train the MMA through (9-10), starting from an initial state W^0 equal to the final state of the sequential training phase 1.

This procedure will usually lead to a global optimum, without too much fine tuning in phase 2. We will call this procedure *cooperative learning* . Such a procedure makes good sense in view of the known results [38,39] stating that computing time, number of required examples and discrepancy between learning and generalization errors can be decreased by controlling the complexity of the network.

3.2 Waveforms

Let us apply the previous formalism to the waveforms problems introduced in section 2.2. We use the MLP+LVQ architecture described previously: we sequentially train each individual module and then cooperatively train the overall MMA: results are shown in figure 7. They show that the cooperation mechanism improves the performances of the sequentially trained architecture [7]. In this example, the cost function C used was a nearest neighbour cost function $\| x - W_c \|^2$, where W_c is the weight vector of the LVQ reference closest to example χ^t and of the same class, and x is the input vector to the LVQ module (i.e. the MLP hidden layer activity vector). We give in the next section various examples of applications where a similar approach was used and led to improved performances.

Method Performance	LVQ	MLP	MLP+LVQ	MLP+LVQ _coop
Problem 1	84.6±1.03	81.6±1.10	83.8±1.05	85±1.02
Problem 2	77±1.19	80.5±1.12	81.1±1.10	82.4±1.08

Figure 7: Results of individual modules MLP, LVQ and MMA, sequentially and cooperatively trained, for `problem1` (top) and `problem2` (bottom).

3.3 Conclusion

The framework we have given in this section is very general and can apply to any architecture (with NN modules or others), provided a global cost function. The particular way to train such an architecture in two successive phases (sequential and then cooperative) requires in addition that each module be separately trainable, through the minimization of a local cost function.
We will now show in the next sections that this method allows to solve real-size applications to excellent performances levels. Some of these applications had never been solved before with simple NNs or other methods; other applications had been using complex large NNs (e.g. in OCR). The versatility of our methodology is in fact its strength: it provides a very general design principle, which shows the benefit of complex architectures when dealing with real world problems.

4 Face Recognition

In many problems of scene analysis, one has to locate and identify pre-specified objects: obstacles in robot path planning, manufactured parts in inspection tasks, cells of a certain type in biological samples analysis... The usual approach in image analysis is to first have a segmentation process for isolating the objects and then a recognition process to identify them. However, one can easily realize that, when faced with such problems in real life, animals tend to locate and identify the objects of relevance to their life (either threats or edible objects) in a unique process: hypothesis about location are generated and then tested through recognition; if the result is not satisfying, new hypothesis are generated and identified... We thus need to have ways to perform Integrated Segmentation Recognition.

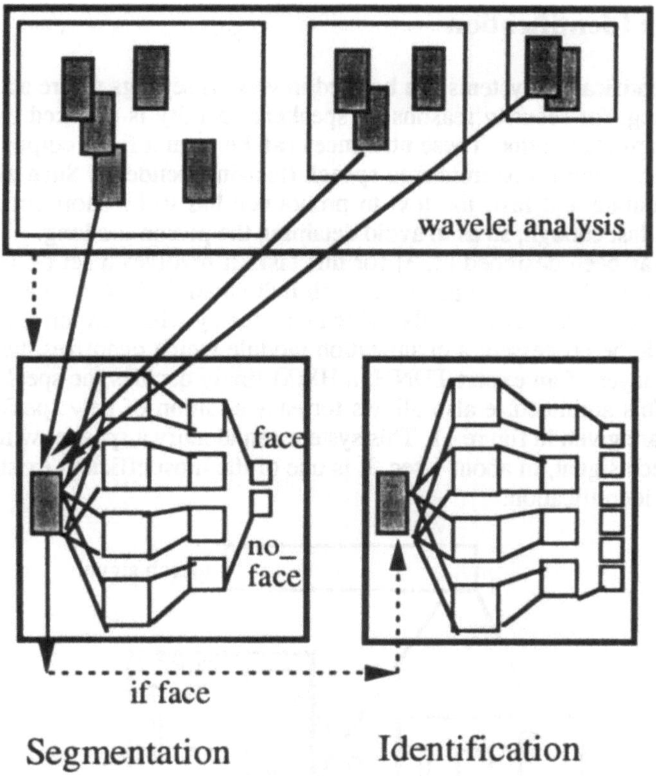

Figure 8: Architecture for face localization/recognition.

We have designed such a process, integrating 2 NNs, for a task of localization-identification of persons in a natural home environment scene [11, 20, 40]. Various data bases were generated, using a video camera: `DataBase1` contains face images of 20 different persons, with about 100 different images of each; `DataBase2` contains 250 scene images, with various persons standing or sitting in their home.
The architecture of the MMA we used is shown in figure 8: it has a pre-processing module, by a wavelet transform analysis [18], followed by a TDNN trained to perform segmentation (classification in *face/no_face*) and then a TDNN (with the same architecture as the segmentation TDNN except for the last layer) to perform the identification (one output neuron per person to identify). Trained on 100 scene images and tested on 120 different scenes, the system gave the performances shown in figure 9 [41].

Non-detection	False detection	Identification error
2.7 %	0.5 %	3.0 %

Figure 9: Performances of the face localization/recognition system.

5 Speaker Identification

Speaker identification systems can be used in various settings where access must be restricted, e.g. for security reasons. A speaker's identity is checked by using sentences he is made to utter. These utterances can be from a fixed corpus (in text-dependent identification) or from free-speech (text-independent). Such systems must be both accurate and fast: the text to pronounce has to be short enough and the recognition fast enough, so as to avoid detaining the person too long.
A system has been designed [2, 3] for this task: it involves a set of TDNNs, each trained on a speakers sub-population (each individual TDNN is an *expert* for that type of speakers); a gating TDNN, which decides by which expert a given speech signal should be processed; a quantization module which quantizes the state of the last hidden layer of an expert TDNN; a HMM finaly decides the speaker's identity (fig. 10). This architecture also allows for easy addition of new speakers. Its performances are given in figure 11. This system can identify a speaker with less than 1 sec. of speech signal, in about 1 sec. It is one of the most efficient existing systems for speaker identification.

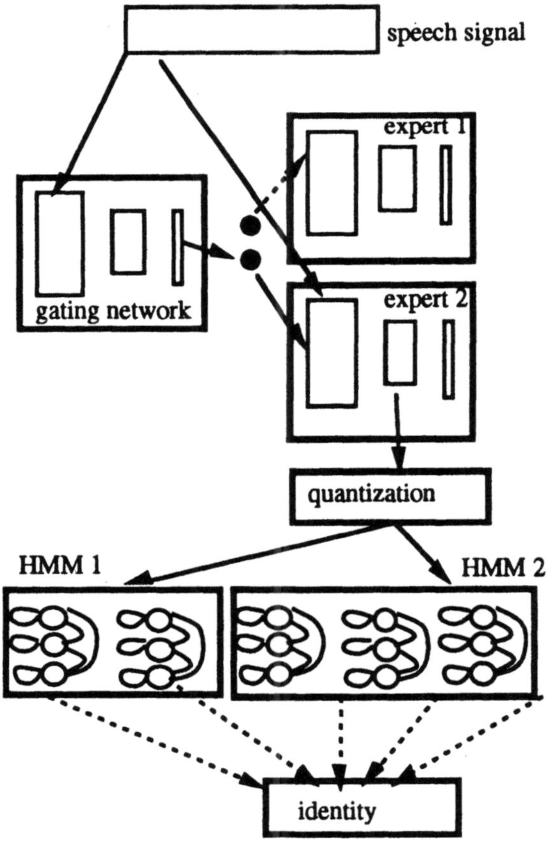

Figure 10: Speaker identification system architecture

Population Architecture	10F	10M	15F	22M
HMM	99.8	99.8		
TDNN	99.8	99.8	82.8	77
TDNN+HMM	99.8	99.8	99.85	99.9

Figure 11: Performances of speaker identification system.

6 Optical Character Recognition

Optical Character Recognition (OCR) has been a benchmark for NN techniques. Many algorithms have been proposed, first to recognize isolated hand-written characters [28], or printed characters [29]; more recently, systems have been designed for recognition of connected characters, integrating both segmentation and recognition [16, 32, 33].

In such systems, a module is trained to identify characters, and is then fed with a window scanning a field containing characters. If the system has a positive answer when the window is centered on a character, the recognition network can be used for segmentation-recognition. One can use a special output to enforce this property [32], or a process to accumulate the answers through the field [16, 33]. Another method is to have some mechanism to ensure that the recognition module correctly rejects non-characters, i.e. outliers.

We have designed such an architecture (fig. 12): it first has a MLP encoder with local connections in the first layer [20]; a RBF network, with 20 references per class, is then trained on the hidden layer of the MLP. This MMA has been cooperatively trained on digits from the NIST database [21] *hsf_0*. It has about 25 000 connections, as compared to *LeNet* [28] which has around 100 000. Cooperative training was performed as described in section 2.2. Performances are shown in figure 13 [20]: the MMA has performances slightly less than the TDNN LeNet. However, its rejection abilities are better, as can be seen on rejection rates of data bases Zarbi, which is a set of letters from *hsf_0*, and Random, a set of random white noise patterns. This rejection ability is linked with the locality information provided by the RBFs [10].

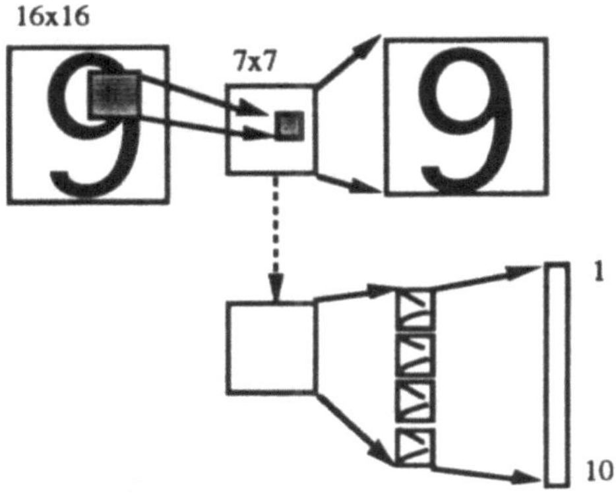

Figure 12: Architecture for Optical Character Recognition

Data Base	*hsf0_eval*		*hsf0_test*		*Zarbi*	*Random*
Architecture	reject	error	reject	error	reject	reject
Le Net	0 0.8	1.4 1	0 0.8	1.4 1	0 27	0 12
MMA	0 1.8	1.9 1	0 1.8	2.0 1.2	0 48	0 59

Figure 13: Perfomances of MLP+RBF compared to LeNet.

When the two networks are fed with inputs coming from a sliding window on a digit field, the error of the system is given by:

$$e = p\,(1-r_g)\,e_g + (1-p)\,(1-r_b) \qquad (11)$$

where p is the percentage of the window positions which are centered onto a digit, r_g (resp. r_b) is the rejection rate of digits (resp. non digits) and e_g is the digit recognition error [20].

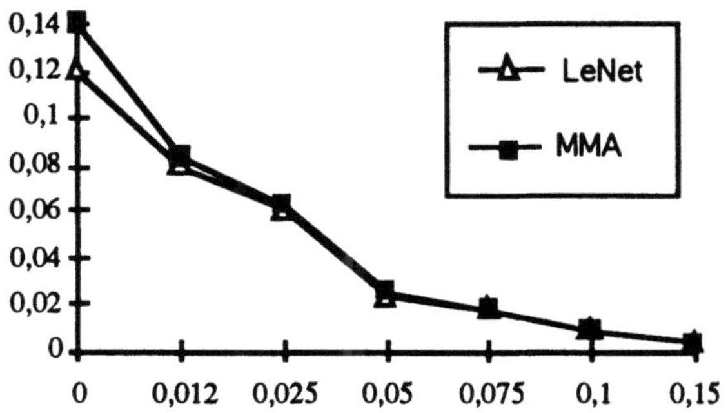

Figure 14: non detection as a function of error rate for MMA (MLP+RBF) compared to LeNet, on a database with p=90 % of digits.

Figure 14 shows the non detection rate (rate of digits rejected by the system) as a function of the global error rate e, for a percentage p=.9 of "good" patterns presented to the system. Clearly, at admissible rejection rates, the two systems have equivalent performances: however, the MMA is 8 times faster (because it has about 10 times less connections). When the rate p is even lower, which would happen if the system were fed with a rather inefficient segmenter, the curves for LeNet and our MMA are indistinguishable.
A similar type of architecture, with a MLP followed by a RBF, cooperatively trained, has been used in an application in High Energy Physics, and allowed an increase of performances of about 2 % with respect to previous single-module architectures [36].

7 Speech Recognition

It is probably in speech processing that the necessity to use multi modular hybrid systems was first acknowledged: propositions have been made to have systems composed of separately trained TDNNs "glued" together [42], a MLP followed by a Dynamic Time Warping module [13] or a TDNN followed by a DTW, cooperatively trained [17]. More recently, HMM models have been integrated with Neural Networks [1, 12].

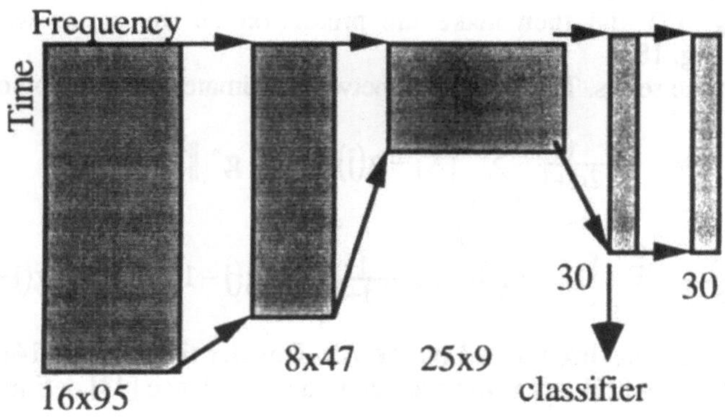

Figure 15: TDNN for feature extraction, followed by classifier.

In the ESPRIT project PYGMALION, a speech database was recorded in an office environment: 30 words (from a word processor command vocabulary) were pronounced 10 times by 10 different speakers. Various techniques were evaluated [17], when used on the speech signal either straight after coding (bark-scale coefficients) either after feature extraction by a TDNN (fig. 15). Results are shown in figure 16. The best performances are obtained when a Dynamic Programming (DP) algorithm is used on the signal coded in the last hidden layer of the TDNN. A TDNN cannot code for the dynamic structure of speech, which is here achieved by the DP algorithm.

Architecture	DP	MLP	TDNN	F-TDNN	RNN	LVQ
SMA	86.7	-	96.5	97	96	83
MMA	98.8	96.5	-	-	96.5	97.75

Figure 16: performances of various classifiers for isolated word recognition (SMA is the Single Module Architecture, where the classifier is trained on the speech signal, MMA is a Multi Modular Architecture: a TDNN is first trained to perform feature extraction, a classifier is then used on the speech signal as coded in the last hidden layer of the TDNN). F-TDNN has filters in frequency and time, RNN is a recurrent network.

8 Time series prediction

A simple, fully connected NN, with no hidden layer implements an AR model. To obtain improved performances, various pre-processings have to be incorporated: e.g. removal of the seasonality, estimation of the trend... These pre-processings can be done "by hand" or can be obtained from a NN module. A multi-modular architecture has been developped [24] to automatically estimate the trend in a first module (fig. 17) and then make the prediction on the series with the trend substracted (fig. 18).

Let X_t be a time series. The smoothing network estimates the trend by minimizing:

$$E\lambda = \frac{1}{2d+1}\sum_{j=-d}^{d}\left[X_j - g(j)\right]^2 + \lambda \| g'' \|^2 \qquad (12)$$

$$\approx \frac{1}{2d+1}\sum_{j=-d}^{d}\left[X_j - g(j)\right]^2 + \lambda \frac{1}{2d+1}\sum_{j=-d}^{d}\left[g(j-1) - 2g(j) + g(j+1)\right]^2$$

This architecture has been tested on the Air-Traveler time series [14]. Results are shown in figure 19 [25]. arv is the average relative variance [43] defined as:

$$arv(S) = \frac{\sum_{t\in S}\left(X_t - \hat{X}_t\right)^2}{\sum_{t\in S}\left(X_t - m_X\right)^2} \qquad (13)$$

where $\hat{X}_t$ is the prediction and m_X is the estimated average of X on set S.

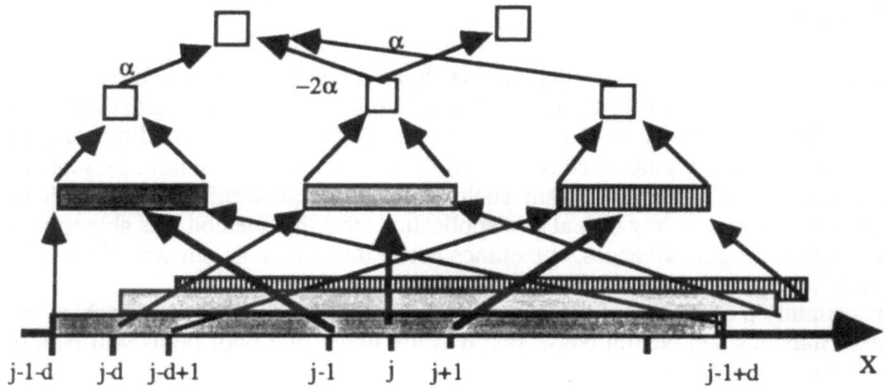

Figure 17: smoothing network

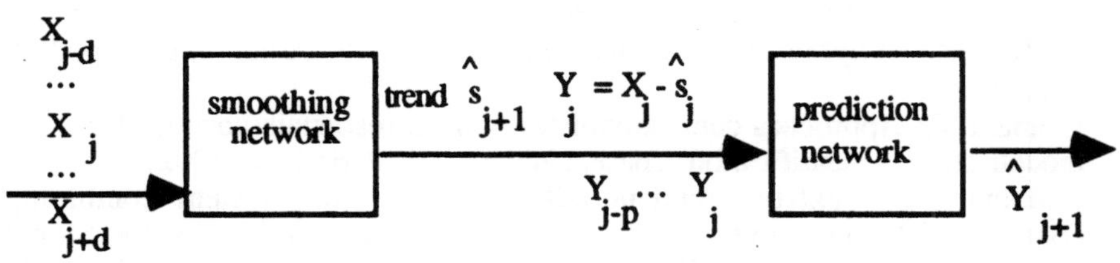

Figure 18: multi-modular architecture for time-series prediction

method	ARIMA	MLP on pre-processed data				MMA
perfor-mances		*log* X_t	∇ *log* X_t	$\nabla_{12}\nabla$ *log* X_t	- trend	
learning	0.0064	0.015 ±0.0012	0.0068 ±0.00068	0.0052 ±0.00083	0.0040 ±0.00065	0.0048 ±0.00041
test	0.0066	0.017 ±0.0017	0.0071 ±0.00063	0.0054 ±0.00060	0.0051 ±0.00061	0.0049 ±0.00047

Figure 19: performances of various techniques for the prediction of the air-traveler time series.

These results clearly show that using simple NNs can sometimes lead to performances much worse than conventional techniques (see for example here the performances of the ARIMA model). However, including pre-processings performed in conventional way can help (MLP on pre-processed data). The Multi-Modular approach (MMA) again does better than any other method, and a lot better than conventional techniques.

9 Conclusions

We have shown in this paper that simple, fully connected, "unstructured" Neural Networks were not any better (if not worse!) than main stream Statistical techniques. The main advantage of NNs comes from the possibility of building complex architectures, from various modules, carefully interconnected. We have presented a framework which allows to train such Multi Modular architectures and have demonstrated on a variety of real size applications that this method was able to produce high level performances, sometimes better than main stream statistical techniques.
It is certainly a challenge of the next years to better elucidate the relationships between Statistics and Neural Networks; it is my belief that both fields will benefit from closer interactions.

References

1. Bengio Y., De Mori R.: Global optimization of a neural network-Hidden Markov Model hybrid. IEEE Trans. on Neural Networks, vol. 3, n° 2, pp252-259, (1992).
2. Bennani Y.: Approches connexionnistes pour la reconnaissance du locuteur: modélisation et identification. Thèse, Université de Paris-Sud, (1992).
3. Bennani Y.: Text-Independent talker identification system combining connectionist and conventional models. In Neural Networks for Signal Processing, II, Proc. of IEEE-SP'92 workshop, S.Y. Kung, F. Fallside, J.A. Sorenson, C.A. Kamm eds, IEEE pub., 131-138, (1992).
4. Bollivier de M., Gallinari P., Thiria S.: Cooperation of neural nets for robust classification. IJCNN 90, San Diego, vol. I, 113-120, (1990).
5. Bollivier de M., Gallinari P., Thiria S. : Neural nets and task decomposition. ICANN'91, Artificial Neural Networks, T. Kohonen, K. Mäkisara, O. Simula, J. Kangas eds, North Holland, vol. II, 1655-1658, (1991).
6. Bollivier de M., Gallinari P., Thiria S.: Cooperation of neural nets and task decomposition. IJCNN'91, Seattle, vol. II, 573-576, (1991).
7. Bollivier de M.: Incorporation de la modularité dans les réseaux connexionnistes par décomposition de tâche. Thèse Université de Paris Sud, (1992).
8. Bottou L.Y., Gallinari P. : A formalism for neural net algorithms. Neuro-Nîmes'91, EC2 ed., 655-669, (1991).
9. Bottou L.Y., Gallinari P. : A framework for the cooperation of learning algorithms. In "Neural Information Processing Systems", NIPS'90, R.P. Lippmann, J.E. Moody, D. S. Touretzky eds., Morgan Kaufmann, vol. 3, 781-788, (1991).
10. Bottou L., Vapnik V.: Local learning algorithms. Neural Computation, vol. 4, 888-900, (1992).
11. Bouattour H., Fogelman Soulie F., Viennet E.: Solving the human face recognition task using neural nets. In Artificial Neural Networks, I. Aleksander, J. Taylor eds, vol. 2, Elsevier; ICANN'92, Brighton. 1595-1598, (1992).

12. Bourlard H., Morgan, N.: A continuous speech recognition system embedding MLP into HMM. NIPS'89, D. Touretsky ed., Morgan Kaufman, vol.2, 186-193 , (1990).
13. Bourlard H., Wellekens C.J.: Multilayer perceptrons and automatic speech recognition. In IEEE 1st ICNN, San Diego, M. Caudill, C. Butler eds, IEEE catalog n° 87TH0191-7, vol. IV, 407-416, (1987).
14. Box G.E.P., Jenkins G.M.: Time series analysis, forecasting and control. Holden-Day, (1970).
15. Breiman L., Friedman J., Olshen R., Stone C.: Classification and regression trees. Wadsworth Int. Group. (1984).
16. Burges C.J.C., Matan O., Le Cun Y., Denker J.S., Jackel L.D;, Stenard C.E., Nohl C.R., Ben J.I.: Shortest path segmentation: a method for training a neural network to recognize character strings. IJCNN'92, Baltimore, vol. III, 165-172,0, (1992).
17. Driancourt X., Bottou L. Y., Gallinari P.: Learning Vector Quantization, Multi-layer perceptron and dynamic programming: comparison and cooperation. IJCNN'91, Seattle, vol. II, 815-819, (1991)
18. Feauveau J.C.: Analyse multi-résolution pour les images avec un facteur de résolution $\sqrt{2}$. Traitement du Signal. vol.7, n°2, 117-128. (1990).
19. Finnoff W., Hergert F., Zimmermann H.G.: Improving model selection by nonconvergent methods. Neural Networks, vol. 6, n° 6, 771-783, (1993).
20. Fogelman Soulie F., Lamy B., Viennet E.: Multi-modular neural network architectures for pattern recognition: applications in optical character recognition and human face recognition. Int. Jl Pattern Recognition and Artificial Intelligence, special issue on Advances in Pattern recognition using neural network technologies; I. Guyon, P. Wang eds, vol. 7, n° 4, (1993). (also published as a book, with same title, World Scientific Pub.)
21. Garris M.D., Wilkinson R.A.: NIST Special Database 3: handwritten segmented characters. NIST document, (1992). The NIST database can be obtained by writing at: NIST, 221/A323 Gaithersburg, MD 20899, USA.
22. Geman S., Biennenstock E., Doursat R.: Neural Networks and the Bias/Variance dilemma. Neural Computation, vol. 4, 1-58, (1992).
23. Jordan M.I., Jacobs R.A.: Hierarchical mixtures of experts and the EM algorithm. MIT Tech. Report 9301, (1993).
24. Kouam A., Thiria S., Badran F., Gallinari P.: Modélisation et prévision des séries temporelles univariées par réseaux connexionnistes. 1er Colloque Africain sur la recherche en Informatique, Yaoundé, 14-20 octobre 1992, INRIA, vol. 2, 591-603, (1992).
25. Kouam A.: Approches connexionnistes pour la prévision des séries temporelles. Thèse, Université de Paris-Sud, (1993).
26. Lang K.J., Waibel A.H., Hinton G.E. : A time delay neural network architecture for isolated word recognition. Neural Networks, vol. 3, n° 1, 23-44, (1990).
27. Le Cun Y.: Generalization and network design strategies. In "Connectionism in Perspective", R. Pfeifer, Z. Schreter, F. Fogelman Soulié, L. Steels eds, Elsevier, 143-155, (1989).

28. Le Cun Y., Boser B., Denker J.S., Henderson D., Howard R.E., Hubbard W., Jackel L.D.: Handwritten digit recognition with a backpropagation network. In "Neural Information Processing Systems", NIPS'89, D. Touretzky ed., Morgan Kaufmann, vol. 2, 396-404, (1990).
29. Loncelle J., Derycke N., Fogelman Soulie F.: Optical character recognition and cooperating neural networks techniques. In Artificial Neural Networks, I. Aleksander, J. Taylor eds, vol. 2, Elsevier; 1591-1594, (1992).
30. McKay D.J.C.: Bayesian interpolation. Neural Computation, vol. 4, 415-447, (1992).
31. McKay D.J.C.: Bayesian non-linear modeling for the energy prediction competition. Tech. Rep., University of Cambridge, (1993).
32. Martin G.L.: Centered-object integrated segmentation and recognition of overlapping handprinted characters. Neural Computation, vol. 5, n° 3, 419-429, (1993).
33. Matan O., Burges C.J.C., Le Cun Y., Denker J.S.: Multi-digit recognition using a space displacement neural network. In "Neural Information Processing Systems", NIPS'91, J.E. Moody, S.J. Hanson, R.P. Lippmann eds., Morgan Kaufmann, vol. 4, 488-495, (1992).
34. Mezard M., Nadal J.P. : Learning in feed-forward layered networks: the tiling algorithm. J. Phys. A: Math. Gene., vol. 22, 2191-2203, (1989).
35. Nowlan S.J., Hinton G.E.: Simplifying neural networks by soft weight-sharing. Neural Computation, vol. 4, 473-493, (1992).
36. Proriol J.: MLP-RBF: a cooperative multi-modular neural network. ICANN'93, S. Gielen, B. Kappen eds, Springer Verlag, 894-897, (1993).
37. Thodberg H.H.: Ace of Bayes; application of neural networks with pruning. Tech. Rep. n°1132E, Danish Meat Res. Inst., (1993).
38. Vapnik V.N.: Estimation of dependences based on empirical data. Springer Verlag, (1982).
39. Vapnik V.N.: Principles of risk minimization for learning theory. In "Neural Information Processing Systems", NIPS'91, J.E. Moody, S.J. Hanson, R.P. Lippmann eds., Morgan Kaufmann, vol. 4, 831-838, (1992).
40. Viennet E., Fogelman Soulie F.: Scene segmentation using Multiresolution analysis and MLP. In Artificial Neural Networks, I. Aleksander, J. Taylor eds, vol. 2, Elsevier; 1599-1602, (1992).
41. Viennet E.:Architectures Connexionnistes Multi-Modulaires: Application à l'Analyse de Scènes. Thèse Université de Paris Sud, (1993).
42. Waibel A.: Modular construction of time-delay neural networks for speech recognition. Neural Computation, vol.1, 39-46. (1989).
43. Weigend A.S., Rumelhart D.E., Huberman B.A.: Generalization by weight elimination with application to forecasting. In "Neural Information Processing Systems", NIPS'90, R.P. Lippmann, J.E. Moody, D. S. Touretzky eds., Morgan Kaufmann, vol. 3, 875-882, (1991).

Cooperative Decision Making Processes and Their Neural Net Implementation

J. Kittler
Department of Electronic and Electrical Engineering
University of Surrey
Guildford GU2 5XH, United Kingdom

1 Introduction

One of the most important functionalities of human perception is the ability to recognise patterns. Not surprisingly, over the last four decades, a considerable effort has been invested in attempts to emulate this functionality in a machine perception system. Recently, much of this activity has been motivated by developments in the field of artificial neural networks (ANN). Good overviews of these algorithms are available in [1], [2], [4] and [6]. One important characteristic of neural network classifiers is that network outputs provide estimates of aposteriori class probabilitities [11] required in a Baysian minimum error classifier [3]. Indeed, if we view neural networks as a universal methodology for function approximation, then in the case of pattern classification problems the functions to be approximated during training are the aposteriori class probabilities.

The function approximation view point has recently thrown light on empirical behaviour of neural networks [5], [7], [8], [9]. The findings have particularly dramatic implications on large scale problems (inputs of high dimensionality). Such problems notably arise in image and vision processing but even more modest applications raise the question of practicability of gaining an effective control over the approximation and estimation errors. The pragmatist's answer to these issues is to resort to heuristics in arbitrarily breaking the classification problem into a multistage process with simple architectures servicing each stage. Such an approach is likely to compromise the optimality of the performance. In any case it does not avoid the requirement for interminable training efforts to reach a reasonable solution and for a multitude of architectural alternatives to be considered in order to gain confidence in the network being able to extract all the relevant information.

These drawbacks are conspicuous in contrast with the functional characteristics of the human nervous system which can learn a pattern from one or a small number of training samples. The learnt model is refined gradually only to cope with pattern class overlaps and ambiguity. The relative importance of stimuli in class definition is rapidly established and presumably reflected in the synaptic strengths.

In parallel with the developments of artificial neural network methodology for pattern classification, the field of statistical pattern recognition witnessed dramatic developments in particular in the area of contextual classification methods. The conventional techniques base the decision about class membership of an object simply on the information contained in the measurements. However, objects by definition do not exist in isolation. Thus the distinguishing feature of object labelling problems in machine perception is that we deal with a large network of objects which interact with each other. The a priori world knowledge or context can be used to help to disambiguate decisions based simply on noisy features of individual objects. For instance in text recognition individual characters are an integral part of larger objects such as words or sentences formed by character groups. Word dictionary and rules of grammar dictate which combinations of characters and implicitly which individual characters are possible. In contextual labelling we effectively associate with each object a decision making process which attempts to combine evidence from observations made on the object together with the contextual information conveyed by the other objects in the network to deduce which label assignment is most appropriate from the point of view of the available measurement information, local constraints and global labelling consistency. A labelling solution is obtained by means of cooperation between these decision making processes.

This the idea of contextual decision making is to formulate the classification problem as one of maximizing the aposteriori probability of labelling of pattern primitives representing single objects given all the observational evidence. One of two basic formulations of the problem can be adopted. In *object centered* labelling [27] the focus is on interpreting a single object at a time. The *message centered* labelling [30] aims to find a joint labelling of pattern primitives. The novel idea of representing complex patterns in terms of primitives has two important implications. First of all it helps to identify the relevant relations between primitives and consequently allow to specify measurements characterising these relations. Making the relational measurements explicit in the formulation is a crucial step in the cooperative decision making approach. It is equivalent to retaining the spatial or temporal structure of stimuli preserved by the human nervous system. This structure is invariably lost by conventional schemes for representing stimuli in artificial neural networks and it then has to be later recovered by means of tedious and unnecessarily complex function approximation procedures.

The second advantage stems from the considerable simplification of the statistical description of the measurement process the use of pattern primitives is expected to afford. The nature of the measurement (stimuli) distribution conditioned on pattern primitives is relatively simple in comparison with unconditional distributions.

Most importantly, the pattern classification processes developed in the paper will be shown to map on conventional artificial neural network architectures. The implication of the relationship appears to be far reaching. We believe that it can offer an analytical route to designing neural networks as far as the number of nodes and layers, node interconnection, the choice of nonlinearity for the activation function and feedback mechanisms are concerned.

Starting from the classification problem formulation, the aposterior probability functions of pattern primitive labelling will be first developed by means of the probability calculus. Thus in contrast to conventional ANN design approaches these aposteriori probability functions will not be approximated directly. Instead, these functions will be expressed in terms of simple components that will define and map on a neural net architecture. In our earlier work it has been shown that specific formulations of the classification problem yield a Hopfield net [42]. In this paper we demonstrate that other formulations lead to a multilayer perceptron-like structure.

The paper is organised as follows. First, two basic formulations of the problem of labelling networks of objects are introduced in Section 2. In Section 3 the recent literature addressing cooperative decsion making processes is reviewed. The various contextual decision making schemes that can be developed from the *object centered* formulation are overviewed in Section 4. Their *message centered* counterparts are presented in Section 5. In Section 6 we outline how object centered labelling schemes map on a multilayer perceptron-like architecture. Finally, Section 7 concludes with a summary of the paper.

2 Problem Formulation

Let us consider a set of measurement vectors $\mathbf{x}_j$, representing respectively objects $a_j, j = 1, ..., N$ arranged in a network with a particular neighbourhood system. Each component of vector $\mathbf{x}_j$ denotes one of three types of measurements:

1. Binary relation measurements A^k_{ji}, $k = 1, 2, ..., m$ between the jth and i^{th} objects.

2. Unary relation measurements y^l_j, $l = 1, 2, ..., r$ from which the binary relations are derived.

3. Unary relation measurements v^i_j, $i = 1, 2, ..., n$ which augment the observational evidence about node j but do not serve as a basis for deriving binary relation measurements A^k_{ji}.

Let us arrange these measurements into vectors as follows:

$$\mathbf{A}_j = \begin{bmatrix} \mathcal{A}_{j1} \\ . \\ . \\ \mathcal{A}_{j(j-1)} \\ \mathcal{A}_{j(j+1)} \\ . \\ . \\ \mathcal{A}_{jN} \end{bmatrix} \tag{1}$$

where

$$\mathcal{A}_{ji} = [A_{ji}^1, ..., A_{ji}^m]^T. \tag{2}$$

For the unary relations we have

$$\mathbf{y}_j = [y_j^1, ..., y_j^r]^T \tag{3}$$

and

$$\mathbf{v}_j = [v_j^1, ..., v_j^n]^T \tag{4}$$

Thus $\mathbf{x}_j$ is an $[m(N-1)+r+n]$ dimensional vector which can be written as

$$\mathbf{x}_j = \begin{bmatrix} \mathbf{v}_j \\ \mathbf{y}_j \\ \mathbf{A}_j \end{bmatrix} \tag{5}$$

We wish to assign each object a_j a label θ_j. Following the conventional Bayesian approach object a_i would be assigned to class ω_r based on the information conveyed by measurement vectors $\mathbf{v}_i$ and $\mathbf{y}_i$ according to the minimum error decision rule [11]. In contrast here we wish to decide about label θ_i using not only the information contained in unary relation measurements relating to object a_i but also any context conveyed by the network. In other words we wish to utilise also the binary relation measurements, i.e. the full measurement vector $\mathbf{x}_i$ plus all the information about the other objects in the network contained in $\mathbf{x}_j$, $\forall j \neq i$. This is a general statement of the problem but in order to develop contextual labelling schemes our formulation will have to be somewhat more precise.

The first important issue to settle is whether we wish to aim at *object centered* or *message centered* interpretation. In object centered interpretation the emphasis is on one node at a time. Contextual information is used to reduce the ambiguity of labelling a single object. Note that object centered interpretation does not guarantee that the global interpretation makes sense. For example, individually most likely object categories in a character recognition problem will not necessarily combine into valid words. The use of context merely reduces the chance of the global labelling being inconsistent.

In contrast, message centered interpretation is concerned with getting the message conveyed by sensory data right. In our text recognition problem the main objective of message centered labelling would be to label characters so that each line of text gives a sequence of valid words.

The choice between object centered and message centered interpretation will depend in the first instance on the application in hand. For example, if we search for a specified object in an image without requiring to understand the entire content of the image, object centered interpretation might be most appropriate. On the other hand, if global understanding of sensory data is at stake, the labelling task should be posed as a message centered interpretation problem.

Generally speaking, in message centered interpretation we search for a joint labelling $\theta_1 = \omega_{\theta_1}, \theta_2 = \omega_{\theta_2}, ..., \theta_N = \omega_{\theta_N}$ which explains observations $\mathbf{x}_1, \mathbf{x}_2, ..., \mathbf{x}_N$ made on the objects in the network. The most appropriate measure of fit between data and interpretation (but by no means the only one) is the aposteriori probability $P(\theta_1 = \omega_{\theta_1}, ..., \theta_N = \omega_{\theta_N}|\mathbf{x}_1, ..., \mathbf{x}_N)$. For the sake of brevity we shall denote this probability function as $P(\theta_1, ..., \theta_N| \mathbf{x}_1, \mathbf{x}_2, ..., \mathbf{x}_N)$ whenever this short hand notation does not compromise the clarity of exposition. The Bayesian approach of maximizing aposteriori probability (MAP) of joint labelling which is referred to in the literature as MAP estimation amounts to the following decision rule:

$$\begin{aligned} &assign \qquad \theta_1 \rightarrow \omega_{\theta_1}, ..., \theta_N \rightarrow \omega_{\theta_N} \qquad if \\ &P(\theta_1 = \omega_{\theta_1}, ..., \theta_N = \omega_{\theta_N}|\mathbf{x}_1, ..., \mathbf{x}_N) = \\ &\qquad = max_{\Omega_1,..,\Omega_N} P(\theta_1, ..., \theta_N|\mathbf{x}_1, ..., \mathbf{x}_N) \end{aligned} \tag{6}$$

where Ω_i is the set of labels admitted by object a_i. For simplicity we shall assume that

$$\Omega_i = \{\omega_0, \omega_1, \ldots, \omega_M\} = \Omega \qquad \forall i$$

where ω_0 is the null label used to label objects for which no other label is appropriate.

The object centered counterpart computes instead the probability $P(\theta_i = \omega_{\theta_i}|\mathbf{x}_1, \mathbf{x}_2, ..., \mathbf{x}_N)$, the aposteriori probability of label θ_i given all the observations. The main difference between message and object centered interpretation can be brought out by expressing both probabilities using the Bayes formula. Starting with the aposteriori probability of joint labelling

$$P(\theta_1, ..., \theta_N|\mathbf{x}_1, \mathbf{x}_2, ..., \mathbf{x}_N) = \frac{p(\mathbf{x}_1, ..., \mathbf{x}_N|\theta_1, ..., \theta_N)P(\theta_1, ..., \theta_N)}{p(\mathbf{x}_1, ..., \mathbf{x}_N)} \tag{7}$$

we note that for given observations the joint probability density function value in the denominator is fixed and therefore the left hand side is proportional to the product in the numerator. The first term of the product, the conditional joint probability density function of measurement vectors $\mathbf{x}_1, ..., \mathbf{x}_N$ models the measurement process whereas the second term embodies our a priori knowledge of the likelihood of various combinations of labels occurring. It is our global, world model.

For the object centered labelling we can write

$$P(\theta_i = \omega|\mathbf{x}_1, ...,\mathbf{x}_N) = \frac{p(\mathbf{x}_1, ...,\mathbf{x}_N|\theta_i = \omega)\hat{p}\,(\theta_j = \omega)}{p(\mathbf{x}_1, ...,\mathbf{x}_N)} \tag{8}$$

where $\hat{p}\,(\theta_j = \omega)$ is the a priori probability of label θ_i taking value ω. Again the denominator in (8) can be dismissed. Expanding the first term of the numerator over all possible labellings in the usual fashion, i.e.

$$\begin{aligned} p(\mathbf{x}_1, ...,\mathbf{x}_N|\theta_i = \omega) &= \sum_{\Omega_1} .. \sum_{\Omega_j} .. \sum_{\Omega_N} p(\mathbf{x}_1, ...,\mathbf{x}_N, \theta_1, ..\theta_j .., \theta_N|\theta_i = \omega) \\ &= \sum_{\Omega_1} ... \sum_{\Omega_N} p(\mathbf{x}_1, ...,\mathbf{x}_N|\theta_1, ..\theta_i = \omega .., \theta_N) P(\theta_1, ..\theta_j .., \theta_N|\theta_i = \omega) \end{aligned} \tag{9}$$

we find

$$\begin{aligned} &P(\theta_i = \omega|\mathbf{x}_1, ...,\mathbf{x}_N) = \\ &= \frac{\sum_{\Omega_1} \cdots \sum_{\Omega_N} p(\mathbf{x}_1, ...,\mathbf{x}_N|\theta_1, ..\theta_i = \omega .., \theta_N) P(\theta_1, ..\theta_i = \omega .., \theta_N)}{p(\mathbf{x}_1, ...,\mathbf{x}_N)} \end{aligned} \tag{10}$$

Thus computing the probability of a particular label ω on a single object a_i amounts to scanning through all the possible combinations of labels $\theta_1, ...,\theta_N$ with label θ_i set to ω and summing up the corresponding products of the respective joint measurement and label probabilities.

The inspection of the expressions for $P(\theta_1, ...,\theta_N|\mathbf{x}_1, \mathbf{x}_2, ...,\mathbf{x}_N)$ and $P(\theta_i = \omega|\mathbf{x}_1, ...,\mathbf{x}_N)$ in (7) and (11) respectively reveals that they are both defined in terms of the same ingredients, namely the a priori probability distribution of joint labelling, $P(\theta_1, ...,\theta_N)$ and the conditional probability density function $p(\mathbf{x}_1, ...,\mathbf{x}_N|\theta_1, ...,\theta_N)$. It is apparent that for any practical value of N and M it will not be feasible to apply techniques of statistical inference to estimate these probability distributions.

It is evident that to obtain workable models some assumptions will have to be introduced which will allow us not only to specify these global probability distributions functions but also to use them for solving practical problems. An important role in this respect is the assumption of Markov property which permits characterization of global dependence in terms of local interactions. More specifically, let without any loss of generality, $\xi_i, i = 1, ..., N$ be a discrete random variable associated with the i-th node of a network of objects with neighbourhood system $I_i, i = 1, ..., N$. The Markov property states that

$$p(\xi_i|\xi_j, \forall j \neq i) = p(\xi_i|\xi_j, \forall j \in I_i^*)$$

where I_i^* denotes the index set of the immediate neighbours to ξ_i, i.e. set I_i with the ith node removed. In other words, the conditional probability of a particular outcome or state of variable ξ_i given all the other observations $\xi_j, \forall j \neq i$ is completely determined by the values of ξ_i's neighbours. This assumption facilitates the maximization of (2) by means of local updates of the object labels.

Alternatively, one may employ a dictionary of label configurations. The approach exploits the fact that the number of permissible label configurations on a network of objects is usually very small in comparison with the number of all combinatorial labellings. If the size of the dictionary is reasonable, an exhaustive scan through all its items becomes feasible.

Finally, an important and physically realistic assumption regarding the unary measurement process distribution is that the outcomes of measurements are conditionally independent.

$$p(\mathbf{v}_1, \mathbf{y}_1 ...., \mathbf{v}_N, \mathbf{y}_N | \theta_1, ..\theta_i, .., \theta_N) = \Pi_{i=1}^{N} p(\mathbf{v}_i, \mathbf{y}_i | \theta_i = \omega_{\theta_i}) \quad (11)$$

For binary relations, on the other hand, we assume that

$$p(\mathcal{A}_{i1}, ..., \mathcal{A}_{iN} | \theta_1, ..\theta_i, .., \theta_N) = \prod_{j \neq i} p(\mathcal{A}_{ij} | \theta_i, \theta_j) \quad (12)$$

All the contextual classification methods that have been developed commence from one of the above formulations and a choice of model for the prior world knowledge and the measurement process. They are briefly reviewed in the following section.

3 Literature Review

In the message centered interpretation category, the deterministic methods exploiting the Markov random field models include the iterative conditional modes technique (ICM) of Besag [12], Blake [17], Blake and Zisserman [18], Koch, Marroquin and Yuille [19], and Witkin, Terzopoulos and Kass [20]. Their stochastic optimization counterpart is represented by the method developed by Geman and Geman [13] which is based on the simulated annealing technique [15]. More recent are the attempts to use the mean field theory [14] to simplify and speed up the discrete optimization process.

The message centered approach combined with the dictionary representation of the prior world knowledge leads to the classical discrete relaxation algorithm of Waltz [29]. However, the seminal qualities of Waltz's algorithm were not matched by practical utility because of its computational complexity (effectively requiring an exhaustive search in a combinatorial optimization space). A computationally feasible technique of discrete relaxation has been developed by Hancock and Kittler [30] which introduces the idea of a label error process to cope with the two fundamental problems of the original algorithm [29]: i) inadmissible label configurations introduced by initial object labelling and ii) the optimization process deadlock, which was the consequence of the (binary) labelling performance criterion used by Waltz.

For the object centered formulation linked with the Markovian assumption, only Markov models of special type can be employed to develop effective contextual classification techniques. Haslett [31] resorted to the Pickard random field model and Devijver [32] succeeded in developing a recursive compound decision scheme for images that can be modelled by a Markov mesh process.

Finally, the object centered formulation combined with the dictionary model of the world knowledge are the germ of a family of algorithms known as probabilistic relaxation. The method was conceived by Rosenfeld, Hummel and Zucker [21] in 1976 and since its publication it has attracted sustained interest. The effectiveness of the approach has been demonstrated on numerous applications including line and edge detection [33], [34]. For a comprehensive list of applications the reader is referred to the review article of Kittler and Illingworth [23].

Notwithstanding its practical potential, the early applications of probabilistic relaxation unveiled many theoretical problems, including inherent bias of the updating process which was exhibited in no information experiments, questions relating to convergence, interpretation of the computed probabilities, and the specification of the compatibility coefficients and support functions [41], [36], [37]. A detailed account of the attempts to overcome these problems can be found in [23]. Most of these problems were overcome in two key papers published in the nineteen eighties [24], [25]. In [24] Hummel and Zucker laid down the theoretical foundations of probabilistic relaxation by formally defining the notion of consistency and by showing that under certain assumptions the optimization of a simple functional was synonymous with improving the consistency of object labelling. They also developed a constrained optimization procedure to optimize the functional by extending the work of Faugeras and Berthod [22].

In spite of this progress the relaxation process design methodology remained very heuristic until the publication of the work of Kittler and Hancock [25] which was aimed at providing theoretical underpinning of probabilistic relaxation using the Bayesian framework. It led to the development of an evidence combining formula which fuses observations and a priori contextual information in a theoretically sound manner. The polynomial combinatorial complexity of the approach has been avoided by means of introducing and developing the concept of label configuration dictionary. The methodology has been validated on problems of edge and line postprocessing [26], [38].

The outstanding criticisms of probabilistic relaxation, namely that

1. the process does not utilise measurement information with the exception of the initialisation stage where observations are used to compute the initial, noncontextual probabilities for the candidate labels at each object, and

2. the richest source of contextual observational information contained in object relations (binary relations) has never been tapped,

have been overcome most recently [28], [27]. The approach has been demonstrated to have wide applicability from relaxation problems on a lattice [40] to graph matching problems [39]. An interesting approach has recently been proposed by Haralick who argues for the use of belief functions rather than likelihood functions in contextual decision making [41].

In the remaining part of the paper we shall concentrate the discussion on dictionary based methods. As already indicated the two fundamental formulations of the labelling problem in this case lead to cooperative decision making processes known as probabilistic relaxation and discrete relaxation respectively. In Section 4 we briefly review probabilistic relaxation algorithms. Section 5 is devoted to a summary of discrete relaxation cooperative decision making processes.

4 Probabilistic Relaxation

Under some mild conditional independence assumptions concerning measurements $\mathbf{x}_j$, $\mathbf{y}_j$ and $\mathcal{A}_{ij}$, $\forall j$ the object centered labelling formulation (11) leads to an iterative probability updating formula [27]

$$P^{(n+1)}(\theta_i = \omega_{\theta_i}) = \frac{P^{(n)}(\theta_i = \omega_{\theta_i})\, Q^{(n)}(\theta_i = \omega_{\theta_i})}{\sum_{\omega_\lambda \in \Omega} P^{(n)}(\theta_i = \omega_\lambda)\, Q^{(n)}(\theta_i = \omega_\lambda)} \tag{13}$$

where $P^{(n)}(\theta_i = \omega_{\theta_i})$ denotes the probability of label ω_{θ_i} at object a_i at the nth iteration of the updating process and the quantity $Q^{(n)}(\theta_i = \omega_\alpha)$ expresses the support the label $\theta_i = \omega_\alpha$ receives at the nth iteration step from the other objects in the scene, taking into consideration the binary relations that exist between them and object a_i. After the first iteration (n=1) the computed entity is the contextual aposteriori class probability $P(\theta_i = \omega_{\theta_i} | \mathbf{x}_1, \mathbf{x}_2, \ldots\ldots, \mathbf{x}_N)$. With the increasing value of n the updating scheme drives the probabilistic labelling into a hard labelling.

The support $Q^{(n)}(\theta_i = \omega_{\theta_i})$ is defined as

$$Q^{(n)}(\theta_i = \omega_{\theta_i}) = \tag{14}$$

$$\sum_{\omega_{\theta_j}, j \in N_i} \frac{1}{\hat{p}(\theta_i = \omega_{\theta_i})} \left\{ \prod_{j \in N_i} \frac{P^{(n)}(\theta_j = \omega_{\theta_j})\, p(\mathcal{A}_{ij} | \theta_i = \omega_{\theta_i}, \theta_j = \omega_{\theta_j})}{\hat{p}(\theta_j = \omega_{\theta_j})} \right\} \times$$

$$\times P(\theta_j = \omega_{\theta_j}, \forall j \in N_i)$$

where $p(\mathcal{A}_{ij} | \theta_i = \omega_{\theta_i}, \theta_j = \omega_{\theta_j})$ is the compatibility coefficient quantifying the mutual support of the labelling $(\theta_i = \omega_{\theta_i}, \theta_j = \omega_{\theta_j})$. N_i denotes the index set of all nodes exluding the node i, i.e.

$$N_i = \{1, 2, \ldots i-1, i+1, \ldots, N\} \tag{15}$$

It is worth noting that when binary relations are not used the support function (14) becomes the standard evidence combining formula developed in [25], i.e.

$$Q^{(n)}(\theta_i = \omega_{\theta_i}) = \tag{16}$$

$$\sum_{\omega_{\theta_j}, j \in N_i} \frac{1}{\hat{p}(\theta_i = \omega_{\theta_i})} \left\{ \prod_{j \in N_i} \frac{P^{(n)}(\theta_j = \omega_{\theta_j})}{\hat{p}(\theta_j = \omega_{\theta_j})} \right\} \times P(\theta_j = \omega_{\theta_j}, \forall j \in N_i)$$

On the other hand, when no additional unary relation measurements are available apart from the set used for generating the binary measurements, the support reduces to

$$Q^{(n)}(\theta_i = \omega_{\theta_i}) = \tag{17}$$

$$\sum_{\omega_{\theta_j}, j \in N_i} \frac{1}{\hat{p}(\theta_i = \omega_{\theta_i})} \left\{ \prod_{j \in N_i} p(\mathcal{A}_{ij} | \theta_i = \omega_{\theta_i}, \theta_j = \omega_{\theta_j}) \right\} P(\theta_j = \omega_{\theta_j}, \forall j \in N_i)$$

The probability updating rule (13) in this particular case will act as an inefficient maximum value selection operator. Thus the updating process can be terminated after the first iteration, the maximum contextual aposteriori label probability selected and set to unity while the probability of all the other labels to zero.

The support function (14) exhibits exponential complexity. In practice its use, depending on application, could be limited only to a contextual neighbourhood in the vicinity of the object being interpreted. Such a measure is appropriate for instance in the case of edge and line postprocessing where the objects to be labelled are pixel sites. A small neighbourhood, say a 3 by 3 window may be sufficient to provide the necessary contextual information. In any case by iteratively updating the pixel label probabilities using formula (13) contextual information would be drawn from increasingly larger neighbourhoods of each pixel.

A more dramatic, complementary reduction in the computational complexity is achieved by noting that in practice many potential label configurations in the contextual neighbourhood of an object are physically inadmissible. By listing the admissible labellings in a dictionary, the above support function can be evaluated by summing up only over the entries $\left(\theta_j = \omega_{\theta_j}^k, \forall j \in N_i\right)$, $\forall k$ in the dictionary, i.e.

$$Q^{(n)}(\theta_i = \omega_{\theta_i}) = \tag{18}$$

$$\sum_{k=1}^{Z(\omega_{\theta_i})} \frac{1}{\hat{p}(\theta_i = \omega_{\theta_i})} \left\{ \prod_{j \in N_i} \frac{P^{(n)}\left(\theta_j = \omega_{\theta_j}^k\right) p\left(\mathcal{A}_{ij} | \theta_i = \omega_{\theta_i}, \theta_j = \omega_{\theta_j}^k\right)}{\hat{p}\left(\theta_j = \omega_{\theta_j}^k\right)} \right\} \times$$

$$\times P\left(\theta_j = \omega^k_{\theta_j}, \forall j \in N_i\right)$$

where $Z(\omega_{\theta_i})$ denotes the number of dictionary entries with label θ_i set to ω_{θ_i}.

In many labelling problems neither of the above simplifications of the support function is appropriate. For instance, in correspondence matching tasks or object recognition all features of an object interact directly with each other. Moreover, without measurements, no labelling configuration is a priori more likely than any other. Then it is reasonable to assume that the prior probability of a joint labelling configuration can be expressed as

$$P\left(\theta_j = \omega_{\theta_j}, \forall j \in N_i\right) = \prod_{j \in N_i} \hat{p}\left(\theta_j = \omega_{\theta_j}\right) \tag{19}$$

Substituting (19) into (14) and noting that each factor in the product in the above expression depends on the label of only one other object apart from the object a_i under consideration, we can simplify the support computation as

$$Q^{(n)}(\theta_i = \omega_\alpha) = \prod_{j \in N_i} \sum_{\omega_\beta \in \Omega} P^{(n)}\left(\theta_j = \omega_\beta\right) p\left(\mathcal{A}_{ij} \mid \theta_i = \omega_\alpha, \theta_j = \omega_\beta\right) \tag{20}$$

It is interesting to note that through this simplification the exponential complexity of the problem is eliminated.

The iteration scheme can be initialised by considering as $P^{(0)}(\theta_i = \omega_{\theta_i})$ the probabilities computed by using the unary attributes only, *i.e.*

$$P^{(0)}(\theta_i = \omega_{\theta_i}) = P(\theta_i = \omega_{\theta_i} | \mathbf{v}_i, \mathbf{y}_i) \tag{21}$$

We discuss this initialisation process in detail elsewhere [27].

5 Discrete Relaxation

For message centered labelling we start from the aposteriori probability of joint labelling given all the measurements in (6). The main difference between the previous approach and the current formulation is that each object is assigned one hard label. The problem is to devise a mechanism for switching the labels so that a global maximum of the probability (6) is attained. To develop an iterative scheme for maximizing this probability, the usual approach is to investigate the effect on this function of changing the label on one object in the network at a time. The use of the same assumptions regarding the measurement process, namely (11) and (12) leads to the following expression:

$$\frac{P(\theta_i = \omega, \theta_j,\ \forall j \in N_i | \mathbf{x}_j,\ \forall j)}{P(\theta_i = \lambda, \theta_j,\ \forall j \in N_i | \mathbf{x}_j,\ \forall j)} = \tag{22}$$

$$= \frac{p(\mathbf{v}_i, \mathbf{y}_i | \theta_i = \omega) \left\{ \prod_{j \neq i} p(A_{ij} | \theta_i = \omega, \theta_j = \omega_{\theta_j}) \right\} P(\theta_i = \omega, \theta_j, \ \forall j \in N_i)}{p(\mathbf{v}_i, \mathbf{y}_i | \theta_i = \lambda) \left\{ \prod_{j \neq i} p(A_{ij} | \theta_i = \lambda, \theta_j = \omega_{\theta_j}) \right\} P(\theta_i = \lambda, \theta_j, \ \forall j \in N_i)}$$

The problem with formula (22) is that if most of the nodes are incorrectly labelled the maximization of the aposteriori probability of joint labelling by label switching will lead to a local optimum corresponding to an incorrect labelling. Thus the method is heavily dependent on initial labelling which in the case where binary relations play a crucial role cannot be achieved using unary information alone.

The situation is somewhat different when we know a priori what labelling configurations are physically admissible. This applies, for instance, to many labelling problems on pixel lattices. One can then consider inadmissible labellings as arising from a label corruption process which can be modelled and used for measuring the congruency of current labels with admissible label configurations. Object labels can be then updated so as to maximize their average congruency with dictionary items. The measure of congruency is assumed to be related to the aposteriori probability of joint labelling.

For the scheme to be computationally manageable, the dictionary of admissible labelling configurations should be defined on a relatively small neighbourhood, I_i of each object a_i. Guided by [30], the following label replacement rule can be derived from (22):

$$assign \ \theta_i \ to \ \omega \ if$$

$$p(\mathbf{v}_i, \mathbf{y}_i | \theta_i = \omega) \left\{ \prod_{j \neq i} p(A_{ij} | \theta_i = \omega, \theta_j = \omega_{\theta_j}) \right\} \times$$
$$\times F(\theta_i = \omega | \theta_l, \forall l \in \cup_j I_j, j \in I_i, j \neq i) =$$
$$= \max_{\alpha \in \Omega} p(\mathbf{v}_i, \mathbf{y}_i | \theta_i = \alpha) \left\{ \prod_{j \neq i} p(A_{ij} | \theta_i = \alpha, \theta_j = \omega_{\theta_j}) \right\} \times$$
$$\times F(\theta_i = \alpha | \theta_l, \forall l \in \cup_j I_j, j \in I_i, j \neq i) \quad (23)$$

where

$$F(\theta_i = \alpha | \theta_l, \forall l \in \cup_j I_j, j \in I_i, j \neq i) = \quad (24)$$
$$= b|I_i| \sum_{j=1}^{|I_i|} \sum_{\Lambda_{ij}^{k\alpha}} a^{K(i,j,k)} P(\theta_i = \alpha, \theta_l = \lambda_{\theta_l}^k, \forall l \in I_j^*)$$

In (24) I_j^* is the index set I_j with index j removed and $\Lambda_{ij}^{k\alpha}$ denotes the kth item in the dictionary of admissible labellings for neighbourhood I_j with the label configuration $(\theta_i = \alpha, \theta_l = \lambda_{\theta_l}^k, \forall l \in I_j^*)$. $a = \frac{P_e}{(1-P_e)}$ is defined by the probability P_e of an admissible label being corrupted and $b = P_e^{|I_i|}$. Finally,

$K(i,j,k)$ is a measure of congruency between $\Lambda_{ij}^{k\alpha}$ and the actual labelling $(\theta_l = \hat{\omega}_{\theta_l}, \forall l \in I_j)$ specified as

$$K(i,j,k) = \epsilon(\hat{\omega}_{\theta_i}, \alpha) + \sum_{\forall l \in I_j^*} \epsilon(\hat{\omega}_{\theta_l}, \lambda_{\theta_l}^k)$$

with $\epsilon(r,s) = 0$ if $r = s$ and $\epsilon(r,s) = 1$ if $r \neq s$.

The label replacement rule (23) provides a viable mechanism for iterative improvement in the consistency of labelling objects in a network. It has been applied successfully to the problem of edge labelling in [30]. Note that as a result of label replacement the label error probability P_e decreases. A suitable schedule for reducing its value as a function of iteration number is required. Alternatively this probability can be estimated from the data.

6 Neural Net Implementation

The aim of this section is to demonstrate how the cooperative processes discussed in Section 4 and Section 5 can be mapped on neural net architectures. The purpose of the mapping is at least twofold. First of all, neural net computation has inspired and motivated considerable activity in specialist hardware and software architecture design and implementation. Software, and hardware systems, including VLSI chips, have been developed to implement various families of neural networks. A successful mapping of contextual decision making processes on such systems would facilitate their wide applicability.

The second, and perhaps more significant purpose is to argue that the mapping process could offer a route to neural network design which is not plagued by the typical problems associated with the development of neural network solutions to pattern classification tasks: lack of guidelines for the choice of architecture and node connectivity, lack of data, unacceptably long training phase, and the last but not the least, the lack of criteria for the selection of the node activation functions and for the weight initialization.

Rather than attempting a comprehensive coverage of all the cooperative processes discussed in the paper, we shall illustrate the basic ideas on a specific contextual labelling algorithm. In particular, we shall consider the probabilistic ralaxation scheme in (13) with the support function given in formula (20). The neural network performing the same computation is presented in Figure 1. It is basically a multilayer perceptron with two main layers and an auxilary layer which performs a normalisation computation to maintain the network outputs in the zero - one range and ensuring that the outputs representing label excitation for each object primitive sum up to a unity. There are only N such auxilary units as there are N object primitives to be labelled. The inputs P_{ij} to the multilayer perceptron are computed by a noncontextual artificial neural network which at its input is stimulated by

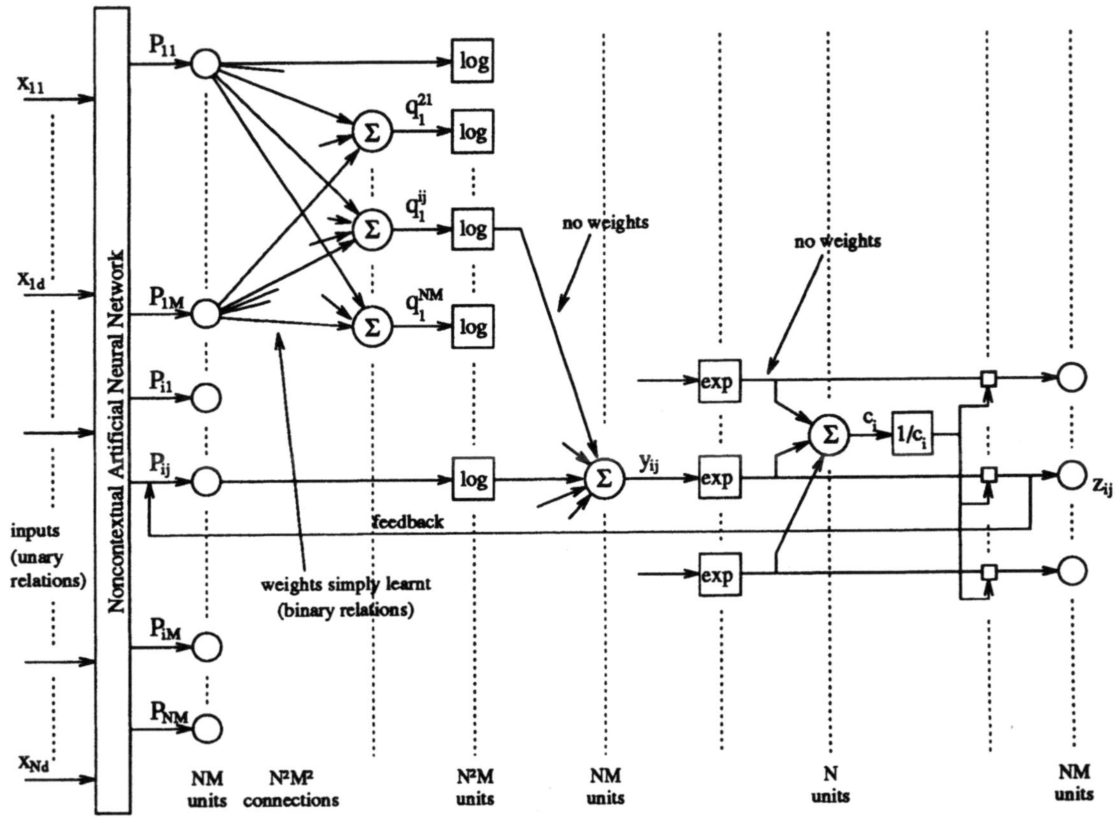

Figure 1: Multilayer Perceptron implementation of the probabilistic relaxation scheme with support function (20)

unary relation measurements observed for each object primitive. We shall not dwell on the the methodology that can be used for designing such a neural network as the number of unary measurements one deals with is normally relatively small and therefore the neural net design problems identified earlier are not applicable. The outputs P_{ij} of this initializing network correspond to the aposteriori (noncontextual) label probabilities for the object primitives based on the unary relations.

The main network has the normal characteristics of a typical multilayer perceptron design. The number of units in the second layer expands wheras for the final layer it contracts. In our design the number of output units is the same as the number of input units to the network with a separate unit for each object primitive/label combination.

The weights applied to the links between the input nodes and the nodes of the second layer are defined by the binary relation probabilities which can be easily estimated during training by techniques of statistical inference rather than weight adaption. The output of each node q_i^{jk} represents the support for label k on object primitive j from object primitive i. Note that the activation function of the units in the second layer is the *log* function and not the usual sigmoid. The connections from the second layer to the third layer have no weights associated with them. The activation function of the units in this third layer is the exponential function.

A distinguishing characteristic of the network is the feedback link from the normalised output to the input. If this link is broken, the output units generate the contextual probabilities of object primitive labelling corresponding to a single iteration of the label updating process in (13). The feedback forces one of the outputs associated with each object primitive to a unity and all the others to a zero.

We have thus demonstrated that a neural network for a complex pattern classification problem can be designed by analysing the nature of the problem first. The analysis makes it possible to incorporate realistic assumptions into the solution of the problem. This in turn often facilitates a dramatic reduction in complexity of the classification problem. Thus instead of having to approximate aposteriori probability functions in high dimensional observation spaces for which a massive architecture of unknown node connectivity would be required, one can express these aposteriori probabilities in terms of functions of simple components. This explicitly specifies the required architecture of the neural network, node connectivity and the functional form of the activation functions. But even more importantly, the training of such a network becomes a simple task of inferring the probability distributions of the relevant measurements in low dimensional spaces. A first guess of these distributions can easily be made from the presentation of very few prototypical patterns to the system. In this sense the training capability of the proposed approach emulates closely that of the human central nervous system which also can learn complex patterns very efficiently from just a few experiences.

7 Conclusions

In the paper cooperative decision making processes for pattern recognition in machine perception have been discussed. Two basic formulations of the problem of labelling networks of pattern primitives were introduced. We then focused on the development of cooperative decision making processes which employ dictionary models for representing the prior world knowledge regarding labelling constraints and configurations. A review of recent results in probabilistic relaxation labelling processes which incorporate observations on relational information concerning the interacting objects was then presented and the discrete equivalent of these cooperative decision making processes was discussed. Finally, it was demonstrated that probabilistic relaxation labelling processes can be mapped onto a neural net architecture, in particular the multilayer perceptron. This has the important implication that cooperative decision making schemes can provide an approach to designing artificial neural networks with the benefit of simple training, and of the ANN architecture and activation functions being uniquely specified. The design approach appears to offer an attractive alternative to the conventional ANN design techniques.

Acknowledgements

This work was supported by the Science and Engineering Research Council, UK (GR/F36316).

References

[1] R P Lippmann, An introduction to computing with neural nets, *IEEE ASSP Magazine*, **4**, 4-22, 1987.

[2] D R Hush and B G Horne, Progress in supervised neural networks, *IEEE Signal Processing Magazine*, **10**, 8-39, 1993.

[3] M D Richard and R P Lippmann, Neural network classifiers estimate Bayesian aposteriori probabilities, *Neural Computing*, **3**, 461-483, 1992.

[4] G A Carpenter and S Grossberg, A self-organizing neural network for supervised learning, recognition and prediction, *IEEE Communications Magazine*, 38-49, 1992.

[5] J E Moody, The effective number of parameters: An analysis of generalization and regularization in nonlinear learning systems, in *Advances in Neural Information Processing Systems 4*, J E Moody, S J Hanson and R P Lippmann, eds., Morgan Kaufmann, San Mateo, CA, 1992.

[6] F Fogelman Soulie, B Lamy and E Viennet, Multi-modular neural network architectures for pattern recognition: Applications in optical character recognition and human face recognition, *Int. Jnl of Pattern Recognition and Artificial Intelligence*, 1993.

[7] J Friedman, Multivariate adaptive regression splines, *Annals of Statistics*, **19**, 1-141, 1991.

[8] H White, K Hornik, M Stinchcombe, Multilayer feedforward networks as universal approximators, in *Artificial Neural Networks*, H White, eds., 13-28, Blackwell, 1992.

[9] A R Barron, Approximation and estimation bounds for artificial neural networks, in *Proc 4th Workshop on Computational Learning Theory*, 243-249, 1992.

[10] P A Devijver and J Kittler, Pattern recognition: A statistical approach, Prentice-Hall, Englewood Cliffs, NJ, 1982.

[11] P A Devijver and J Kittler, Pattern recognition: A statistical approach, Prentice-Hall, Englewood Cliffs, NJ, 1982.

[12] J Besag, On the satatistical analysis of dirty pictures, *Journal Royal Statist. Society*, **48**, Series B, 259-302, 1986.

[13] S Geman and D Geman, Stochastic relaxation, Gibbs distributions and the Bayesian restoration of images, *IEEE Trans. Pattern Analysis and Machine Intelligence*, **PAMI-6**, 721-741, 1984.

[14] D Geiger and F Girosi, Parallel and deterministic algorithms from MRF's: Surface reconstruction, *IEEE Trans. Pattern Analysis and Machine Intelligence*, **PAMI-13**, 181-188, 1991.

[15] S Kirkpatrick, C D Gellatt and M P Vecchi, Optimization by simulated annealing, *Science*, **220**, 671-680, 1983.

[16] B Chou and R Raman, On relaxation algorithms based on Markov random field models,*Technical Report 212*, University of Rochester, Computer Science Dept, 1987.

[17] A Blake, The least disturbance principle and weak constraints, *Pattern Recognition Letters*, **1**, 393-399, 1983.

[18] A Blake and A Zisserman, Visual reconstruction, MIT Press, Cambridge MA, 1987.

[19] C Koch, J Marroquin and A Yuille, Analog neuronal networks in early vision, *Proc Nat. Academic Science*, **83**, 4263-4267, 1986.

[20] A Witkin, D Terzopoulos and M Kass, Signal matching through scale space, *Intern. Journal Computer Vision*, 133-144, 1987.

[21] A Rosenfeld, R Hummel and S Zucker, Scene labeling by relaxation operations, *IEEE Trans System Man and Cybernetics*, **SMC-6**, 420-433, 1976.

[22] O Faugeras and M Berthod, Improving consistency and reducing ambiguity in stochastic labeling, *IEEE Trans. Pattern Analysis and Machine Intelligence*, **PAMI-3**, 412-423, 1981.

[23] J Kittler and J Illingworth, A review of relaxation labelling algorithms, *Image and Vision Computing*, **3**, 206,216, 1985.

[24] R Hummel and S Zucker, On the foundations of relaxation labeling process, *IEEE Trans. Pattern Analysis and Machine Intelligence*, **PAMI-5**, 267-286, 1983.

[25] J Kittler and E R Hancock, Combining evidence in probabilistic relaxation, *Intern. Journal of Pattern Recognition and Artificial Intelligence*, **3**, 29-51, 1989.

[26] E R Hancock and J Kittler, Edge labeling using dictionary-based relaxation, *IEEE Trans. Pattern Analysis and Machine Intelligence*, **PAMI-12**, 165-181, 1990.

[27] J Kittler, W J Christmas and M Petrou, Probabilistic relaxation for matching problems in computer vision, *Proc 4th Intern. Conference on Computer Vision*, 666-673, Berlin, 1993.

[28] J Kittler, P Papachristou and M Petrou, Combining evidence in dictionary based probabilistic relaxation *Proc 8th Scandinavian Conference on Image Analysis*, 785-793, Tromso, 1993.

[29] D L Waltz, Understanding line drawings of scenes with shadows, in *The Psychology of Computer Vision*, P H Winston, ed., McGraw-Hill, New York, 1975.

[30] E R Hancock and J Kittler, Discrete relaxation, *Pattern Recognition*, **23**, 711-733, 1990.

[31] J Haslett, Maximum likelihood discriminant analysis on the plane using a Markovian model of spatial context, *Pattern Recognition*, **18**, 287-296, 1985.

[32] P A Devijver, Probabilistic labelling in a second order Markov mesh, in *Pattern Recognition in Practice, Vol. 2*, E S Gelsema and L Kanal, eds., North Holland, 1986.

[33] S Peleg and A Rosenfeld, Determining compatibility coefficients for curve enhancement relaxation processes, *IEEE Trans Systems, Man and Cybernetics*, **SMC-8**, 548-555, 1978.

[34] S Zucker, R Hummel and A Rosenfeld, An application of relaxation labelling to line and curve enhancement, *IEEE Tranc Computers*, **C-26**, 394-404, 1977.

[35] R M Haralick, An interpretation of probabilistic relaxation, *Computer Vision, Graphics and Image Processing*, **22**, 388-395, 1983.

[36] R L Kirby, A product rule relaxation method, *Computer Graphics and Image Processing*, **13**, 158-189, 1985.

[37] S Peleg, A new probabilistic relaxation scheme, *IEEE Trans. Pattern Analysis and Machine Intelligence*, **PAMI-2**, 362-369, 1980.

[38] E R Hancock and J Kittler, Relaxation refinement of intensity ridges, *Proc 11th Internat. Conference on Pattern Recognition*, 459-463, 1992.

[39] J Kittler, W J Christmas and M Petrou, Probabilistic relaxation for matching of symbolic structures, *Proc Workshop on Syntactic and Structural Pattern Recognition*, H Bunke ed, 471-480, World Scientific, Singapore, 1993.

[40] J Kittler, P Papachristou and M Petrou, Probabilistic relaxation in line postprocessing, *Proc Workshop on Statistical Methods in Pattern Recognition*, 1-2, Tromso, 1993.

[41] R M Haralick, Contextual decision making with degress of belief, *Proc 11th Intern Conf on Pattern Recognition*, 105-111, The Hague, 1992.

[42] E R Hancock and J Kittler, An improved error criterion for neural networks, *Proc 7th Scandinavian Conference on Image Analysis*, 1094-1101, Aalborg, Denmark, 1991.

Associative Memory Networks and Sparse Similarity Preserving Codes

Günther Palm[1], *Friedhelm Schwenker*[1] *and Friedrich T. Sommer*[2]

[1] University of Ulm, Department of Neural Information Processing, 89069 Ulm, Germany
[2] University of Düsseldorf, C. und O. Vogt Institut für Hirnforschung, Moorenstr. 5, 40225 Düsseldorf, Germany

Abstract This paper addresses the following main topics:

- Definition of the associative memory tasks, auto-association and hetero-association.
- Use of neural networks and local learning rules for the realization of associative memory.
- Derivation of the information capacity as an evaluation criterion.
- Comparision and optimization of local learning rules for associative memory.
- Sparse, distributed, similarity preserving data representation.

For auto-association and hetero-association the most plausible implementation of an associative memory by means of a neural network with modifiable connections is presented.

The evaluation of the memory's performance in storing and retrieving information is discussed and the information storage capacity is defined. With respect to this criterion one can optimize the local rules for synaptic modification and the statistical format of the patterns to be stored.

The result is that the patterns should be sparse (i.e. they should contain mostly zeros) and the learning rule should be Hebbian. In the optimal case one can achieve a storage capacity of about 0.7 bit/synapse in hetero-association and 0.35 bit/synapse in auto-association. The second value can not be reached with realistic iterative retrieval procedures, but in practice values of 0.18 bit/synapse can be achieved for auto-association and above 0.6 bit/synapse for hetero-association. We derive some of these results mathematically and present some simulation studies illustrating the asymptotic mathematical calculations.

Finally we present some basic ideas on the construction of sparse, distributed, similarity preserving representation of data.

1 Introduction

From a theoretical point of view, an artifical neural network implements a mapping F between an input space X and an output space Y, so one can distinguish three different kinds of mappings, corresponding to different applications:

- Both, the input and output space are continuous spaces.
- F is a mapping from a continuous set into a finite set, this divides the input space into a finite number of regions.
- Both, the input and the output space are discrete.

Typical applications for neural networks realizing mappings between continuous inputs and outputs are tasks for control, navigation, robotics, or prediction of time series. Neural networks which are used for this kind of application have to be *approximative* or *interpolative* which means: $F(x^k + \epsilon) = y^k + \delta$ for small ϵ and δ, suppose (x^k, y^k) to be an input-output relation from the *training set*, for which $F(x^k) = y^k$ is known.

Neural networks representing a mapping F from a continuous input space into a set of finite elements, are employed for classification or pattern recognition. For tasks like these the behavior of the mapping F should be different: A new input pattern $x^k + \epsilon$, close to an input x^k from the the learning set should be classified to $y^k = F(x^k) = F(x^k + \epsilon)$ which is the desired output corresponding to the input x^k.

By a mapping between discrete input and output spaces a memory task can be realized. On this topic we will focus in this paper.

An associative memory is a single-layer neural network that maps a set of input patterns $X = \{x^1, \ldots, x^M\}$ into a set of output patterns $Y = \{y^1, \ldots, y^M\}$, in such a way that each input pattern x^k is associated with exactly one output pattern y^k. In 1958 by K. Steinbuch the 'Lernmatrix' network was invented, illustrated in his famous book *Automat und Mensch* [19]. The idea of the Lernmatrix network was to implement a mapping that associates binary input patterns with binary output patterns by a Hebbian learning process which produces binary synaptic weights. Steinbuch's idea was to build the Lernmatrix with very simple elements, such as resistors and wires. The performance of this associative memory network has been studied by D. Willshaw [24] and later by G. Palm [10] in terms the number of storable patterns, error probability of retrieved output patterns and memory capacity.

In the sixties and beginning seventies the architecture of the linear associative memory network was introduced by many authors; the canonical references on the subject are the papers by J. Anderson [2] and T. Kohonen [7, 8]. A linear associative memory is a single-layer neural network with a matrix of synaptic weights W. The task is to store a set of M pairs or associations $(x^k, y^k) \in \mathbb{R}^n \times \mathbb{R}^m$ and to retrieve y^k exactly or at least with just a few errors, if the input x^k is presented to the network. This association is done by a linear mapping

$$\tilde{y}^k = x^k W. \tag{1}$$

By using this notation one alludes to the interpretation of w_{ij} as the strength or weight of the directed connection from input or neuron i to neuron j.

Note that the linear associative network (1) realizes an approximative mapping, whereras an associative memory of the Lernmatrix type is not approximative. The analysis tools for linear associative memory are based on results derived from linear algebra. Linear associative memories are not subject of this paper. We will concentrate on the storage and retrieval of *binary learning patterns* from a neural associative memory consisting of *threshold neurons*.

The paper is organized as follows: In the second section we introduce the basic ideas of neural associative memory, describe the different storage and retrieval procedures, derive evaluation criteria and state some of the main results. Many of these results are asymptotical for growing number of neurons, $n \longrightarrow \infty$, whereas in section 3 we show results for finite size associative memory, achieved by computer simulations and analytical treatment as well. Finally we discuss some ideas on the construction of sparse, distributed, similarity preserving representations of data.

2 Basic Concepts of Neural Associative Memory

It is the goal of this section to present an overview of the results on neural associative memory (e.g. , see C.E. Shannon [17] containing A.M. Uttley's papers [22] and [23], G. Palm [11], or the reprint collection[18] edited by G. Shaw and G. Palm). In the recent scientific literature one can find many models for neural associative memory, very similar in their basic architecture, but different in many details.

One possible categorization of neural associative memory is into *feedforward* and *feedback*. In a feedforward network, as shown in Fig. 1, an input vector x is presented to a single layer of n neurons. In a single processing step an output vector $\tilde{y}$ is evaluated. In a feedback associative memory the output signals of the neurons, or just a part of those, are fed back to the input (see Fig. 2). Processing of the currently appeared output pattern as a new input, the network shows a new activity pattern at the output. The idea of feedback associative memory is that the activity pattern of the neurons converge to a stable state which represents the final output of the memory.

Another classification of neural associative memory with respect to the performed task is into *hetero-association* and *auto-association*. In hetero-association the memory is storing a mapping $x \longrightarrow y$, where the content y is

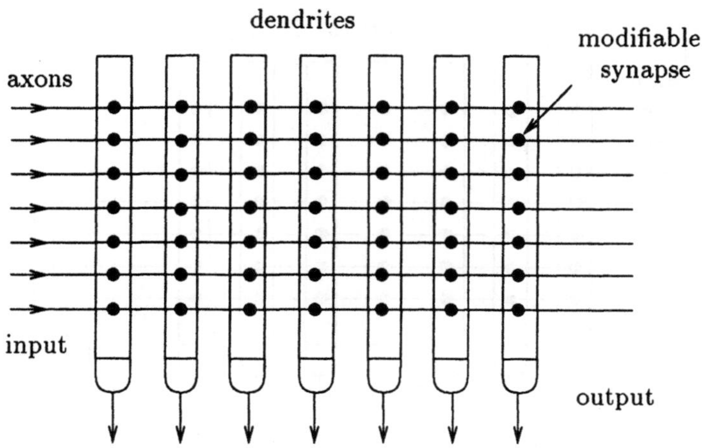

Figure 1: Associative memory consisting of axons, dendrites, and modifiable synapses.

addressed by a key or address x; we call this *pattern mapping*. In an auto-associative memory the address pattern is assumed to be equal to the content. Associating x with itself as in auto-association, it is possible to retrieve the patterns by means of *fault-tolerant self-addressing* or *pattern completion*. It is also an interesting approach to use feedback in an auto-associative memory to perform iterative retrieval.

An artifical neural network is composed of a large number of processing elements called neurons. Each neuron comprises a large number of adjustable synapses connecting it to other neurons.

It was W.A. Little [9] who introduced the analogy between Ising spin systems and neural network models. Methods developed in statistical physics were introduced to analyze the behavior of the feedback retrieval process in large neural associative memories. An Ising spin system consists of a set of coupled basic elements, each able to take the two states 'up' and 'down', respectively corresponding to states 'active' and 'silent' of a binary neuron. In the spin glass literature the neural states are often modelled as -1 and $+1$. The spin-to-spin interactions correspond to the synaptic weights of the neural network. The textbooks by Amit [1] and Hertz, Krogh, and Palmer [5] give a resonably deep insight into the field of attractor networks.

We assign these two neural states the real numbers 'a' and '1' with $a \in [-1, 0]$. The type of binary patterns we are dealing with are *distributed patterns*. A distributed binary pattern includes more than one 1-component per state, whereas in a *singular pattern* exactly one position is set to '1' and the

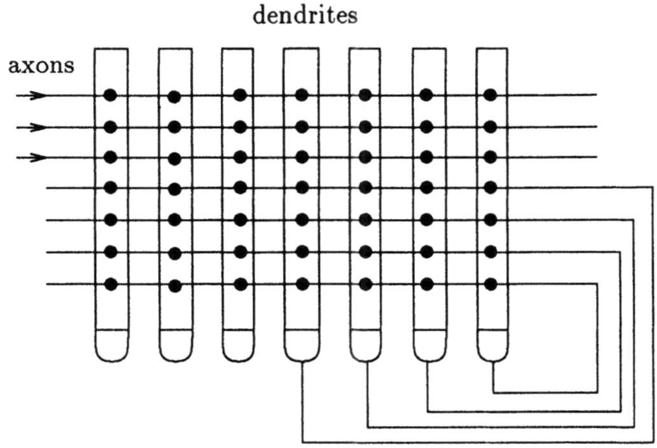

Figure 2: An auto-associative memory consisting of threshold neurons with feedback connections.

others are set to 'a'. We call the pairs of associations,

$$S = \{(x^k, y^k) : k = 1, \ldots, M\} \tag{2}$$

the set of *learning patterns* or the set of *memory patterns*.

We distinguish two different neural information processing steps, namely the *retrieval process* and the *storage* or *learning process*. During the storage process the learning patterns are stored by means of adjusting the synaptic weights, whereas in the retrieval process an input pattern is propagated through the network, which leads to a new acitivity of each neuron, thus resulting in an estimate for one of the stored patterns y^k.

In this section and also in section 3 the learning patterns are assumed to be randomly generated. All components of x^k and y^k are generated independently: with the same probability $p := prob[x_i^k = 1]$ for all input patterns, and with probability $q := [y_j^k = 1]$ for all output patterns.

2.1 Learning in Associative Memory

In the learning process each pair $(x^k, y^k) \in S$ is presented to the neural associative memory; the address pattern x^k at the input and the content pattern y^k at the output (see Fig. 1). This provides a pre- and postsynaptic signal at every synapse. According to these two signals the synaptic weight is changed. A prescription which determines the synaptic change by the post- and presynaptic signals we call *local learning rule* or *local two-term rule*. A local learning rule $R(x, y)$ with presynaptic signal x and postsynaptic signal y can be described by a 2×2 matrix, or a vector $R(x, y) = (r_1, r_2, r_3, r_4)$ (see Fig. 3) .

In this paper we focus on local learning rules for the synaptic modification, whereas in many artifical neural networks three-term learning rules are often used together with supervised learning. A very typical class of three-term learning rules is the *delta rule* type, for example the perceptron learning rule. Here the synaptic weight modification is proportial to the presynaptic signal x and the difference $y - t$ between the actual output y and the teacher signal t.

Furthermore, we use *one-step learning* for synaptic modification, in which each pattern is presented just one time. Network models with more flexible retrieval behavior often need time consuming learning procedures presenting the learning set many times.

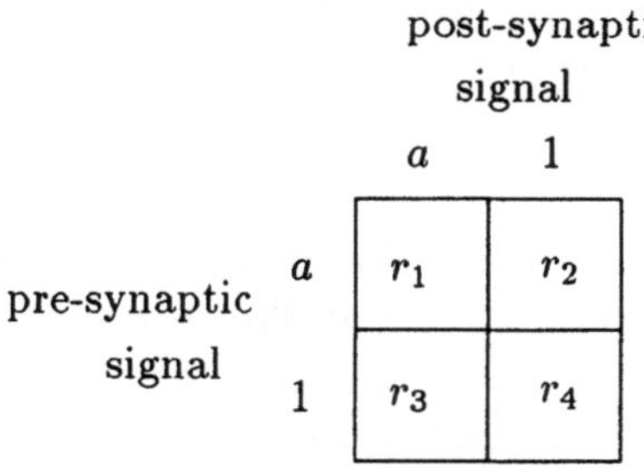

Figure 3: Amount of synaptic modification by a two-term learning rule $R(x, y)$, depending on the pre- and postsynaptic signal.

We will focus on the following learning rules that are very common in the literature:

- The *Hebb rule* or asymmetric coincidence rule $H := (0, 0, 0, 1)$ increases the synaptic value for pre- and postsynaptic activity, corresponding to '1'. This rule for synaptic modification between pairs of firing nerous cells has been postulated by D. Hebb [4].

- The *agreement rule* or symmetric coincidence rule $A := (1, -1, -1, 1)$ increases the synaptic value for agreeing pre- and postsynaptic signals and decreases the synaptic value for disagreeing states. This rule is used in the Hopfield model [6], therefore it is often called Hopfield rule.

- The *correlation rule* $C := (pq, -p(1-q), -(1-p)q, (1-p)(1-q))$ builds up the correlation between activity states of the pre- and postsynaptic neurons over the set of learning patterns. It depends on the probabilities p and q of having a '1' as pre- and postsynaptic signal, respectively.

In hetero-association the set of learning patterns $S = \{(x^k, y^k) : k = 1, \ldots, M\}$ is stored by forming the synaptic connectivity matrix W with a two-term learning rule R:

$$W = w_{ij} = \sum_k R(x_i^k, y_j^k). \tag{3}$$

The connectivity matrix in auto-association, where a set $S = \{x^k : k = 1, \ldots, M\}$ is stored, becomes

$$W = w_{ij} = \sum_k R(x_i^k, x_j^k). \tag{4}$$

Since the final synaptic strength is reached by M single updates we call this an *incremental learning rule.* In *binary learning* the synaptic weight matrix $\bar{W}$ is obtained by a highly nonlinear operation called *clipping*:

$$\bar{w}_{ij} = \text{sgn}(w_{ij}) \tag{5}$$

with the definition sgn(0) := 0. Obviously, in auto-association the connectivity matrix becomes symmetric for all three learning rules H, A, and C.

2.2 Retrieval from Associative Memory

In the retrieval phase an address pattern is applied to the input of the network. The input signals are propagated through the synaptic connections w_{ij} to all neurons at the same time. Each neuron j transforms the input signals into its *dendritic potential* d_j, which is the sum of inputs weighted by the corresponding synaptic strenght:

$$d_j := \sum_i w_{ij} x_i. \tag{6}$$

The new activity $\tilde{y}_j$ of neuron j is determined by a nonlinear operation called *threshold detection*:

$$\tilde{y}_j = f_j(d_j - \theta_j) \tag{7}$$

In almost all neural network models the function f_j is a monotonously increasing function, the *transfer function*; in our models it is chosen constant $f_j = f$ for all neurons, also the *threshold value* θ_j is adjusted globally to $\theta_j = \theta$ for all j. Because we are dealing with binary input and output patterns, the neural transfer function f is binary valued with $f(x) = 1$, for $x \geq 0$ and $f(x) = a$ for $x < 0$, corresponding to the neural states 'active' or 'firing' and 'silent' or 'not firing', respectively.

In *one-step* retrieval the output pattern is evaluated from the incoming address pattern by a single synchronous processing step of all neurons in parallel. In the spin glass literature on auto-association *iterative retrieval* is considered, where the output pattern feeds back to the input until a fixed point is reached. Two different updating modes of the neural activity are distinguished: By *synchronous updating* a complete processing step as in one-step retrieval is performed by all neurons at the same time. Here the new input pattern can be different from the previous input pattern at all positions (e.g., see [6]). In neural network models with *asynchronous updating*, only for a single randomly selected neuron the new output activity is calculated. The new input pattern differs at most in this component from the preceeding input (e.g., see [9]).

2.3 Evaluation Criteria

In the last two subsections we described storage and recall of learning patterns by the use of simple retrieval strategies. We are dealing with distributed binary patterns also leading to a distributed storage of the pattern in the memory. With the Hebbian rule A as learning rule a single pattern (x^k, y^k) stored by (3) or (5) modifies all synapses w_{ij} with $x_i^k = 1$ and $y_j^k = 1$.

It is the basic idea of associative memory to allow noisy address patterns $\hat{x}$ to retrieve the desired output; e.g., for pattern completion with auto-association. But, a memory which allows errors in the addressing will probably make some errors in the output pattern. With binary learning patterns two types of errors occur. These *retrieval error probabilities* can be expressed by the conditional probabilities:

$$e_1 = prob[\tilde{y}_j^k = a \mid y_j^k = 1], \qquad e_a = prob[\tilde{y}_j^k = 1 \mid y_j^k = a]. \tag{8}$$

In this context a couple of questions arise, which we try to answer in the following subsections:

- How many learning patterns can be stored in a network and retrieved with resonably low errors?
- With how many wrong bits in the address the content can be retrieved from the memory?
- How many components per pattern should be set to '1'?
- What is the best local learning rule?
- Does incremental learning improve binary learning?
- Does iterative retrieval improve one-step retrieval?

These questions need evaluation criteria for evaluation and comparision of different learning rules and retrieval procedures. In many cases simply the

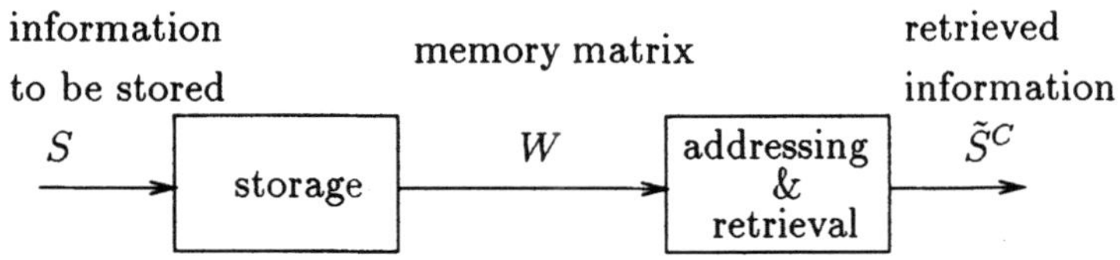

Figure 4: The information channel.

number of storable patterns, or the ratio $\alpha = M/n$ of patterns per neuron, is considered as an evaluation criterion. But, if one tries to compare different models, e.g., for different activity values per pattern, one needs evaluation criteria based on information theory.

For a set of randomly generated learning patterns $S = \{(x^k, y^k) : x^k \in \{a,1\}^n,\ y^k \in \{a,1\}^m, k = 1, \ldots, M\}$ where each component is choosen independently from the others with $p = prob[x_i^k = 1]$ and $q = prob[y_j^k = 1]$, the *mean information* contained in a single content pattern y^k is given by the product $I(y^k) := mi(q)$ where $i(q)$ is the *Shannon information* defined as:

$$i(q) := -\left(q\ \mathrm{ld}[q] + (1-q)\ \mathrm{ld}[(1-q)]\right). \tag{9}$$

For the set of content patterns $S^C := \{y^k : k = 1, \ldots, M\}$ the mean information is

$$I(S^C) := M mi(q). \tag{10}$$

The *pattern capacity* compares the mean information of the content patterns with the size of the $n \times m$ synaptic weight matrix W:

$$P := \max_M I(S^C)/nm = M^* i(q)/n, \tag{11}$$

where M^* equals the maximum number of stored patterns for a given retrieval quality criterion limiting the number of error in the retrieved patterns. The pattern capacity measures the amount of information that can be stored in a memory, but takes not into accout the information loss due to the retrieval errors.

During the storage process the synaptic weight matrix is created. In the retrieval process the stored information is read out by addressing the content patterns $y \in S^C$ with its corresponding address pattern $x \in S^A$ with $S^A := \{x^k : k = 1, \ldots, M\}$. This leads to the set of retrieved output patterns $\tilde{S}^C = \{\tilde{y}^k : k = 1, \ldots, M\}$, probably containing errors as defined in (8).

Measuring the information that can be obtained through the whole information channel (see Fig. 4), the information necessary to correct the errors of the retrieved output patterns should be subtracted from the information of the content patterns. In information theory the capacity of the whole channel is the *transinformation* $T(\tilde{S}^C, S^C)$, measuring the information of the channel's output $\tilde{S}^C$ about the channel's input S^C:

$$T(\tilde{S}^C, S^C) = I(S^C) - I(S^C \mid \tilde{S}^C), \tag{12}$$

where the *conditional information* $I(S^C \mid \tilde{S}^C)$ describes the amount of information necessary to correct the errors in the patterns of $\tilde{S}^C$ to achieve the correct output patterns.

This leads to the definition of *memory capacity* or *association capacity*

$$A := \max_M T(\tilde{S}^C, S^C)/nm \tag{13}$$

which becomes for randomly generated binary patterns to

$$A := (M^*/n) \left[i(q) - I(y_i^k \mid \tilde{y}_i^k) \right], \tag{14}$$

with the *conditional information* per component

$$I(y_i^k \mid \tilde{y}_i^k) = p[\tilde{y}_i^k = 1] \cdot i(p[y_i^k = a \mid \tilde{y}_i^k = 1]) + p[\tilde{y}_i^k = a] \cdot i(p[y_i^k = 1 \mid \tilde{y}_i^k = a]), \tag{15}$$

which can be expressed in terms of the probability q and the error probabilities e_a and e_1.

In auto-association the retrieval results in an output pattern $\tilde{x}$ by taking a noisy version $\hat{x}$ of a learning pattern x as an address pattern. Measuring the performance of the pattern completion task the information of the address pattern $\hat{x}$ about the content pattern x should also be taken into account. This could be done by the transinformation $T(\hat{S}^C, S^C)$, where $\hat{S}^C$ is the set of address patterns, representing incomplete or noisy versions of S^C. This leads to the definition of the *completion capacity*:

$$\begin{aligned} C &:= \max_{\hat{S}^C} \left[T(\tilde{S}^C, S^C) - T(\hat{S}^C, S^C) \right] /n^2 && (16) \\ &= \max_{\hat{S}^C} \left[I(S^C \mid \hat{S}^C) - I(S^C \mid \tilde{S}^C) \right] /n^2 && (17) \\ &= \max_{\hat{x}^k} (M^*/n) \left[I(x_i^k \mid \hat{x}_i^k) - I(x_i^k \mid \tilde{x}_i^k) \right]. && (18) \end{aligned}$$

2.4 Some Asymptotic Results

In this section we review some asymptotic results on the memory capacity of very large associative matrices (see also [13]). To understand the flavour of the arguments leading up to these results, let us consider the special case of binary Hebbian learning with $a = 0$ and hetero-association. Storing a set of M randomly generated patterns (x^k, y^k), approximatively

$$p_0 = (1 - pq)^M \approx exp(-Mpq) \tag{19}$$

is the probability for an arbitrary synaptic weight w_{ij} to stay at $w_{ij} = 0$. Thus a fraction of approximatively $p_1 = 1 - p_0$ of the synaptic weights switch from 0 to 1. With a part $\hat{x}^k$ of the memory pattern as input, and with the threshold choice $\theta = \sum_i \hat{x}_i^k$, the retrieved output contains all 1's of the content y^k and some additional 1's. Thus $e_1 = 0$ whereas $e_0 \neq 0$ depends on the density of 1's in the synaptic weight matrix. If the matrix W is randomly filled with probability $p_1 = prob[w_{ij} = 1]$, then the error probability e_0 is $e_0 = p_1^\theta$. Thus e_0 increases with p_1 and also with M. In order to achieve a high memory capacity it turns out that the entries of the synaptic weight matrix should be balanced, that means $p_1 = p_0 = 0.5$ (see [24] or [10]). To achieve $p_1 \leq 0.5$, i. e.

$$Mpq = -\ln[p_0] \leq \ln[2], \tag{20}$$

it is necessary to keep the product Mpq low which can be achieved by using sparse address and content patterns. Then it is possible to store a large set of patterns ($M \gg n$) in the memory, leading to an asymptotical memory capcity of $A = \ln[2] \approx 0.69$ (see [10]).

In auto-association and pattern completion with one-step retrieval a completion capacity $C = \ln[2]/4 \approx 0.173$ can be achieved with sparse content patterns by using half of the content as address pattern. In [15] the upper bound for the maximal reachable completion capacity with fixed point retrieval was determined to $\ln[2]/2 \approx 0.35$. This bound can not be reached with effective iterative retrieval strategies starting from an incomplete or noisy version of the content pattern (see section 3 and [16]).

For incremental learning rules and threshold detection as retrieval strategy it turns out by a *signal-to-noise analysis* that for hetero-association the optimal memory capacity of $A = 1/(2\ln[2]) \approx 0.72$ can be achieved with the correlation rule $C := (pq, -p(1-q), -(1-p)q, (1-p)(1-q))$ – where p and q are respectively the fractions of ones in the address and content patterns. The signal-to-noise analysis shows that for any local learning rule R the best choice of p is given by the *zero average* input condition:

$$\mu := p + (1-p)a = 0, \tag{21}$$

which determines the optimal relation between a and p in the address pattern, see [14]. If the zero average input condition is not fulfilled for a learning rule R, different from the correlation rule C, then its asymptotic memory capacity is zero. For $p = 1/2$ the zero average input condition implies $a = -1$, and for sparse input patterns, i.e. $p \rightarrow 0$ asymptotically, the zero input activity is asymptotically fulfilled for $a = 0$.

For the choice $p = q = 1/2$ and $a = -1$, which is very common in the spin glass literature, the correlation rule becomes $(1/4, -1/4, -1/4, 1/4)$ which is equivalent to the Hopfield rule A. For the Hopfield rule this choice is optimal.

Furthermore, it turns out that retrieval with the *high fidelity* requirement

$$e_1 \rightarrow 0 \qquad e_a/q \rightarrow 0, \tag{22}$$

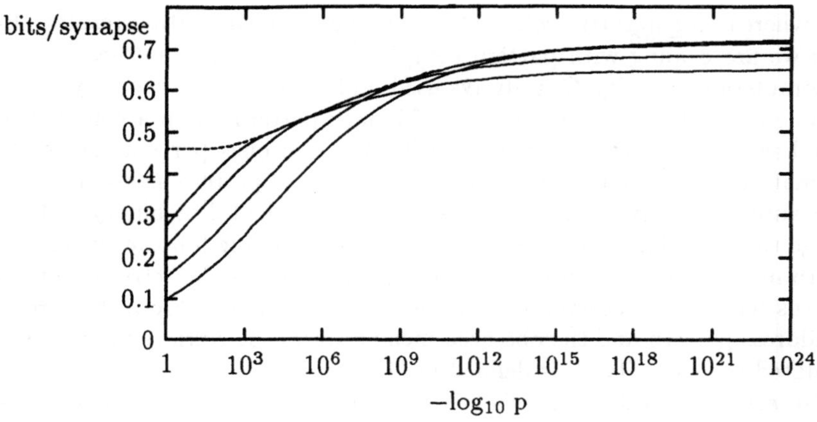

Figure 5: Asymptotic capacity ($n \to \infty$ and $p, q \to 0$) for the incremental Hebbian learning rule for different retrieval fidelity requirements ($e_0 \leq 0.1\%, 1\%, 5\%, 10\%$). The dashed line shows the local learning bound. The correlation rule shows very similar behavior, differing only in the range of nonsparse activity.

can only be achieved for sparse content patterns ($q \to 0$ asymptotically). For small p and q the correlation rule is very similar to the Hebbian learning rule. Therefore, the asymptotical capacities of the correlation rule and the Hebb rule, shown in Fig. 5, are for sparse learning patterns also very similar. Thus for sparse address and content patterns ($p, q \to 0$) a memory capacity of $A = 1/(2ln2)$ can be achieved with high retrieval accuracy by using the Hebbian learning rule.

For incremental learning auto-association and pattern completion with sparsely coded patterns a completion capacity of $C = 1/(8 \ln[2]) \approx 0.18$ can be achieved with one-step retrieval. For fixed point retrieval an upper bound for the completion capacity has been determined as $1/(4 \ln[2])$, see [15]. It seems that the value for fixed point retrieval can not be achieved by realistic retrieval strategies starting from a part of the memory pattern.

3 Results for Finite Size Associative Memory

In this section we focus on the storage and retrieval of sparsely coded binary memory patterns (with $a = 0$) from an auto-associative memory using one-step, two-step and iterative retrieval. The results for one-step and two-step retrieval are obtained by computer simulation and theoretical treatment as well, whereas for iterative retrieval we present only simulation results. Because we are dealing with pattern completion by means of auto-association the completion capacity C is always used and simply called capacity.

In our computer simulations a set of binary patterns with a constant activity has been generated randomly with $k << n$ ones per pattern, so the information per memory pattern is very low. These pattern sets were stored in an auto-associative memory by using the incremental or binary Hebbian storage rule H defined in (4) and (5) respectively. Using a noisy version $\hat{x}$ of a learning pattern x as an input pattern, the errors of the retrieved output patterns have been observed during the retrieval process. From the error in the address pattern and the observed mean error of the retrieved patterns we calculated the capacity C as defined in (18).

In iterative retrieval the threshold θ has to be adjusted in each retrieval step and the end of the iteration loop has to be determined. Such a procedure we call a ***threshold control strategy***, see [16] for further details. In section 3.2 we describe the strategy TK+ which has been used in our computer simulations.

3.1 Incremental versus Binary Hebbian Learning

In computer simulations the binary Hebbian learning rule shows always better performance than the incremental Hebbian learning rule; Fig. 6 shows the simulation results for an associative memory with $n = 1900$ neurons. Incremental learning achieves a capacity of approximatly 7% for one-step retrieval, and approximately 9% for iterative retrieval. Almost the double capacity values, namely 14.5 % and 18% can be obtained with binary Hebbian learning. However, for incremental learning $C \approx 18\%$, and for binary learning $C \approx 17.3\%$ can be achieved asymptotically.

It can be observed in Fig. 6 that the capacity for iterative retrieval goes back to the capacity values for one-step retrieval, if only a few or many patterns were stored in the memory. Only in an intermediate range iterative retrieval yields higher capacity values. In Fig. 6 the effective storage ranges for iterative retrieval are $2000 < M < 7000$ for incremental, and $5000 < M < 14000$ for binary learning. The effective storage range is a typical property of iterative retrieval, it also can be observed by means of retrieval time. In this range the retrieval time rises from $t = 1$ up to $t \approx 3$, but is in all models very short.

For the incremental Hebbian learning rule the completion capacities which can be achieved with realistic memory sizes (up to $n \approx 10^4$) are far below the asymptotic bound of $1/(8 \ln[2])$. The rate of convergence to the asymptotic completion capacity seems to be much faster for the binary Hebbian learning rule, so that it is possible to achieve reasonably high completion capacities with memory sizes in the range form $n = 10^3$ to $n = 10^4$.

Since additive Hebbian learning is apparently inferior to binary Hebbian learning on all interesting counts (capacity, iteration time, storage requirements) we will focus on binary Hebbian learning in the remainder of this section.

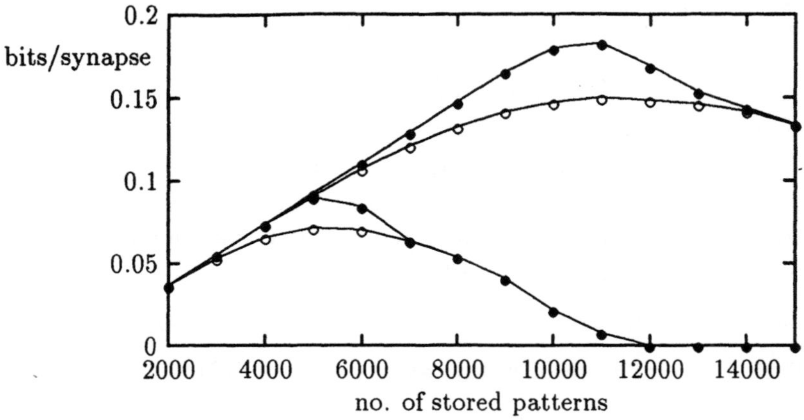

Figure 6: The capacity C of the incremental and binary learning rule are plotted for one-step retrieval and for iterative retrieval (8th retrieval step). The activities of the memory and address patterns are set to $k = 13$ and $l = 6$, respectively.

3.2 Analytical Results on Two-step Retrieval

In this subsection we present a calculation of the error probabilities for one-step and two-step retrieval with the binary Hebbian learning rule for patterns of constant activity based on statistical methods introduced by Palm in [10].

As an address pattern in the first retrieval step an incomplete version $\hat{x}$ of a learning pattern x with $l < k$ ones is used. We set the threshold to $\theta = l$ in the first retrieval step, which guarantees that the retrieved output pattern constists of two parts:

- the whole learning pattern x
- a few number of additional ones which are wrong bits

Thus $e_1 = 0$ and the the probability to obtain a wrong bit is determined by

$$e_0 = 1 + \sum_{h=1}^{l} \binom{l}{h} (-1)^h \left[\frac{n-k}{n} + \frac{k}{n-h} \cdot T(n,k,h) \right]^{M-1}, \tag{23}$$

where we use for brevity

$$T(n,k,i) := \prod_{h=0}^{i-1} \frac{n-k-h}{n-h}, \tag{24}$$

(see [10] for details). Therefore, in the mean $\tilde{m}_{off} := (n-k)e_0$ additional ones appear in the retrieved output pattern $\tilde{x} =: \tilde{x}(1)$ after the first retrieval step. Using $\tilde{x}(1)$ as new input pattern and setting $\theta = k$, an output pattern $\tilde{x}(2)$ with the following properties can be retrieved:

(a) Each zero-component of $\tilde{x}(1)$ stays at this value in $\tilde{x}(2)$.

(b) Each one-component of x stays at this value in $\tilde{x}(2)$.

Property (a) can be achieved by a logical ANDing between $\tilde{x}(1)$ and the pattern retrieved by threshold detection with $\theta = k$. This logical ANDing guarantees convergence of the retrieval process to a fixed point.

Again, we abtain $e_1 = 0$ after the second retrieval step. For the error probability e_0 of $\tilde{x}(2)$ we abtain the approximation:

$$e_0 = e^{-\tilde{m}_{off}} \sum_{j=1}^{n-k} \frac{\tilde{m}_{off}^j}{j!} \sum_{i=0}^{j} \binom{\tilde{m}_{on}+j-1}{j-i} (1-p_0)^{\tilde{m}_{on}+i-1} p_0^{j-i}, \tag{25}$$

with $\tilde{m}_{on} := k - l$ for brevity. Taking into account the dependencies between different matrix elements the expression $(1-p_0)^u p_0^v$ in (25) should be exchanged by the probability

$$p_{uv} := p\left[w_{1q} = w_{2q} = \cdots = w_{uq} = 1 \wedge w_{(u+1)q} = \cdots = w_{(u+v)q} = 0\right], \tag{26}$$

which is approximately the product of p_A and p_B with

$$p_A = 1 + \sum_{h=1}^{u} \binom{u}{h} (-1)^h \left[1 - \left(\frac{k\,T(n,k,v)}{n-v} - \frac{k\,T(n,k,v+h)}{n-v-h}\right)\right]^{M-1} \tag{27}$$

$$p_B = \left[1 - \frac{k}{n}\{1 - T(n-1,k-1,v)\}\right]^{M-l}. \tag{28}$$

The relations (26) to (28) result from an analysis of the binary storage process with learning patterns of fixed activity k (see [21] or [16] for further details).

3.3 Iterative Retrieval Procedures

In Fig. 7 the capacities for one-step, two step, and iterative retrieval for the binary Hebbian learning rule are shown; here $M = 10,000$ patterns with $k = 13$ have been stored in an auto-associative memory with $n = 1,900$

neurons. The retrieval process started from an incomplete or noisy version of a stored pattern. The parameter l denotes the number of ones in the address pattern. Here $l < k$ corresponds to an address pattern which is a part of a stored pattern, and $l > k$ to an address pattern which is a stored pattern with some additional ones.

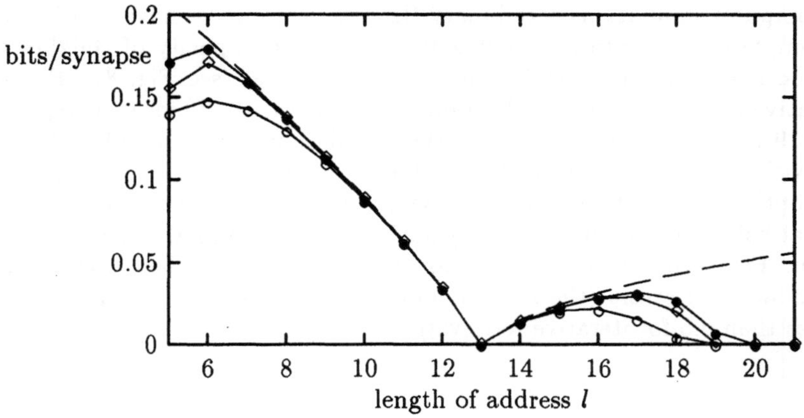

Figure 7: The capacity of one-step, two-step, and iterative retrieval (8th step) for different address patterns; the dashed line shows the completion capacity for error free retrieval.

The dashed line in Fig. 7 represents the missing information in the address. This is a bound for the completion capacity which could be achieved by an errorfree retrieval procedure. Near the errorfree address the curves almost coincide, but if the errors in the address pattern increases the errors in the retrieved output pattern increases as well, and therefore the capacities for one-step, two-step, and iterative retrieval stays below this bound.

For $l \approx k/2$ the curves of the capacities reach their maximum. This type of diagram is M-shaped for all models, with two local maxima. It is obviously clear that the capacity for all models is zero when we use the stored patterns without any distortions as address patterns, therefore the curves in Fig. 7 go back to capacity $C = 0$ for $l = k = 13$. The right maximum of the capacity curve for $l > k$ is always smaller than the left one due to the following reasons:

- Because of the sparsity of the learning patterns, it is much easier to correct an additional 1 (detection of the wrong 1 among the $k + 1$ ones), then to correct a missing 1 (detection of the wrong 0 among $n - (k - 1)$ zeros) of a stored pattern.

- The models show more fault tolerance against missing ones than against additional ones in the address pattern.

For small M (suboptimal memory load) the completion capacity coincide over a larger range with the capacity achieved by errorfree retrieval. In this case the maximum of these curves can be reached for address patterns with $l < k/2$ ones, where more than half the information of the stored pattern has to be completed.

In computer simulations with binary Hebbian learning we have even obtained completion capacities exceeding the asymptotic capacity of $\ln[2]/4 \approx 0.173$ both with iterative and with two-step retrieval (see Fig. 8). For an associative memory with 18,000 neurons we achieved 17.9% for two-step and about 19% for iterative retrieval. In this simulation more than 500,000 patterns with a constant activity of $k = 19$ had been stored.

The optimal completion capacity values for one-step, two-step, and iterative retrieval have been reached by using half of the learning pattern as address pattern. Furthermore these completion capacities were reached with a very small number of errors (the mean number of errors is about 2 for two-step and less than 0.5 for iterative retrieval).

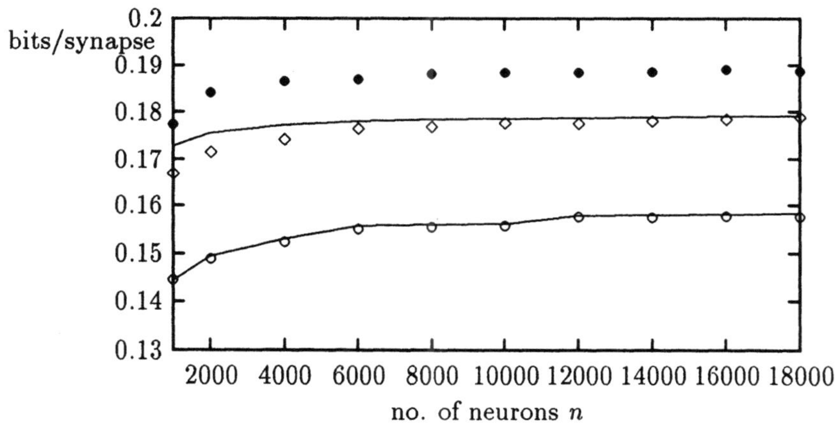

Figure 8: Optimal completion capacities (M, k and l optimized) for one-step and two-step retrieval, and the simulation results for iterative retrieval (8th step).

3.4 Concluding Remarks

Although incremental Hebbian learning reaches asymptotically a slightly higher completion capacity value than binary Hebbian learning, for realistic memory sizes binary Hebbian learning is superior in one-step, two-step, and iterative retrieval.

The completion capacity values for binary Hebbian learning exceed the asymptotic capacity of $\ln[2]/4$ for associative memories with $1,900$ neurons, with iterative and two-step retrieval as well.

By theoretical analysis one can find out that the optimal completion capacity for two step-retrieval reaches its absolute maximum (which is slightly larger than the capacity value for $n = 18,000$) for a matrix size of about $n = 200,000$ and than goes down towards the asymptotic value of $\ln[2]/4 \approx 17.32\%$; it appears that the same is true for iterative retrieval.

The completion capacity values for one-step, two-step, and iterative retrieval have been reached by using half of the learning pattern as address pattern.

These completion capacities can be reached with a very small number of errors (e.g., for the simulation with $n = 18,000$ neurons the error ratio e_0/k is less than 1% for iterative retrieval).

The retrieval process takes a very short time; the mean iteration time was less than five steps in computer simulation.

These properties, together with the fact that only one bit per synapse is needed for the storage matrix, suggest the auto-associative memory with the binary Hebbian learning rule suitable for applications.

4 Sparse Similarity Preserving Codes

An associative memory can efficently be used for tasks like fault tolerant information retrieval. But the patterns to be stored have to be binary valued. Thus, a coding procedure is needed that transforms patterns of any input space into binary coded patterns.

In order to get a high memory capacity of the associative memory, the patterns have to be sparse (see section 2.4 or [12]). On the other hand a similarity preserving coding procedure is necessary to render the fault tolerance in the information retrieval task.

In many applications it is easy to achieve sparsely coded binary patterns. Let us briefly discuss an example: Assume, we have to store a large set of strings, e.g., names of cities, in an associative memory in such a way that allows to ignore typographical errors. Coding a word, e.g. 'SYDNEY', according to the triplets of consecutive letters leads to a sparse binary pattern. For our example we detect the seven triplets '#SY', 'SYD', 'YDN', 'DNE','NEY','EY.'. For the post-processing of the retrieval result, it is useful to add 2 extra symbols (the beginning of a string '#' and the ending of a string '.') to the alphabet. Ekeberg studied slightly different coding schemes for text-retrieval from associative memory in [3].

For example, the DARWIN–dictionary with approximatively 300,000 German words with in the mean $k = 10.75$ characters per pattern, contains about $n = 9,000$ different triplets. Each component of a code vector represents exactly one of the n possible triplets. A component is set to 1, if the corresponding triplet occurs in the word to be coded, this is leading to a mean activity of k/n. This coding procedure is similarity preserving for many similarity or distance measures which are defined in the set of strings. A very common distance measure between two strings A and B is the *Levenstein distance* measuring the minimal number of replacements, insertions, and deletions to obtain B from A.

4.1 General Strategy for Similarity Preserving Coding

Let us assume that a set of data points $\{v^1, \ldots, v^M\}$ is a subset of an input space X with a metric $d : X \times X \longrightarrow \mathbb{R}$. Of course, the Hamming distance between binary pattern is an integer value. Therefore it is impossible to preserve the exact distances during the binary coding procedure. But the coding procedure we are going to describe is able to preserve the ordering of the distances.

The input to our coding algorithm is a distance matrix $D \in \mathbb{R}^M \times \mathbb{R}^M$. Corresponding to this distance matrix we define distance classes by collecting similar entries of the distance matrix into the same distance class. Between classes we define integer valued distances in such a way that the ordering of the real distances is preserved. This procedure gives an $M \times M$ distance matrix with integer valued entries. Before running the coding algorithm this distance matrix has to be transformed into an overlap matrix. This transformation of a Hamming distance into an overlap is done by using:

$$d_{ij} = l_i + l_j - 2 \cdot o_{ij}, \tag{29}$$

where d_{ij}, o_{ij}, l_i, and l_j denote the Hamming distance, the overlap, the number of ones in binary vector c^i, and the number of ones in c^j, respectively. Furthermore the equation (29) shows that, the distances d_{ij} have to be even.

The coding algorithm generates a set of binary code vectors $c^1, \ldots, c^M$ from the overlap matrix O.

The basic concept of the coding procedure is quite straightforward: The initial code sequences are arranged line by line into a matrix with n rows. In the beginning these code sequences are empty. They are successively filled column by column from left to right. Adding the column vector $e_i + e_j$ to the already existing code sequences leads to an overlap of 1 for the code vectors c^i and c^j and does not change all other overlaps. Here e_i denotes the i–th unit vector. Proceeding in this way one is able to generate code sequences $c^1, \ldots, c^M$, which have the same overlaps as given by the overlap matrix O.

Sometimes these code vectors can become very long. Generating the code vectors as described before, the length L of each code vector becomes

$$L = \sum_i \sum_{j>i} o_{ij}. \tag{30}$$

In each of the code vectors c_i there are

$$Z_i = \sum_{j \neq i} o_{ij} \tag{31}$$

components set to 1. It is often possible to achieve shorter code vectors. This could be realized by adding the column $e_i + e_j + e_k$. This column gives overlaps between the code vectors c^i and c^j, c^j and c^k, and c^i and c^k. So we get three overlaps in comparision to only one overlap. This line of thought leads to a minimization problem concerning the length of the code vectors, which is computationally hard, but reasonable suboptimal solutions can be found by heuristic strategies. In [20] Stellmann described several methods for optimizing binary code vectors in detail.

Acknowledgement

This work has been partially supported by the BMFT.

References

[1] D. J. Amit. *Modelling Brain Function.* Cambridge University Press, Cambridge, 1989.

[2] J. A. Anderson. A simple neural network generating an interactive memory. *Mathematical Biosciences*, 14:197–220, 1972.

[3] Ö. Ekeberg. Robust dictionary lookup using associative networks. *Int. Journal Man-Machine Studies*, 28:29–43, 1988.

[4] D.O. Hebb. *The Organization of Behavior.* Wiley, New York, 1949.

[5] J. Hertz, A. Krogh, and R. G. Palmer. *Introduction to the Theory of Neural Computation.* Addison Wesley, New York, 1991.

[6] J.J. Hopfield. Neural networks and physical systems with emergent collective computational abilities. *Proceedings of the National Academy of Sciences, USA*, 79, 1982.

[7] T. Kohonen. Correlation matrix memory. *IEEE Transactions on Computers*, C-21(4):353–359, 1972.

[8] T. Kohonen. *Associative Memory.* Springer, Berlin, 1977.

[9] W.A. Little. The existence of persistent states in the brain. *Mathematical Biosciences*, 19:101–120, 1974.

[10] G. Palm. On associative memory. *Biological Cybernetics*, 36:19–31, 1980.

[11] G. Palm. *Neural Assemblies.* Springer, Berlin, 1982.

[12] G. Palm. Local synaptic rules with maximal information storage capacity. *Neural and synergetic Computers*, 42:100–110, 1988.

[13] G. Palm. Memory capacities of local rules for synaptic modification. *Concepts in Neuroscience*, 2:97–128, 1991.

[14] G. Palm. On the information storage capacity of local learning rules. *Neural Computation*, 1992.

[15] G. Palm and F. T. Sommer. Information capacity in recurrent McCulloch-Pitts networks with sparsely coded memory states. *Network*, 3:1–10, 1992.

[16] F. Schwenker, F. T. Sommer, and G. Palm. Iterative retrieval of sparsely coded associative memory patterns. *submitted to Neural Networks*, 1993.

[17] C.E. Shannon and I. Mc Carthy, editors. *Automata Studies.* University Press, Princeton NJ, 1956.

[18] G.L. Shaw and G. Palm, editors. *Brain Theory*, volume 1 of *Advanced Series in Neuroscience.* World Scientific, Singapore, 1988.

[19] K. Steinbuch. *Mensch und Automat.* Springer, Heidelberg, 1961.

[20] U. Stellmann. *Ähnlichkeitserhaltende Codierung.* PhD thesis, University of Ulm, 1992.

[21] F. T.Sommer. *Theorie neuronaler Assoziativspeicher: Lokales Lernen und iteratives Retrieval von Information.* PhD thesis, University of Düsseldorf, 1993.

[22] A. M. Uttley. Conditional probability machines and conditioned refexes. In *Automata Studies*, pages 237–252. University Press, Princeton NJ, 1956.

[23] A. M. Uttley. Temporal and spatial patterns in a contitional probability machine. In *Automata Studies*, page 277ff. University Press, Princeton NJ, 1956.

[24] D. J. Willshaw, O. P. Buneman, and H. C. Longuet-Higgins. Nonholographic associative memory. *Nature*, 222:960–962, 1969.

Multistrategy Learning and Optimal Mappings

H. Wechsler
Professor of Computer Science
George Mason University
Fairfax, VA 22030, USA wechsler@cs.gmu.edu

Abstract. Future advances on the connectionist front concern both modeling and learning and require (i) awareness of existing analogies between neural networks and related statistical disciplines, and (ii) the development of functional and hybrid learning schemes. The unified framework provided by statistics, spectral analysis, information theory and evolutionary computation provides both insights and solutions to difficult problems concerning network performance, local learning, novelty detection and rejection handling, and functional approximation using optimal bases. The most important result established in this chapter is the significance of proper sampling (corresponding to 'Nyquist frequency') and the tradeoffs between signal localization and detail of representation (corresponding to the uncertainty principle from signal processing and information theory) on overall network performance.

1 Introduction

Neural networks research should draw inspiration from many disciplines if one considers their goals and the corresponding brain metaphors from computational neurosciences. Both (task and) functionality, and brain structure and metaphor suggest that hybrid learning systems are most appropriate. The neural complexity suggested by brain research and the wide range of tasks involved in cognitive processing require a relatively large repertoire of intelligent modules driven by specific learning (adaptation and estimation) schemes. It is then to the advantage of any intelligent system to develop and implement hybrid adaptation modules driven by multistrategy learning schemes.

The basic tasks neural networks have to cope with involve learning adaptive mappings for functional approximation, solving inverse problems within the framework provided by regularization, and learning to represent (sensory) inputs through functional decomposition using optimal (kernel) bases ('receptive fields'). The last task, that of finding 'optimal' representations is fundamental to any meaningful biological function, as recognition surely is, and by most accounts it is even more important than higher level ('cognitive') learning.

Several theoretical results, starting with the one due to Kolmogorov, reestablished neural networks as a respectable scientific discipline when they showed that multilayer feedforward networks are universal approximators (Hecht-

Nielsen, 1990). Specifically, Kolmogorov's theorem was able to prove that for any given continuous function $f : [0, 1]^n \text{---} \mathbf{R}^m$, $f(x) = y$, f can be implemented exactly by a three-layer feedforward neural network having n fanout processing elements in the first (**x** - input consisting of elements p = 1, n) layer, (2n + 1) processing elements in the middle ('hidden') layer, and m processing elements in the top (**y** - output) layer. The processing elements of the hidden layer implement the following transfer function:

$$z_k = \Sigma^n \lambda^k \varphi (x_p + k\varepsilon)$$

The m top layer processing elements (*output units*) have the following transfer functions:

$$y_i = \Sigma^{2n+1} g_i (z_k)$$

Even that Kolmogorov's result is theoretical rather than constructive it still holds much relevance for neural networks research by showing that the mapping of arbitrary continuous functions from the n - dimensional cube $[0, 1]^n$ to the real numbers R in terms of functions of only one variable is possible. Kolmogorov's theorem also provided the answer to the Hilbert's 13th problem (wrongly) conjecturing that 'there are continuous functions of three variables not representable as superpositions of continuous functions of two variables'.

Neural networks (NN) solutions for inverse problems expanded on their applicability when NN were shown to be equivalent to statistical (MAP) estimation. Finally, it is most exciting to know that there is growing interest to emulate the evolution of lattices of receptive fields towards the development of optimal (kernel) bases suitable for functional decomposition and signal representation. Such kernel bases would amount to optimal 'dictionaries' consisting of those (word) primitives able to express best and in a compact form a wide range of meaningful inputs characteristic to some sensory environment.

Most of the brain metaphors that have been suggested so far are motivated by the desire to explain mental function in terms of those devices or paradigms dominating either technology or science during some extended time interval. The clock (for Descartes), the steam engine and the hydraulic pump (for Freud), and the telegraph were at some time suggested as models of brain function (Daugman, 1990). More recently, and starting with the cybernetic revolution due to Wiener, Shannon, and Von Neumann, brain function has been modeled using the computer paradigm. Other recent models revolve around statistical mechanics, which actually preceded and led to information theory, quantum mechanics (Penrose, 1989), chaos (Freeman, 1992), holography (Pribram, 1991), and to evolution and Darwinism (Edelman, 1987). The reader should note also the thoughtful observation made by Albert Szent - Gyorgi that *the brain is not an organ of thinking but an organ of survival, like claws and fangs. It is made in such a way as to make us accept as truth that which is only advantage. It is an exceptional, almost pathological constitution one has, if one follows thoughts logically through, regardless of consequences. Such people make martyrs, apostles, or scientists, and mostly end on the stake, or in a chair, electric or academic* '. Different metaphors for brain function could thus be considered and adopted as long as one takes into account task functionality and evaluates whether the resulting behavior is beneficial or not.

2 Statistical Pattern Recognition and Adaptive Control

Fundamental links have been established recently between statistical pattern recognition and neural networks when the network outputs were shown to possess specific statistical significance. As an example, if backpropagation (BP) learning is defined over the error surface: $e(f) = \Sigma [y_i - f(x_i)]^2$, Geman, Bienenstock and Doursat (1992) have shown that among all the functions of *x*, the regression is the best prediction of *y* given *x* in the Minimum Square Error (MSE) sense , i.e., $E [(y - f(x))^2 | x] \geq E [(y - E(y | x))^2 | x]$. Another recent but related result due to Richard and Lippmann (1991) states that MSE approximation estimates Bayesian probabilities according to the degree to which the training data reflect true likelihood distribution and a priori probabilities.

MSE fitting corresponds to Maximum Likelihood (ML) estimation and also to the Maximum a Posteriori (MAP) estimation for uniform a priori on the original data sought. As an example, using MSE estimation one gets the sample mean as an unbiased estimator whose variance is bounded by the ratio between the noise variance and the number of samples used in estimation. Note also the well known fact from statistics that the error function e(f) can be represented as e(f) = 'bias' + 'variance' and that smoothing introduces bias as details of the 'true' regression function are lost - neural networks enjoy low bias at the price of large variance.

There are obvious functional similarities between backpropagation (BP) and the Kalman filter widely used in control. Both estimation models, within their own computational framework, employ the same paradigm: predict and update. Note, however, that the Kalman filter is recursive and it allows for incremental/iterative estimation as stochastic information is gathered while backpropagation lacks the superposition ability. Most recently there is a growing interest in fuzzy (logic) control systems. Fuzzy control systems are appropriate for those situations involving continuous variables, close analytical formula are lacking, simple sensors and actuators are highly desirable, noise is a problem and robustness is sought, expertise is readily available, and explanation facilities and incremental maintenance are required. The components of a fuzzy system include a fuzzifier ('crisp' to 'fuzzy' mapping) to establish the degree of membership, fuzzy rules possibly implemented using fuzzy associative memories, fuzzy (parallel) inference engine, and a defuzzifier ('fuzzy' to 'crisp') to decide on some specific course of action. There are obvious analogies between fuzzy and connectionist models - both can be used as universal approximators. Fuzzy membership functions can be actually derived using neural learning. Further insights are gained if one realizes that the fuzzy membership functions are analogous to the way the Gaussian functions weight the closeness of a new input to any of the kernels employed by the radial basis functions (RBFs) schemes.

3 Spectral Analysis and Adaptive Signal Processing

Connectionist models attempt to implement 'optimal' mappings between input - output pairs. The representational aspect, as important as the actual learning taking place, involves data compression schemes such as Karhunen-Loeve Transform (KLT) / Principal Component Analysis (PCA), Singular Value Decomposition (SVD), and/or higher order encoding schemes. The usual framework for optimization is that provided by inverse problems. Optimization involves, among other things, Bayesian estimation of the Maximum a Posteriori (MAP) or Maximum Likelihood (ML) kind, regularization using pseudo and generalized inverse solutions, and restoration using maximum entropy criteria. We further observe that if degraded observations ('measurements') are linearly transformed subject to white noise then the MAP estimate is the Wiener filter output for zero mean white noise, while the ML estimate is the least squares estimate. One final note concerns analogies between minimum norm least squares solutions, implementations using pipeline FIR like filters, and novelty ('innovation') filters.

Connections can be easily established between (2nd order) statistics ('covariance'), geometry and curvature ('Hessian' - ∇^2), and spectral signatures. The motivation for such connections comes from the fact that the Fourier transform of the autocorrelation function is the power spectrum. The link between neural networks and adaptive signal processing can be firmly established through the use of optimization in terms of cost functions involving minimum square error (MSE) estimation leading to solutions such as the generalized Wiener filters. As a simple example one can easily show that the Wiener-Hopf derivation is conceptually similar to that involving radial basis functions (RBFs). Assume that e_i, d_i, y_i stand for the error at the output, and the desired and observed outputs, respectively. The Wiener - Hopf derivation following Widrow and Stearns (1985) is,

$$e_i = d_i - y_i$$
$$e_i = d_i - X^T{}_i W = d_i - W^T X_i$$

where X and W are the input and the synaptic weight matrix defining the feedforward network. It is easy to show that

$$E(e_i)^2 = E(d_i)^2 + W^T E(X_i X^T{}_i)W - 2E(d_i X^T{}_i)W$$
$$MSE = E(e_i)^2 = E(d_i)^2 + W^T RW - 2P^T W = \text{quadratic }(W)$$
$$\nabla = 2RW - 2P \text{ and } \nabla^2 = R > 0$$
$$\nabla = 0 = 2RW^* - 2P$$
$$W^* = R^{-1}P \text{ and } MSE = E(d_i)^2 - P^T W^*$$

where W* represents the optimal MSE solution. The RBF solution can be easily derived as

$$Y = \Phi(\,||X - m||\,)$$
$$R = E(Y_i Y^T_i) \text{ and } P = E(d_i Y^T_i)$$
$$W^* = R^{-1}P$$

where the kernels *m* are found using k - means, linear vector quantization (LVQ), and/or adaptive mixtures, and Φ are Gaussian weighting functions. The conceptual similarity between the Wiener - Hopf and RBF thus revolves around (i) the inclusion of covariance (2nd order statistics) to describe functional characteristics (as it is the case for most of neural networks) and (ii) solving for the optimal solution of inverse problems using matrix algebra.

4 Network Performance

Hush and Horne (1993) review recent theoretical results concerning the capabilities and limitations of neural networks. Multilayer perceptron (MLP) have been shown capable of approximating arbitrary nonlinear mappings. The practical concerns involving MLP revolve around choosing the network size, complexity of learning, and the ability of the network to generalize. As an example, one can show that the number of hidden layer nodes should be less than the number of training samples in order to avoid overfitting. Theoretical results like the Vapnik-Chervonenkis dimension (VC-dimension) would measure the capacity of the system and give some indication on the size of the network needed to make the generalization error bounded and eventually arbitrary small. Generalization can be improved through complex regularization by incorporating the model complexity as one of the penalty factors driving up the overall error. Such a criterion often referred to as the Minimum Description Length (MDL) stands behind optimization methods labeled as weight sharing and employing pruning of similar weights.

We mention some of the major results for predicting generalization performance before making some obvious statements whose origin comes from signal analysis and information theory. For systems which contain f(x) in their set of implementable functions and are linear in the parameters, Moody (1992) has shown that the corresponding PSE (Predicted mean-Squared-Error) is given by

$$PSE = MSE + 2\sigma^2 N_{eff} / P$$

where MSE is the mean-squared-error experienced during training, N_{eff} is the effective number of parameters in the network (usually much less than the actual number of parameters), P is the number of training samples, and σ^2 is the variance of the noise. The estimate for the variance is

$$\text{est}(\sigma^2) = (MSE)\, P / (P - N_{eff}).$$

Approximation and estimation bounds for artificial networks have been derived by Barron (1994) using complexity regularization and statistical risk. Barron has specifically shown that the mean squared error between the estimated network and a target function f is bound by

$$O\,(C^2_f\ /\ n) + O\,(nd\ \log N\ /\ N)$$

where n is the number of nodes, d is the input dimension of the function, N is the number of training observations, and C_f is the first absolute moment of the Fourier magnitude distribution of f. The two contributions to this total risk are the approximation error and the estimation error. The approximation error refers to the distance between the target function and the closest neural network function of a given architecture while the estimation error refers to the distance between this ideal network function and an estimated network function. For the case $n \sim C_f\ (N\ /\ (d\ \log N))^{1/2}$ the order of the bound on the mean integrated squared error is optimized to be $O\ (C_f\ ((d/N)\ \log N)^{1/2})$. The approximation bounds thus estimate the performance of the network in terms of the spectral characteristics of the data being analyzed.

Minimal background in signal analysis and information theory is required for one to qualitatively confirm Barron's results and to further expand on them for the benefit of gaining insights regarding network performance. The concepts required for this task, those of (i) aliasing and Nyquist frequency, and (ii) uncertainty are defined first and their implication for proper and optimal network design is discussed next.

The Shannon *sampling theorem* sets the minimum rate for sampling a bandwidth-limited continuous signal so it can be uniquely recovered from its samples. The theorem states that the sampling frequency f_N must be at least twice the bandwidth of the signal f_s (i.e., the largest frequency in the signal). The sampling frequency, called the Nyquist frequency, obeys thus the relationship $f_N = 2f_s$. If the sampling theorem is not obeyed, phenomena associated with aliasing would result. This occurs when a continuous signal is sampled at such a rate that the translated versions of its spectrum (created by the sampling process) overlap in the frequency domain. This prevents recovery of the (continuous) original signal from the (discrete) sampled signal. To avoid aliasing, one must thus sample at twice the rate of the highest frequency in the continuous signal, i.e., the sampling should be performed at the Nyquist rate. One way to decrease the sampling (Nyquist) rate is to blur ('smooth') the original signal so its bandwidth decreases. If the large bandwidth was caused by noise then blurring speeds up computation and makes the whole process more robust. If, however, the large bandwidth is due to actual signal information residing at high frequencies, smoothing will cause loss of information, and as a consequence the network performance will degrade. The conclusion to be drawn is that one should first properly analyze the spectral information and thus become able to discriminate 'noise' from 'information' before reliable predictions about future network performance could be made.

The next fundamental concept bearing on network performance comes from information theory and is due to Gabor (1946). The famous by now concept, known as the uncertainty principle, revolves around the resolution of information simultaneously in (2D) spatial and spectral terms, and it is closely related to the choice of optimal lattices of receptive fields (kernel bases) for representing ('decomposing') some underlying signal. As recounted by Daugman (1990), Gabor pointed out that there exists a "quantum principle" for information, which he illustrated through the construction of a spectrogram-like information diagram. The information diagram, a plane whose axes correspond to time (or space) and frequency, must necessarily be grainy, or quantized, in the sense that it is not possible for any signal or filter (and hence any carrier or detector of information) to occupy less than a certain minimal area in this plane. This minimal or quantal area, which reflects the inevitable trade-off between time (space) resolution Δt (Δs) and frequency resolution $\Delta\omega$ and equals the lower bound on their product, is expressed by the uncertainty relations

$$(\Delta t)\,(\Delta\omega) > 1/4\,\pi \quad \text{and} \quad (\Delta s)\,(\Delta\omega) > 1/4\,\pi$$

Gabor noted that Gaussian-modulated complex exponentials offer the optimal way to encode signals (of arbitrary spectral content) or to represent them, if one wished the code primitives to have a well-defined epoch of occurrence in time (space) as well as well-defined spectral identity. The conclusion to be drawn from the above discussion are better understood and visualized if one were to associate time (space) occurrence with localization while frequency change is associated with the speed at which a signal would change. As a consequence it becomes obvious that one can not achieve at the same time optimal signal localization and also optimally track the details of the changes taking place in spatiotemporal signal patterns. The tradeoffs between signal localization and detail have to be resolved using the conjoint spatiotemporal/spectral representation corresponding to the signal one attempts to map and/or track. The tradeoffs are usually resolved by choosing some specific tessellation of the conjoint representation based on constraints such as compactness of representation in analogy with the well known MDL (minimum length description) constraint from information theory. MDL like constraints are implemented using standard optimization methods or, as we will discuss later on, principles of evolutionary computation.

The wavelet base functions (Mallat, 1989), self-similar, spatially localized, and spatial frequency/orientation tuned kernels provide one possible tessellation of the conjoint spatial/spectral signal domain. The corresponding wavelet hierarchical (pyramid) is obtained as the result of orientation-tuned decompositions at a dyadic (powers of two) sequence of scales. The 2D wavelet representation **W** of the function f(x, y) is then

$$W(a_x, a_y, s_x, s_y) = \iint f(x, y)\,(a_x a_y)^{-1/2}\,\Psi^*\,[(x - s_x)(a_x)^{-1}, (y - s_y)(a_y)^{-1}]$$

where Ψ (x, y) is the "mother" wavelet, a_x and a_y are scale parameters, and s_x and s_y are shift parameters. The self-similar Gabor basis functions **g** are a special case of non-orthogonal wavelets, correspond to sinusoids modulated by a

Gaussian, can be easily tuned to any bandwidth (scale) and orientation, and are defined as

$$g(x, y) = \exp \{ -1/2 [(x / \sigma_x)^2 + (y / \sigma_y)^2] \} \exp \{ j2\pi [f_x x + f_y y] \}$$

where $f_x = f_0 \cos\theta$, $f_y = f_0 \sin\theta$, f_0 is spatial frequency, θ is the angle of spatial orientation, $\sigma_x = c/f_x$, $\sigma_y = c/f_y$, and *c* is a scale factor. The frequency (octave) **B** and orientation Ω (radian) half-peak bandwidths of the "daisy petal" Gabor filters are

$$B = \log [(\pi f \lambda \sigma + \alpha) / (\pi f \lambda \sigma + \alpha)]$$

$$\Omega = 2 \tan^{-1} [\alpha /(\pi f \sigma)]$$

where λ the spatial aspect ratio is $\lambda = \sigma_x / \sigma_y$, $\sigma = \sigma_y$, **f** is the radial center frequency, and $\alpha = 2^{-1/2}$ (Bovik et al, 1990).

Yet another conceptual enhancement of wavelets and/or Gabor functions over the standard quadrature mirror filters (QMF) standard implementations is related to the choice of an optimal base of wavelets and it involves adaptation (See also Sect. 5 on evolutionary computation.) Appropriate bases can then be constructed and they include packets based on least entropy (Coiffman et al, 1992), wavelet networks using stochastic gradient descent akin to backpropagation (BP) (Zhang and Benveniste, 1992), and/or functional approximation in terms of dynamic receptive fields (RFs) using radial basis functions (RBFs) (Ng and Lippmann, 1991) and/or Gaussian bar architectures consisting of semilocal and overlapping units (Hartman and Keeler, 1991). RBFs, related to potential functions, implement adaptation as functional approximation as that involved in sparse surface reconstruction. Given some function f(x), its approximation (decomposition in terms of basis functions) or learned prototype is $< c_i, T_i, R >$ and is found as

$$f(x) = \Sigma c_i N(|| x - T_i ||^2_R)$$

where T_i are kernels (bases) of the function to be learned given in terms of parametrized templates across the space of geometrical (and/or topological) variability and weighted by coefficients c_i. **N** is the Gaussian distribution, **R** is the normalization matrix, and the corresponding norm is defined as

$$|| x - T_i ||^2_R = (x - Ti) R' R (x - Ti)$$

5 Evolutionary Computation and Network Performance

The time and space requirements of any cognitive theory are important determinants of that theory plausibility. Complexity satisfaction provides a major source of constraints on the solution of the problem. Much of past analytical and theoretical work has tacitly assumed that the language of continuous mathematics is equivalent to the language of computation. Mathematical modeling, however, is not equivalent to computational modeling. There are still issues of representation, discretization, sampling, numerical stability, and computational complexity (at least) to contend with (McClelland and Rumelhart, 1986).

The standard mode of theorizing is deductive - it assumes that human agents derive their conclusions by logical processes from complete, consistent and well-defined premises in a given problem using mostly static environments. This works well in simple problems, but it breaks down beyond a "problem complexity boundary" where human computational abilities are exceeded or the assumptions of deductive rationality cannot be relied upon. Beyond this problem complexity boundary, and despite problems becoming ill-defined, humans still continue to reason well, but by using induction rather than deduction (Arthur, 1992). Beyond 'problem complexity boundaries' bounded rationality (Simon, 1982) substitutes for optimal solutions, and simulation substitutes for closed analytical solutions.

Artificial worlds (Lane, 1992) known as large scale artifacts represent visualization means for simulating evolving collective behavior when analytical techniques break down. Artificial worlds predict future behavior, check which properties are arbitrary and which are not, and could possibly suggest means for preventing harmful behaviors from emerging. New conjectures can be tested for and the role that information plays in evolution and innovation can be properly assessed. Deductive rigor needs to be replaced by behavioral rigor based on precise and observed actualities of human behavior (Arthur, 1992). As an example, one of the drives behind intelligent behavior and characteristic of complex systems is the striving for a maximal condition, whereby agents "seek" excitation and "avoid" inhibition (Klopf, 1982). As it is the case for the natural habitat the search for optimal solutions using neural networks could then take advantage from using the evolutionary computation (EC) aspect characteristic of artificial worlds in general, and genetic algorithms (GAs) in particular, and employ (cross breeding and mutation as) selection strategies for behavioral optimization and adaptation.

One could approach functional approximation as learning from examples using the analogy to surface reconstruction from sparse data. It leads to minimization problems characterized by high dimensionality (and thus expensive to solve) and solutions possibly trapped into local minima. Genetic algorithms (GAs) (Goldberg, 1989), as examples of evolutionary computation, are nondeterministic methods, similar to stochastic approximations, that can overcome such problems. Genetic algorithms (GAs) work by maintaining a constant-sized population of candidate solutions known as individuals. The power of a genetic algorithm lies in its ability to exploit, in a highly efficient manner, information about a large number of individuals. The search underlying GAs is such that breadth and depth are balanced according to the observed performance of the individuals evaluated so far. By allocating more reproductive occurrences to above average individual solutions, the overall effect is to increase the population's average fitness. GAs are useful to determine appropriate dynamic receptive fields (RFs) and to speed up the derivation of feature models using optimal adaptive feature extraction methods.

Network performance, as discussed earlier, is closely related to the spectral characteristics of the data being analyzed and it involves well known tradeoffs between (i) signal representation and localization, and (ii) faithfulness for signal detail. Network performance can be enhanced only if one were to carry out a careful and synergetic analysis using (a) conjoint spatiotemporal/spectral signal representations, (b) information theory concepts leading to the development of 'optimal' lattices of receptive fields (LRFs), and (c) evolutionary computation for the realization of optimal LRFs.

Conjoint spatiotemporal/spectral signal representations can be derived using decomposition techniques such as Gabor, wavelets, and/or the Wigner distribution for whom the receptive fields, known as kernels are well defined. Alternatively, one could try to derive the optimal kernels suitable for each task according to specific circumstances and constraints. The uncertainty principle holds as much relevance for signal decomposition and representation as MSE - like cost functions hold for much of the neural learning schemes. Searching for optimal kernels and their adaptive mixtures corresponds to the development of evolutionary lattices of receptive fields. The factors determining the RF structure could include maximum preservation of information from input to output, variance maximization, diversity vs. redundancy of mappings as a function of snr, architecture ('wiring') vs synapses ('weights') tradeoffs, and the degree of compactness and (minimum) entropy of the ensuing code (Linsker, 1988). Alternatively, one could view layered feedforward networks as multistage encoders and assess the performance of both the hidden and output nodes using as a measure the conditional class entropy (Bichsel and Seitz, 1989). As demonstrated by Linsker (1988) Hebbian learning tends to conserve information from the input layer to further layers. Bichsel and Seitz point out, however, that in most problems one is not interested in the complete information of the input patterns, but rather would be interested and benefit most from separating this information from the information concerning the class of the patterns. Therefore, the conditional entropy with respect to the class of the input pattern is a much better performance measure than the conditional entropy with respect to the whole information content in the input patterns and it follows that Hebbian learning is not, in general, optimum.

The overall goal, when one is concerned with developing some optimal network to faithfully represent some given signal, should be to establish 'optimal dictionaries' in analogy to optimal bases and kernel functions (Mallat and Zhang, 1992) using 'matching pursuit' techniques similar to projection pursuit strategies (Friedman, 1987) from statistics. Tracking signals is then similar to deriving optimal but compact functional mappings and the choice of kernels could be done using techniques characteristics of evolutionary computation. Furthermore, the same evolutionary computation could also facilitate local and global tradeoffs to be made and lead to hybrid but unified encoding schemes such as the wavenets (Zhang and Benveniste, 1992) to result if one were to establish formal links between network coefficients and some signal ('wavelet') transform for optimal mapping implementation.

Adaptive analysis schemes suitable to encode and track spatiotemporal patterns of change using the wavelet and/or Gabor signal representations are also motivated by the concept of dynamic receptive fields (RFs). The overall concern is to assess the contributions that adaptive techniques can make to optimal signal representation and that the costs involved are not prohibitive. One should then select the waveforms covering the time-frequency domain that match best the underlying signal structures. For signals as those corresponding to time-varying patterns and thus characterized by a wide range of different spatiotemporal-frequency localizations, adaptive spatiotemporal - frequency transforms are required. Such adaptive transforms can draw much benefit from the availability of suitable "dictionaries" of RFs for compact signal encoding. A signal is said then to be coherent with respect to a dictionary, if most of its energy can be decomposed using only a few elements that belong to the dictionary.

6 Selective Learning Algorithms

The point of departure herein is the recent paper by Bottou and Vapnik (1992) on local learning algorithms. As the training data is seldom evenly distributed in the input space one attempts to locally adjust the capacity of the training system to the properties of the training set in each area of the input space. Uneven data distributions lead to (learning and) classification algorithms that lack in rejecting (i) by ambiguity when there is too much data to consider, and in rejecting (ii) by lack of confidence in the decision boundaries when not enough training examples are available.

Bottou and Vapnik suggest then the following straightforward algorithm for each testing pattern: (a) select the *few* training examples located in the vicinity of the testing pattern; (b) train a neural network with only these few examples; and (c) apply the resulting network to the testing pattern. It is obvious that the power of the algorithm rests in an appropriate choice of some suitable metric for proximity and on how many examples one should actually consider for each pattern using such a metric. One can benefit from studying robust statistics regarding, amongst other things, outliers and consensus methods, or one can consider the arguments advanced by Bottou and Vapnik regarding the existing tradeoffs between locality, capacity, and the number of available training examples. The capacity ('VC-dimension') stands for the maximum number of training examples which can be learned without error for all possible 'binary' labelings. The VC-dimension is in some cases simply given by the number of free parameters of the classifier, but in most practical cases it is quite difficult to determine it analytically. It comes without surprise that the 'local capacity' should match the density of training examples. Guyon et al (1992) address this very problem and have suggested the use of structural risk minimization for tuning the capacity of the classifier to the available amount of training data.

As Bottou and Vapnik go further to elaborate, 'a high capacity learning system is able to model accurately and with high confidence the parts of the decision boundary that are well described by the training examples. In these areas, both rejection and misclassification are rare. The same system, however, produces unreliable high confidence decision boundaries in the poorly sampled areas of the pattern space: rejections are rare, but misclassifications are frequent. Alternatively, a low capacity learning system builds low confidence boundaries in the poorly sampled areas of the pattern space. This system rejects more atypical patterns, but reduces the number of misclassifications. Unfortunately, such a device performs poorly in the well sampled areas. Unable to take profit of the abundant data, it builds poor decision boundaries, and rejects almost everything, because everything looks too ambiguous'. The conclusions drawn suggest that backpropagation (BP) is a nonlocal algorithm, with a comparatively high capacity. BP performance could be improved by introducing locality and by reducing capacity. The kNN classifier is an extremely local algorithm, with a very low capacity. Reducing its locality while increasing its capacity should improve the resulting performance (of the kNN).

One can expand on the analysis provided by Bottou and Vapnik and improve on the performance of learning algorithms when the concept of locality goes beyond the mere distribution in the input space and includes also 'semantic' relatedness based on similarity measures. The motivation for such an expanded concept of locality comes from perception where one can benefit from using active, selective, and functional processing. Enhanced perceptual performance is thus achieved when one is 'active' in deciding 'where' to look, 'selective' in deciding for 'what' to look, and 'functional' when associating task and process. We show next how known relationships between distributed associative memories (DAMs) and regression analysis lead to local, robust, and selective neural processing, and also how one can develop statistically significant (vigilance and) rejection criteria.

The distributed associative memory (DAM) model (Kohonen, 1988) assumes that there are *n* (paired) classes of *m* dimensional ('feature model') vectors that have to be learned by association. This can be written as

$$Ms_i = r_i \qquad \text{for } i = 1, 2, ..., n$$

where s_i and r_i denote the *ith* stimulus and response vectors, respectively. One then seeks to learn the memory matrix *M* such that when the *kth* stimulus target vector s_k is projected onto the space defined by *M* the resulting projection will be the response (identity) vector r_k. Specifically, one has to solve

$$MS = R$$

where *S* and *R* are the corresponding stimulus and response matrices, respectively. A unique solution for the above equation does not necessarily exist for any arbitrary group of associations. The number of associations *n* is usually much less than *m*, the dimension of the vectors. Consequently, the system of equations is underconstrained. The constraint used to seek for a unique matrix M is that of minimizing the norm $||MS - R||^2$ and yields

$$M = RS^+$$

where S^+ is known as the Moore-Penrose generalized inverse (GI) of S (Kohonen, 1988).

The recall operation projects an unknown target vector s onto the memory space M. The projection yields the response vector r,

$$r = Ms = R(S^+s)$$

If the memorized stimulus targets are independent, and the unknown stimulus target s is one of the memorized targets s_k, then the recalled target will be the associated response vector r_k. If the memorized stimulus targets are dependent, then the response recalled by one of the memorized stimulus targets will contain the associated response target, and some *cross-talk* from the other stored response targets. The recall can be viewed as the weighted sum of the response vectors. The recall, using a linear squares classifier, begins by assigning weights according to how well the unknown stimulus vector matches each of the memorized stimuli vectors. The response vectors are multiplied by the corresponding weights (given as S^+s) and summed together to build the recall. The recall is usually dominated by the memorized response target that is closest in representation to the target observed. The DAM provides for interactions between stored associations and thus allows for generalization, quite useful when facing stimuli targets the system has not been trained with beforehand.

The DAM allows for incremental learning and exhibits fault-tolerant behavior with respect to both local and/or internal memory damage (Wechsler, 1990). Furthermore, the recall, as explained above, improves on the signal to noise ratio (snr). Consequently, for the autoassociative case, when a noisy version of a memorized target is presented, the recall is improved by a factor corresponding to the ratio of the number of memorized stimuli vectors n and the dimensionality of the stimulus vector m (Stiles and Denq, 1985). The error correction process can be explained by noting that the DAM is the orthogonal projection matrix for the set of stimulus vectors. The noise vector, if random, will be projected onto the space spanned by the n memorized stimulus-response pairs. The recall, however, is dominated by that response vector that is closest to the unknown stimulus vector. Consequently, the noise corresponds mostly to that axis the recall belongs to, and the amount of noise recalled is thus reduced. The advantages accrued from using DAM include incremental learning and iterative solutions. Incremental learning facilitates learning over time, parallels human performance, and does not require that all the training data is available at once, while iterative (recursive solutions) rather than closed-form solutions facilitate computation.

The distributed associative memory (DAM) realizes thus optimal, in the least-square error (LSE) sense, associative mappings corresponding to classical conditioning. The DAM has been shown to be quite successful in the recognition of noisy and occluded 2D objects, and also in the implementation of efficient and robust indexing techniques for data retrieval. An augmented DAM model (Polzleitner and Wechsler, 1990), using existing relationships between least-square error (LSE) approximation and estimation techniques such as regression analysis, provides for local, robust, and selective neural processing, and also leads to statistically significant (vigilance and) rejection criteria. The selectivity displayed by DAMs during the recall stage, and corresponding to the expanded concept of locality, is based on a sound statistical theory of rejection. The availability of the reject option, the prerequisite for novelty detection, leads to (preattentive and) iterative identification strategies, and eventually enables the memory to decide whether the stimulus is known or novel (unknown).

The relationships between DAM and regression analysis responsible for selective memory recall are quite simple. Assume the autoassociative case where $R = S$ so the build-up memory phase corresponds to $M = SS^+$. The recall phase is thus given by

$$x' = S\,(S^+ x) = Sy$$

and one immediately recognizes $y = (y_1, y_2, .., y_n)$ as regression coefficients (y_k). The significance of regression coefficients can be tested using the student t - test. One can then be selective in (iteratively) discarding from further consideration those classes whose coefficients are statistically insignificant. Such selectivity of recall allows the classifier to decide on those *few* patterns needed to explain and eventually classify the input. The classifier rejects the input pattern as unknown when all the regression coefficients are found insignificant based on a sound statistical measure R^2 known as the coefficient of determination. The coefficient of determination is defined as

$$R^2 = [\,\mathrm{var}(x) - RSS] / \mathrm{var}(x) \quad \text{and} \quad RSS = E(\,||\, x - x' \,||\,)$$

Bias (and cross-talk) due to varying signal averages and noise for stimuli vectors can be eliminated using augmented vectors $S' = [S; 1]$. Note that both normalization and rejection are achieved using a sound statistical theory and that there is no need for arbitrary vigilance factors. The DAM displays selectivity by iteratively filtering out unlikely (model) responses from the recall memory.

7 Conclusions

We discussed existing analogies to connectionism and neural learning from several scientific disciplines involved with signal representation and optimization, statistical pattern recognition, spectral analysis and information theory, and adaptive systems and control. The case was made (a) that many fundamental results in neural networks were already available if one would have surveyed related disciplines and refrain from 'reinventing the wheel', and (b) that further advances in neural networks research thus require careful comparative studies. The most important result established in this chapter is the significance of proper sampling (corresponding to 'Nyquist frequency') and the tradeoffs between signal localization and detail of representation (corresponding to the uncertainty principle from signal processing and information theory) on overall network performance. As our discussion has drawn also from neurosciences and evolution, it should become obvious that neural modeling should be augmented and it should include hierarchical and hybrid learning scheme whose development could be achieved using evolutionary principles of computation.

References

Arthur, W. B. (1992) On learning and adaptation in the economy. TR 92-07-038, Santa Fe Institute.

Barron, A. R. (1992) Neural net approximation. *Proc. 7th Yale Workshop on Adaptive and Learning Systems.*

Barron, A. R. (1994), Approximation and estimation bounds for artificial neural networks. *Machine Learning* (preprint).

Bichsel, M. and Seitz, P. (1989) Minimum class entropy: A maximum information approach to layered networks. *Neural Networks*, **2**, 133-141.

Bovik, A. C., M. Clark, and W. S. Geisler (1990) Multichannel texture analysis using localized spatial filters. *IEEE Trans. on Pattern Analysis and Machine Intelligence*, **12**(1), 55-73.

Bottou, L. and Vapnik, V (1992) Local learning algorithms. *Neural Computation*, **4**, 888-900.

Coiffman, R., Y. Meyer, and V. Wickerhauser (1992) Wavelet analysis and signal processing. In *Wavelets and Their Applications*, ed. M. B. Ruskai, 453-470, Jones and Bartlett Publishers, Boston.

Daugman, J. G. (1990) Brain metaphor and brain theory. In *Computational Neuroscience*, ed E. L. Schwartz, 9-18, MIT Press.

Daugman, J. G. (1990) An information-theoretic view of analog representation in striate cortex. In *Computational Neuroscience*, ed E. L. Schwartz, 403-424, MIT Press.

Edelman, G. (1987) *Neural Darwinism*. Basic Books.

Freeman, W. J. (1992) Tutorial on neurobiology: From single neurons to brain chaos. *Int. Journal of Bifurcation and Chaos*, **2**(3), 451-482.

Friedman, J. H. (1987) Exploratory projection pursuit. *Journal of American Statistical Association*, **82**, 249-266.

Gabor, D. (1946) Theory of communication. *Journal of IEEE*, **93**, 429-459.

Geman, S., E. Bienenstock, and R. Doursat (1992) Neural networks and the bias/variance dilemma. *Neural Computation*, **5**, 1-58.

Goldberg, D. E. (1989) *Genetic Algorithms in Search, Optimization, and Machine Learning*. Addison-Wesley.

Guyon, I., V. N. Vapnik, B. E. Boser, and S. A. Solla (1992) Structural risk minimization for character recognition. In *Advances in Neural Information Processing Systems* **4**, eds J. E. Moody, S. J. Hanson, and R. P. Lippmann, 471-479, Morgan Kaufmann, Denver.

Hartman, E. and J. Keeler (1991) Predicting the future: Advantages of semilocal units. *Neural Computation*, **3**, 566-578.

Hecht-Nielsen, R (1990) *Neurocomputing*. Addison-Wesley.

Hush, D. R. and Horne, B. (1993) Progress in neural networks: What's new since Lippman ? *IEEE Signal Processing Magazine* **1**, 8- 39.

Klopf, A. H. (1982) *The Hedonistic Neuron. A Theory of Memory, Learning, and Intelligence*. Harper and Row, New York.

Kohonen, T. (1988) *Self-Organization and Associative Memories*. Springer-Verlag.

Lane, D. A. (1992) Artificial worlds and economics. TR 92-09-048, Sanata Fe Institute.

Linsker, R. (1988) Self-organization in a perceptual neural network. *Computer*, **21**, 105-117.

Mallat, S. (1989) A theory for multiresolution signal decomposition: the wavelet representation. *IEEE Trans. on Pattern Analysis and Machine Intelligence*, **11**(7), 674-693.

Mallat, S. and Z. Zhang (1992) Matching pursuits with time-frequency dictionaries. TR 619, Computer Science Department, New York University.

McClelland, J. L., D. E. Rumelhart, and the PDP Research Group (Eds.) (1986) *Parallel Distributed Processing*. MIT Press

Moody, J. E. (1991) Note on generalization, regularization, and architecture selection in nonlinera learning systems. In *Neural Networks for Signal Processing: Proc. of the 1991 IEEE Workshop*, eds B. H. Juang, S.Y. Kung, and C. A. Kamm, 1-10, IEEE Press.

Moody, J. E. (1992) The effective number of parameters: An analysis of generalization and regularization in nonlinera learning systems. In *Advances in Neural Information Processing Systems* **4**, eds J. E. Moody, S. J. Hanson, and R. P. Lippmann, 847-854, Morgan Kaufmann, Denver.

Ng, K. and R. P. Lippmann (1991) A comparative study of the practical characteristics of neural networks and conventional pattern classifiers. TR 894, MIT Lincoln Lab.

Penrose, R. (1989) *The Emperor's New Mind*. Oxford University Press.

Polzleitner, W. and H. Wechsler (1990) Selective and focused invariant recognition using distributed associative memories (DAMs). *IEEE Trans. on Pattern Analysis and Machine Intelligence*, **12**(6), 809-814.

Pribram, K. H. (1991) *Brain and Perception*. Lawrence Erlbaum Associates.

Richard, M. D. and R. P. Lippmann (1991) Neural network classifiers estimate Bayesian *a posteriori* probabilities. *Neural Computation*, **3**, 461-483.

Simon, H. (1982) *The Science of the Artificial*. MIT Press.

Stiles, G. S. and D. L. Denq (1985) On the effect of noise on the Moore-Penrose generalized inverse associative memory. *IEEE Trans. on Pattern Analysis and Machine Intelligence*, **7**(3), 358-360.

Wechsler, H. (1990) *Computational Vision*. Academic Press.

Widrow, B. and S. D. Stearns (1985) *Adaptive Signal Processing*. Prentice-Hall.

Zhang, Q. and A. Benveniste (1992) Wavelet networks. *IEEE Trans. on Neural Networks* **3**(6), 889-898.

Self-Organizing Neural Networks for Supervised and Unsupervised Learning and Prediction

Gail A. Carpenter and Stephen Grossberg

Center for Adaptive Systems and
Department of Cognitive and Neural Systems,
Boston University, 111 Cummington Street,
Boston, Massachusetts 02215 USA

Abstract. A neural network architecture for fast, stable, incremental learning of recognition categories and multidimensional maps is described. The architecture, called fuzzy ARTMAP, achieves a synthesis of fuzzy logic and Adaptive Resonance Theory (ART) neural networks. Fuzzy ARTMAP realizes a Minimax Learning Rule that conjointly minimizes predictive error and maximizes code compression. The system automatically learns a minimal number of recognition categories, or "hidden units", to meet accuracy criteria, and the final code can include both fine and coarse categories. At each learning stage, system weights may be translated into a set of if-then rules that characterize the decision making process. Prediction is improved by training the system several times using different orderings of the input set, then voting on the outcomes. ART and ARTMAP networks are being applied to problems such as medical prediction, airplane design, electrocardiogram analysis, seismic recognition, adaptive software, and radar scene analysis.

1 Introduction: Autonomous Learning, Recognition, and Prediction in a Nonstationary World

As we move freely through the world, we can attend to both familiar and novel objects, and can rapidly learn to recognize, test hypotheses about, and learn to name novel objects without unselectively disrupting our memories of familiar objects. This article describes a self-organizing neural network architecture—called a fuzzy ARTMAP—that is capable of fast, yet stable, on-line recognition learning, hypothesis testing, and adaptive naming in response to an arbitrary stream of analog or binary input patterns.

The fuzzy ARTMAP architecture combines a set of computational properties (Table 1) whose unavailability in alternative approaches have limited their ability to function autonomously in a rapidly changing world. These properties enable fuzzy ARTMAP to autonomously learn, recognize, and make predictions about:

AUTONOMOUS LEARNING AND CONTROL IN A NONSTATIONARY WORLD

Need one system that reconciles conflicting properties -
a system that can autonomously learn about:

(A) RARE EVENTS
- need FAST learning

(B) LARGE NONSTATIONARY DATABASES
- need STABLE learning

(C) MORPHOLOGICALLY VARIABLE EVENTS
- need MULTIPLE SCALES of generalization (fine/coarse)

(D) ONE-TO-MANY AND MANY-TO-ONE RELATIONSHIPS
- need categorization, naming, and expert knowledge

To realize these properties, ARTMAP systems:

(E) PAY ATTENTION
- ignore irrelevant data

(F) TEST HYPOTHESES
- discover predictive constraints hidden in data streams

(G) CHOOSE BEST ANSWERS
- quickly select globally optimal solution at any stage of learning

(H) CALIBRATE CONFIDENCE
- measure on-line how well a hypothesis matches the data

(I) DISCOVER RULES
- identify transparent IF-THEN relations at each learning stage

(J) SCALE
- preserve all desirable properties in arbitrarily large problems

Table 1.

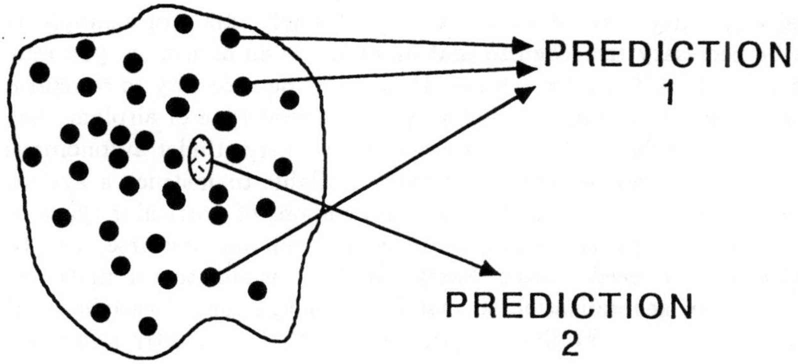

Figure 1. Fuzzy ARTMAP can learn a different prediction for a rare event than for all the similar events that surround it.

(A) Rare Events

A successful autonomous agent must be able to learn about rare events that have important consequences, even if these rare events are similar to a surrounding cloud of frequent events that have different consequences (Figure 1). *Fast learning* is needed to pick up a rare event on the fly. For example, a rare medical case may be the harbinger of a new epidemic. A faint astronomical signal may signify important consequences for theories of the Universe. A slightly different chemical assay may predict the biological activity of a new drug. Many traditional learning schemes use a form of slow learning that tends to average over similar event occurrences. In contrast, fuzzy ARTMAP can rapidly learn a rare event that predicts different consequences than a cloud of similar events in which it is embedded.

(B) Large Nonstationary Data Bases

Rare events typically occur in a nonstationary environment whose event statistics may change rapidly and unexpectedly through time. Individual events may also occur with variable probabilities and durations, and arbitrarily large numbers of events may need to be processed. Each of these factors tends to destabilize the learning process within traditional algorithms. New learning in such algorithms tends to unselectively wash away the memory traces of old, but still useful, knowledge. Using such an algorithm, for example, learning a new face could erase the memory of a parent's face. More generally, learning a new type of expertise could erase the memory of previous expert knowledge. Fuzzy ARTMAP contains a *self-stabilizing memory* that permits accumulating knowledge to be stored reliably in response to arbitrarily many events in a nonstationary environment under incremental learning conditions, until the algorithm's full memory capacity, which can be chosen arbitrarily large, is exhausted.

(C) Morphologically Variable Types of Events

In many environments, some information is coarsely defined whereas other information is precisely characterized. Otherwise expressed, the morphological variability of the data may change through time. For example, it may just be necessary to recognize that an object is an animal, or you may need to confirm that it is your own pet. It may just be necessary to recognize that an object is an airplane, or that it is a particular type of airplane that is flown for a particular purpose by a particular country. Under autonomous learning conditions, no teacher is typically available to instruct a system about how coarse its generalization, or compression, of particular types of data should be. Multiple scales of generalization, from fine to coarse, need to be available on an as-needed basis. Fuzzy ARTMAP is able to automatically adjust its scale of generalization to match the morphological variability of the data. It embodies a Minimax Learning Rule that conjointly *min*imizes predictive error and *max*imizes generalization using only information that is locally available under incremental learning conditions in a nonstationary environment.

(D) Many-to-One and One-to-Many Relationships

Many-to-one learning takes two forms: categorization and naming (Figure 2). For example, during categorization of printed letter fonts, many similar exemplars of the same printed letter may establish a single recognition category, or compressed representation. Different printed letter fonts or written exemplars of the letter may establish additional categories. Each of these categories carries out a many-to-one map of exemplar into category. During naming, all of the categories that represent the same letter may be associatively mapped into the letter name, or prediction. This is a second, distinct, type of many-to-one map. There need be no relationship whatsoever between the visual features that define a printed letter A and a written letter A, yet both categories may need to be assigned the same name due to cultural, not visual, reasons.

One-to-many learning is used to build up expert knowledge about an object or event (Figure 3). A single visual image of a particular animal may, for example, lead to learning that predicts: animal, dog, beagle, and my dog "Rover". A computerized record of a patient's medical check-up may lead to a series of predictions about the patient's health. A chemical assay of a sample of coal or petroleum may lead to many predictions about its uses as an energy source or structural material. In many learning algorithms, the attempt to learn more than one prediction about an event leads to unselective forgetting of previously learned predictions, for the same reason that these algorithms become unstable in response to nonstationary data.

2 The Inadequacy of Error-Based Learning

Error-based learning systems, including the popular back propagation algorithm [1–3], find it difficult, if not impossible, to achieve any of the computational goals (A)–(D). Back propagation compares its actual prediction with a correct prediction and uses the error to change adaptive weights in a

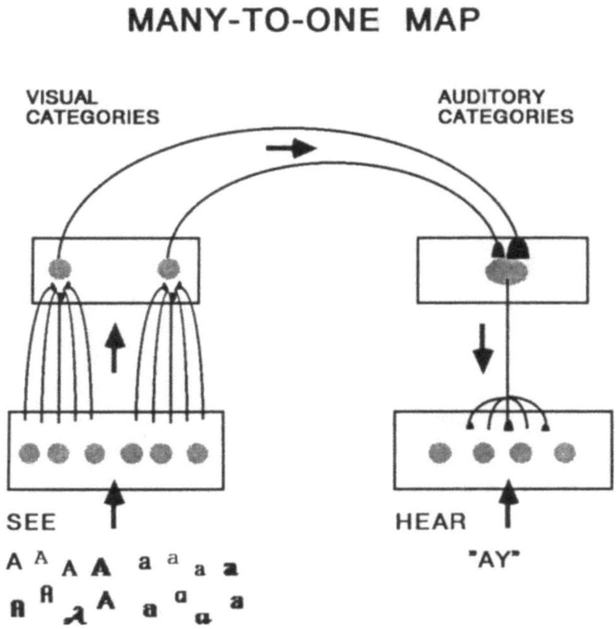

Figure 2. Many-to-one learning combines categorization of many exemplars into one category, and labelling of many categories with the same name.

direction that is error-reducing. Fast learning would zero the error on each learning trial, and therefore cause massive forgetting. Statistical changes in the environment drag the adaptive weights away from their estimates of the previous environment. Longer event durations zero the error more, and thereby destabilize previous memories for the same reason that fast learning does. The selection of a fixed number of hidden units tends to fix a uniform level of generalization. Error-based learning also tends to force forgetting of previous predictions under one-to-many learning conditions, because the present correct prediction treats all previously learned predictions as errors. Ratcliff [4] has noted, moreover, that back propagation fails to simulate human cognitive data about learning and forgetting.

3 Attentive Hypothesis Testing, Match-Based Learning, and Confidence Estimation

Fuzzy ARTMAP exhibits the properties (A)–(D) of Section 2 because it implements a qualitatively different set of heuristics than error-based learning systems. These heuristics are embodied in the following types of processes:

(E) Pay Attention

A Fuzzy ARTMAP system can learn top-down expectations (also called primes, or queries) that can bias the system to ignore masses of irrelevant

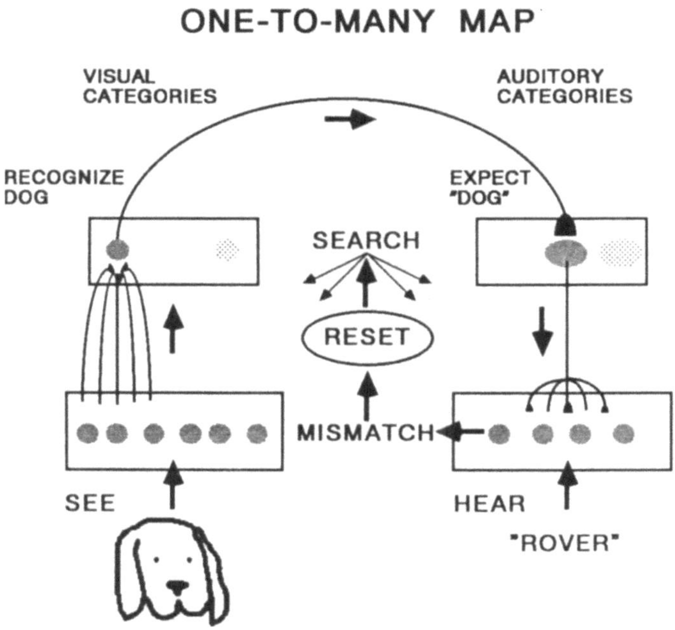

Figure 3. One-to-many learning enables one input vector to be associated with many output vectors. If the system predicts an output that is disconfirmed at a given stage of learning, the predictive error drives a memory search for a new category to associate with the new prediction, without degrading its previous knowledge about the input vector.

data. A large mismatch between a bottom-up input vector and a top-down expectation can drive an adaptive memory search that carries out

(F) Hypothesis Testing and Match-Based Learning

The system actively searches for recognition categories, or hypotheses, whose top-down expectations provide an acceptable match to bottom-up data. The top-down expectation focuses attention upon, and binds, that cluster of input features that it deems to be relevant. If no available category, or hypothesis, provides a good enough match, then selection and learning of a new category and top-down expectation is automatically initiated. When the search discovers a category that provides an acceptable match, the system locks into an attentive resonance whereby the input exemplar refines the adaptive weights of the category based on any new information that it contains.

Thus the fuzzy ARTMAP system carries out match-based learning, rather than error-based learning. A category modifies its previous learning only if its top-down expectation matches the input vector well enough to risk changing its defining characteristics. Otherwise, hypothesis testing selects a new category on which to base learning of a novel event.

(G) Choose Globally Best Answer

In many learning algorithms, as learning proceeds, local minima or less than optimal solutions are selected to represent the data. In fuzzy ARTMAP, at any stage of learning, an input exemplar first selects the category whose top-down expectation provides the globally best match. A top-down expectation hereby acts as a *prototype* for the class of all the input exemplars that its category represents. After learning self-stabilizes, every input directly selects the globally best category without any search. Before learning self-stabilizes, familiar events gain direct access to the globally best category without any search, even if they are interspersed with unfamiliar events that drive hypothesis testing for better matching categories.

(H) Calibrate Confidence

A confidence measure, called *vigilance*, calibrates how well an exemplar matches the prototype that it selects. Otherwise expressed, vigilance measures how well the chosen hypothesis matches the data. If vigilance is low, even poor matches are accepted. Many different exemplars can then be incorporated into one category, so compression and generalization by that category are high. If vigilance is high, then even good matches may be rejected, and hypothesis testing may be initiated to select a new category. In this case, few exemplars activate the same category, so compression and generalization are low. A very high vigilance can select a unique category for a rare event that predicts an outcome different from that of any of the similar exemplars that surround it.

The Minimax Learning Rule is realized by adjusting the vigilance parameter in response to a predictive error. Vigilance is increased just enough to initiate hypothesis testing to discover a better category, or hypothesis, with which to match the data. In this way, a minimum amount of generalization is sacrificed to correct the error. This process is called *match tracking* because vigilance tracks the degree of match between exemplar and prototype in response to a predictive error.

(I) Rule Extraction

At any stage of learning, a user can translate the state of a fuzzy ARTMAP system into an algorithmic set of rules. From this perspective, fuzzy ARTMAP can be interpreted as a type of self-organizing expert system. These rules evolve as the system is exposed to new inputs. This feature is particularly important in applications such as medical diagnosis from a large database of patient records. Table 2 summarizes some medical and other benchmark studies that compare the performance of fuzzy ARTMAP with alternative recognition and prediction models. One of these benchmarks is summarized below. Others are described in [5–6].

(J) Properties Scale

One of the most serious deficiencies of many Artificial Intelligence algorithms is that their desirable properties tend to break down as small toy problems are generalized to large-scale problems. In contrast, all of the de-

ARTMAP BENCHMARK STUDIES

1. Medical database - mortality following coronary bypass grafting (CABG) surgery

    FUZZY ARTMAP significantly outperforms:

    - LOGISTIC REGRESSION
    - ADDITIVE MODEL
    - BAYESIAN ASSIGNMENT
    - CLUSTER ANALYSIS
    - CLASSIFICATION AND REGRESSION TREES
    - EXPERT PANEL-DERIVED SICKNESS SCORES
    - PRINCIPAL COMPONENT ANALYSIS

2. Mushroom database

    DECISION TREES (90-95 % correct)

    ARTMAP (100% correct)
    Training set an order of magnitude smaller

3. Letter recognition database

    GENETIC ALGORITHM (82% correct)

    FUZZY ARTMAP (96% correct)

4. Circle-in-the-Square task

    BACK PROPAGATION (90% correct)

    FUZZY ARTMAP (99.5% correct)

5. Two-Spiral task

    BACK PROPAGATION (10,000 - 20,000 training epochs)

    FUZZY ARTMAP (1-5 training epochs)

Table 2.

sirable properties of fuzzy ARTMAP scale to arbitrarily large problems. It must be emphasized, however, that fuzzy ARTMAP solves a particular type of problem. It is not intended to solve all problems of learning or intelligence. The categorization and prediction problems that ARTMAP does handle well are, however, core problems in many intelligent systems, and have been technology bottlenecks for many alternative approaches.

A summary is now given of Adaptive Resonance Theory, or ART, networks for unsupervised learning and categorization. Then a connection between certain ART systems and fuzzy logic is noted. Fuzzy ART networks for unsupervised learning and categorization are next described. Finally, fuzzy ART modules are combined into a fuzzy ARTMAP system that is capable of supervised learning, recognition, and prediction. A benchmark comparison of fuzzy ARTMAP with genetic algorithms is then summarized.

4 A Review of Unsupervised ART Systems

Adaptive Resonance Theory, or ART, was introduced as a theory of human cognitive information processing [7–8]. The theory has since led to an evolving series of real-time neural network models for unsupervised category learning and pattern recognition. These models are capable of learning stable recognition categories in response to arbitrary input sequences with either fast or slow learning. Model families include ART 1 [9], which can stably learn to categorize binary input patterns presented in an arbitrary order; ART 2 [10], which can stably learn to categorize either analog or binary input patterns presented in an arbitrary order; and ART 3 [11], which can carry out parallel search, or hypothesis testing, of distributed recognition codes in a multi-level network hierarchy. Variations of these models adapted to the demands of individual applications have been developed by a number of authors.

Figure 4 illustrates one example from the family of ART 1 models, and Figure 5 illustrates a typical ART search cycle. Level F_1 in Figure 4 contains a network of nodes, each of which represents a particular combination of sensory features. Level F_2 contains a network of nodes that represent recognition codes which are selectively activated by patterns of activation across F_1. The activities of nodes in F_1 and F_2 are also called short term memory (STM) traces. STM is the type of memory that can be rapidly reset without leaving an enduring trace. For example, it is easy to reset the STM of a list of numbers that a person has just heard once by distracting the person with an unexpected event. STM is distinct from LTM, or long term memory, which is the type of memory that we usually ascribe to learning. For example, we do not forget our parent's names when we are distracted by an unexpected event.

As shown in Figure 5a, an input vector **I** registers itself as a pattern **X** of activity across level F_1. The F_1 output vector **S** is then transmitted through the multiple converging and diverging adaptive filter pathways emanating

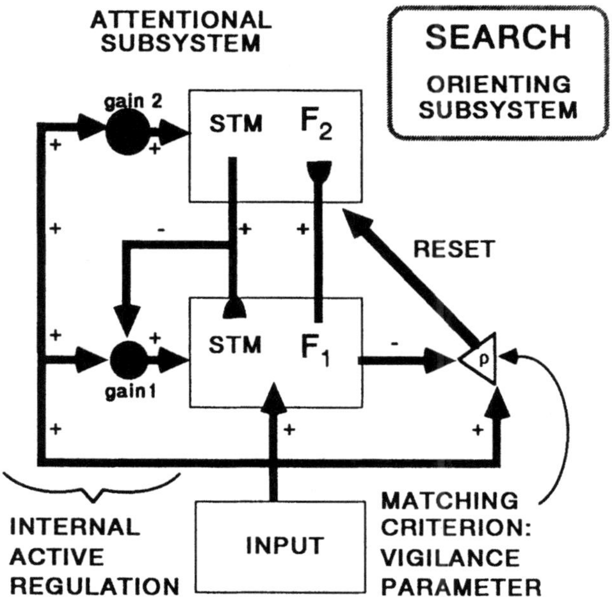

Figure 4. Typical ART 1 neural network [9].

from F_1. This transmission event multiplies the vector **S** by a matrix of adaptive weights, or LTM traces, to generate a net input vector **T** to level F_2. The internal competitive dynamics of F_2 contrast-enhance vector **T**. A compressed activity vector **Y** is thereby generated across F_2. In ART 1, the competition is tuned so that the F_2 node that receives the maximal $F_1 \rightarrow F_2$ input is selected. Only one component of **Y** is nonzero after this choice takes place. Activation of such a winner-take-all node defines the category, or symbol, of the input pattern **I**. Such a category represents all the inputs **I** that maximally activate the corresponding node. So far, these are the rules of a self-organizing feature map, also called competitive learning, self-organizing feature maps, or learned vector quantization. Such models were developed by Grossberg [12–16] and von der Malsburg [17, 18]. Cohen and Grossberg [19–20], Grossberg and Kuperstein [21], and Kohonen [22] have applied them extensively to problems in speech recognition and adaptive sensory-motor control, among others.

Activation of an F_2 node may be interpreted as "making a hypothesis" about an input **I**. When **Y** is activated, it generates an output vector **U** that is sent top-down through the second adaptive filter. After multiplication by the adaptive weight matrix of the top-down filter, a net vector **V** inputs to F_1 (Figure 5b). Vector **V** plays the role of a learned top-down expectation.

Activation of **V** by **Y** may be interpreted as "testing the hypothesis" **Y**, or "reading out the category prototype" **V**. The ART 1 network is designed to match the "expected prototype" **V** of the category against the active input pattern, or exemplar, **I**. Nodes that are activated by **I** are suppressed if they do not correspond to large LTM traces in the prototype pattern **V**. Thus F_1 features that are not "expected" by **V** are suppressed. Expressed in a different way, the matching process may change the F_1 activity pattern **X** by suppressing activation of all the feature detectors in **I** that are not "confirmed" by hypothesis **Y**. The resultant pattern $\mathbf{X}^*$ encodes the cluster of features in **I** that the network deems relevant to the hypothesis **Y** based upon its past experience. Pattern $\mathbf{X}^*$ encodes the pattern of features to which the network "pays attention".

If the expectation **V** is close enough to the input **I**, then a state of *resonance* develops as the attentional focus takes hold. The pattern $\mathbf{X}^*$ of attended features reactivates hypothesis **Y** which, in turn, reactivates $\mathbf{X}^*$. The network locks into a resonant state through the mutual positive feedback that dynamically links $\mathbf{X}^*$ with **Y**. The resonant state persists long enough for learning to occur; hence the term *adaptive resonance* theory. ART systems learn prototypes, rather than exemplars, because the attended feature vector $\mathbf{X}^*$, rather than the input **I** itself, is learned.

This attentive matching process is realized by combining three different types of inputs at level F_1 (Figure 4): bottom-up inputs, top-down expectations, and attentional gain control signals. The attentional gain control channel sends the same signal to all F_1 nodes; it is a "nonspecific", or modulatory, channel. Attentive matching obeys a 2/3 Rule [9]: an F_1 node can be fully activated only if two of the three input sources that converge upon it send positive signals at a given time. The 2/3 Rule shows how an ART system can be "primed" to expect a subsequent event that may or may not occur. A top-down expectation activates to subthreshold levels the F_1 nodes in its prototype. None of the nodes are activated well enough to generate output signals in the absence of their "second third" of the 2/3 Rule. They are nonetheless "primed", or ready, to fire rapidly and vigorously if a bottom-up input does match their prototype well enough. Thus ART systems are "intentional" or "goal-oriented" systems in the sense that their expectations can be primed to selectively seek out data in which they are interested.

The 2/3 Rule also allows an ART system to react to inputs in the absence of prior priming, since a bottom-up input directly activates its target F_1 features and indirectly activates them via the nonspecific gain control channel to satisfy the 2/3 Rule (Figure 5a). After the input instates itself at F_1, leading to selection of a hypothesis **Y** and a top-down expectation **V**, the 2/3 Rule ensures that only those F_1 nodes that are confirmed by the expectation can remain active in STM.

The criterion of an acceptable 2/3 Rule match is defined by a dimensionless parameter called *vigilance*. Vigilance weighs how close the input exem-

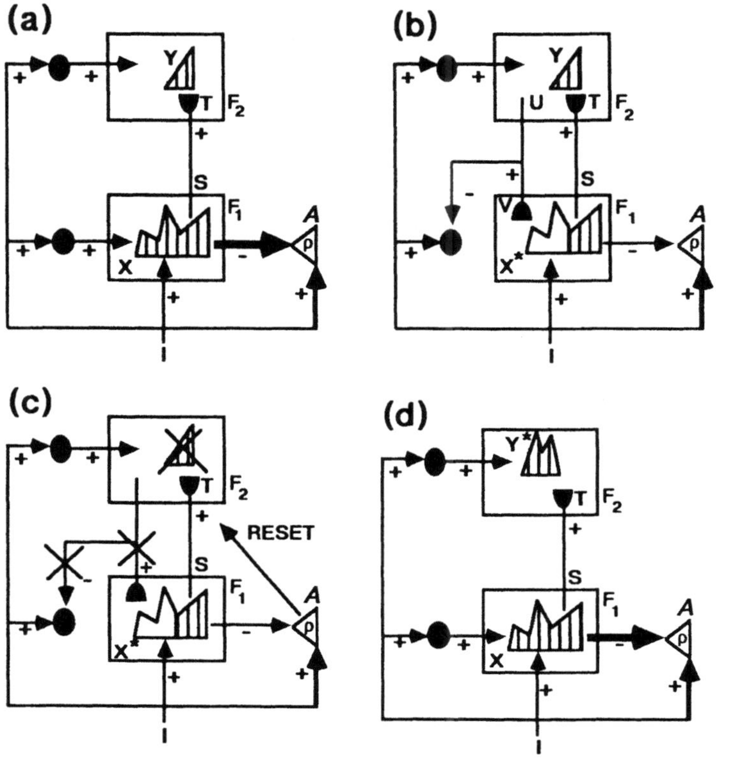

Figure 5. ART search for an F_2 code: (a) The input pattern **I** generates the specific STM activity pattern **X** at F_1 as it nonspecifically activates the orienting subsystem A. Pattern **X** both inhibits A and generates the output signal pattern **S**. Signal pattern **S** is transformed into the input pattern **T**, which activates the STM pattern **Y** across F_2. (b) Pattern **Y** generates the top-down signal pattern **U** which is transformed into the prototype pattern **V**. If **V** mismatches **I** at F_1, then a new STM activity pattern $\mathbf{X}^*$ is generated at F_1. The reduction in total STM activity which occurs when **X** is transformed into $\mathbf{X}^*$ causes a decrease in the total inhibition from F_1 to A. (c) If the matching criterion fails to be met, A releases a nonspecific arousal wave to F_2, which resets the STM pattern **Y** at F_2. (d) After **Y** is inhibited, its top-down prototype signal is eliminated, and **X** can be reinstated at F_1. Enduring traces of the prior reset lead **X** to activate a different STM pattern $\mathbf{Y}^*$ at F_2. If the top-down prototype due to $\mathbf{Y}^*$ also mismatches **I** at F_1, then the search for an appropriate F_2 code continues.

plar **I** must be to the top-down prototype **V** in order for resonance to occur. Because vigilance can vary across learning trials, recognition categories capable of encoding widely differing degrees of generalization, or morphological variability, can be learned by a single ART system. Low vigilance leads to broad generalization and abstract prototypes. High vigilance leads to narrow generalization and to prototypes that represent fewer input exemplars. In the limit of very high vigilance, prototype learning reduces to exemplar learning. Thus a single ART system may be used, say, to recognize abstract categories of faces and dogs, as well as individual faces and dogs. Exemplars can be coded by "grandmother cells" at the same time that abstract prototypes are coded by general categories of the same network. The particular combination of prototypes that is learned depends upon the predictive success of the learned categories in a particular task environment.

If the top-down expectation **V** and the bottom-up input **I** are too novel, or unexpected, to satisfy the vigilance criterion, then a bout of hypothesis testing, or memory search, is triggered. Search leads to selection of a better recognition code, symbol, category, or hypothesis to represent input **I** at level F_2. An *orienting subsystem* mediates the search process (Figure 4). The orienting subsystem interacts with the attentional subsystem, as in Figures 5c and 5d, to enable the attentional subsystem to learn new F_2 representations with which to remember novel events without risking unselective forgetting of its previous knowledge.

The search process prevents associations from forming between **Y** and $\mathbf{X}^*$ if $\mathbf{X}^*$ is too different from **I** to satisfy the vigilance criterion. As shown in Figure 5c, the search process resets **Y** before such an association can form. A familiar category may be selected by the search if its prototype is similar enough to the input **I** to satisfy the vigilance criterion. The prototype may then be refined in light of new information carried by **I**. If **I** is too different from any of the previously learned prototypes, then an uncommitted F_2 node is selected and learning of a new category is initiated. A network parameter controls how deeply the search proceeds before an uncommitted node is chosen.

As inputs that correspond to a particular category are practiced over learning trials, the search process converges upon a stable learned recognition category in F_2. This process corresponds to making the inputs "familiar" to the network. After familiarization takes place, all inputs coded by that category access it directly in a one-pass fashion, and search is automatically disengaged. The category selected is, moreover, the one whose prototype provides the globally best match to the input pattern. Learning can proceed on-line, and in a stable fashion, with familiar inputs directly activating their categories, while novel inputs continue to trigger adaptive searches for better categories, until the network's memory capacity is fully utilized.

These properties of ART systems have been used to explain and predict a variety of cognitive and brain data that have, as yet, received no other theoretical explanation ([23]–[24]). For example, a formal lesion of the orienting subsystem creates a memory disturbance that remarkably mimics properties of medial temporal amnesia ([27]–[28]). These and related data correspondences to orienting properties [28] have led to a neurobiological interpretation of the orienting subsystem in terms of the hippocampal formation of the brain. In applications to visual object recognition, the interactions within the F_1 and F_2 levels of the attentional subsystem are interpreted in terms of data concerning the prestriate visual cortex and the inferotemporal cortex [29], with the attentional gain control pathway interpreted in terms of the pulvinar region of the brain.

From a computer science perspective, ART systems have an interpretation that is no less interesting. The read-out of the top-down expectation $\mathbf{V}$ may be interpreted as a type of hypothesis-driven query. The matching process at F_1 and the hypothesis testing process at F_2 may be interpreted as query-driven symbolic substitutions. From this perspective, ART systems provide examples of new types of self-organizing production systems [30]. This interpretation of ART networks as production systems indicates how they contribute to the program of artificial intelligence, one of whose major goals has been to understand the cognitive operations of human thinking in terms of production systems. The ability of ART production systems to explain many cognitive and neurobiological data that cannot be explained by classical production systems illustrates how ART systems have brought us closer to realizing this major goal of artificial intelligence.

By incorporating predictive feedback into their control of the hypothesis testing cycle, the ARTMAP systems that are described below embody self-organizing production systems that are also goal-oriented. ARTMAP systems are thus a new type of self-organizing expert system which is capable of stable autonomous fast learning about nonstationary environments that may contain a great deal of morphological variability. The fact, as shown below, that fuzzy logic may also be usefully incorporated into ART systems blurs even further the traditional boundaries between artificial intelligence and neural networks.

As indicated in Figure 2, ARTMAP systems are capable of compressing different sorts of information into many distinct recognition categories which may all be used to make the same prediction. The expertise of such an ARTMAP system can be inferred by a direct study of the "rules" whereby it arrives at its predictions. This may be done, moreover, at any stage of the learning process. Suppose, for example, that the input vectors are not letter fonts, as in Figure 2, but are rather vectors of biochemicals, and that the outputs are not letter names, but are rather indices of desired drug effects on behavior. There may be multiple ways in which different biochemicals can achieve the same clinical effect on behavior. Correspondingly, at any point in the learning process, the operator of an ARTMAP system can test how many recognition categories have been detected that give rise to the desired clinical effect. The operator simply needs to check which LTM traces are large in the pathways from learned recognition categories to the desired output node. Within each recognition category, the prototype, or vector of large LTM traces, characterized a particular "rule", or bundle of biochemical features, that predicts the desired clinical effect. The "if-then" nature of the rule derives from the associative nature of ARTMAP predictions; namely, "if the biochemical has features close enough to a particular prototype, then it predicts the desired outcome." A list of all the prototype vectors provides a transparent set of rules whereby one can predict the desired outcome. Many such rules may coexist without mutual interference due to the competitive interactions whereby each hypothesis **Y** in Figure 5 is compressed. Associative networks such as back propagation often mix multiple rules among the same LTM traces because they do not have the competitive dynamics to separate them.

One may also ask if this particular type of rule-based system exhibits aspects of "creativity". Here it is useful to observe, as indicated in Figure 3, that ARTMAP systems, albeit "supervised", do not use the correct answers to directly force changes in LTM traces, as do supervised systems such as back propagation. The ARTMAP system uses the fact that its answers are wrong, along with its present state of knowledge, to test new hypotheses until it discovers on its own new representations that are capable of predicting the correct answers.

ART 1 (BINARY)	FUZZY ART (ANALOG)
CATEGORY CHOICE	
$T_j = \dfrac{\lvert \mathbf{I} \cap \mathbf{w}_j \rvert}{\alpha + \lvert \mathbf{w}_j \rvert}$	$T_j = \dfrac{\lvert \mathbf{I} \wedge \mathbf{w}_j \rvert}{\alpha + \lvert \mathbf{w}_j \rvert}$
MATCH CRITERION	
$\dfrac{\lvert \mathbf{I} \cap \mathbf{w}_J \rvert}{\lvert \mathbf{I} \rvert} \geq \rho$	$\dfrac{\lvert \mathbf{I} \wedge \mathbf{w}_J \rvert}{\lvert \mathbf{I} \rvert} \geq \rho$
FAST LEARNING	
$\mathbf{w}_J^{(new)} = \mathbf{I} \cap \mathbf{w}_J^{(old)}$	$\mathbf{w}_J^{(new)} = \mathbf{I} \wedge \mathbf{w}_J^{(old)}$
$\cap$ = logical AND intersection	$\wedge$ = fuzzy AND minimum

Figure 6. Comparison of ART 1 and fuzzy ART.

5 A Connection Between ART Systems and Fuzzy Logic

Fuzzy ART is a generalization of ART 1 that incorporates operations from fuzzy logic [31]. Although ART 1 can learn to classify only binary input patterns, fuzzy ART can learn to classify both analog and binary input patterns. Moreover, fuzzy ART reduces to ART 1 in response to binary input patterns. As shown in Figure 6, the generalization to learning both analog and binary input patterns is achieved by replacing appearances of the intersection operator ($\cap$) in ART 1 by the MIN operator ($\wedge$) of fuzzy set theory. The MIN operator reduces to the intersection operator in the binary case. Of particular interest is the fact that, as parameter α approaches 0, the function T_j which controls category choice through the bottom-up filter reduces to the operation of fuzzy subsethood [32]. T_j then measures the degree to which the adaptive weight vector $\mathbf{w}_j$ is a fuzzy subset of the input vector $\mathbf{I}$.

In fuzzy ART, input vectors are normalized at a preprocessing stage (Figure 7). This normalization procedure, called complement coding, leads

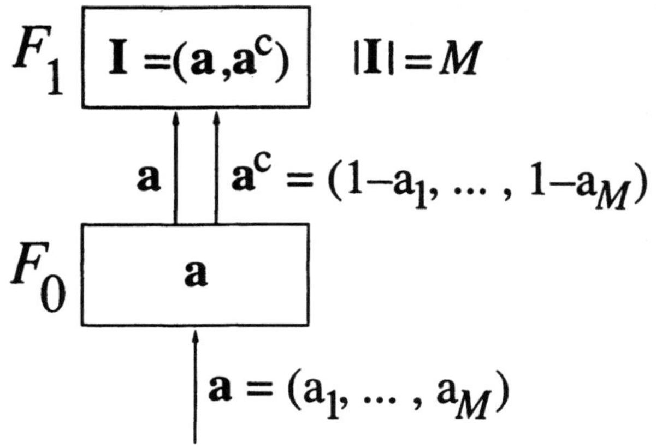

Figure 7. Complement coding uses on-cell and off-cell pairs to normalize input vectors.

to a symmetric theory in which the MIN operator ($\wedge$) and the MAX operator ($\vee$) of fuzzy set theory [33] play complementary roles. The categories formed by fuzzy ART are then hyper-rectangles. Figure 8 illustrates how MIN and MAX define these rectangles in the 2-dimensional case. The MIN and MAX values define the acceptable range of feature variation in each dimension. Complement coding uses on-cells (with activity $\mathbf{a}$ in Figure 7) and off-cells (with activity $\mathbf{a}^c$ in Figure 7) to represent the input pattern, and preserves individual feature amplitudes while normalizing the total on-cell/off-cell vector. The on-cell portion of a prototype encodes features that are critically present in category exemplars, while the off-cell portion encodes features that are critically absent. Each category is then defined by an interval of expected values for each input feature. For instance, we learn by example that men usually have hair on their heads. Fuzzy ART would encode this feature a wide interval ([A, 1]) of expectations of "hair on head" for the category "man". Similarly, since men sometimes wear hats, the feature "hat on head" would be encoded by a wide interval ([0, B]) of expectations. On the other hand, a dog almost always has hair on its head but almost never wears a hat. These features for the category "dog" would thus be encoded by two narrow intervals ([C, 1] for hair and [0, D] for hat) corresponding to narrower ranges of expectations for these two features.

Learning in fuzzy ART is stable because all adaptive weights can only decrease in time. Decreasing weights correspond to increasing sizes of category "boxes". Smaller vigilance values lead to larger category boxes. Learning stops when the input space is covered by boxes. The use of complement coding works with the property of increasing box size to prevent a proliferation of categories. With fast learning, constant vigilance, and a finite input set of arbitrary size and composition, learning stabilizes after just one presenta-

$\wedge$ Fuzzy AND (conjunction)

$\vee$ Fuzzy OR (disjunction)

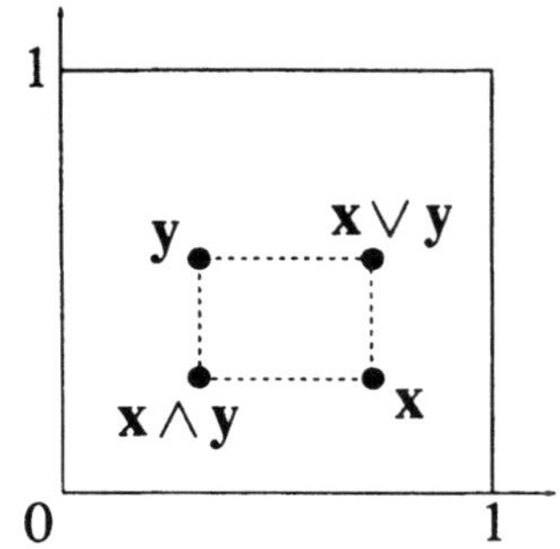

$$\mathbf{x} = (x_1, x_2) \qquad \mathbf{y} = (y_1, y_2)$$
$$(\mathbf{x} \wedge \mathbf{y})_1 = \min(x_1, y_1) \qquad (\mathbf{x} \wedge \mathbf{y})_2 = \min(x_2, y_2)$$
$$(\mathbf{x} \vee \mathbf{y})_1 = \max(x_1, y_1) \qquad (\mathbf{x} \vee \mathbf{y})_2 = \max(x_2, y_2)$$

Figure 8. Fuzzy AND and OR operations generate category hyper-rectangles.

tion of each input pattern. A fast-commit slow-recode option combines fast learning with a forgetting rule that buffers system memory against noise. Using this option, rare events can be rapidly learned, yet previously learned memories are not rapidly erased in response to statistically unreliable input fluctuations. See the Appendix for the equations that define the fuzzy ART Algorithm.

When the supervised learning of fuzzy ARTMAP controls category formation, a predictive error can force the creation of new categories that could not otherwise be learned due to monotone increase in category size through time in the unsupervised case. Supervision permits the creation of complex categorical structures without a loss of stability. We now summarize the main additional ingredients whereby fuzzy ART modules are combined into a fuzzy ARTMAP architecture.

6 Fuzzy ARTMAP

Each fuzzy ARTMAP system includes a pair of fuzzy ART modules (ART_a and ART_b), as in Figure 9. During supervised learning, ART_a receives a stream $\{\mathbf{a}^{(p)}\}$ of input patterns and ART_b receives a stream $\{\mathbf{b}^{(p)}\}$ of input patterns, where $\mathbf{b}^{(p)}$ is the correct prediction given $\mathbf{a}^{(p)}$. These modules are linked by an associative learning network and an internal controller that ensures autonomous system operation in real time. The controller is designed to create the minimal number of ART_a recognition categories, or "hidden units," needed to meet accuracy criteria. As noted above, this is accomplished by realizing a Minimax Learning Rule that conjointly minimizes predictive er-

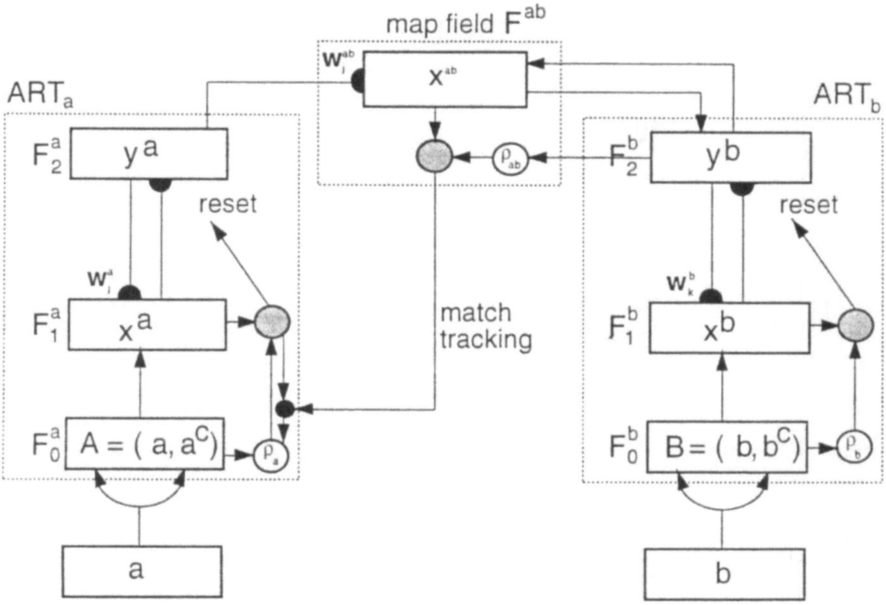

Figure 9. Fuzzy ARTMAP architecture. The ART_a complement coding preprocessor transforms the M_a-vector **a** into the $2M_a$-vector $\mathbf{A} = (\mathbf{a}, \mathbf{a}^c)$ at the ART_a field F_0^a. **A** is the input vector to the ART_a field F_1^a. Similarly, the input to F_1^b is the $2M_b$-vector $(\mathbf{b}, \mathbf{b}^c)$. When a prediction by ART_a is disconfirmed at ART_b, inhibition of map field activation induces the match tracking process. Match tracking raises the ART_a vigilance ρ_a to just above the F_1^a to F_0^a match ratio $|\mathbf{x}^a|/|\mathbf{A}|$. This triggers an ART_a search which leads to activation of either an ART_a category that correctly predicts **b** or to a previously uncommitted ART_a category node.

ror and maximizes predictive generalization. This scheme automatically links predictive success to category size on a trial-by-trial basis using only local operations. It works by increasing the vigilance parameter ρ_a of ART_a by the minimal amount needed to correct a predictive error at ART_b (Figure 10).

Parameter ρ_a calibrates the minimum confidence that ART_a must have in a recognition category, or hypothesis, that is activated by an input $\mathbf{a}^{(p)}$ in order for ART_a to accept that category, rather than search for a better one through an automatically controlled process of hypothesis testing. As in ART 1, lower values of ρ_a enable larger categories to form. These lower ρ_a values lead to broader generalization and higher code compression. A predictive failure at ART_b increases the minimal confidence ρ_a by the least amount needed to trigger hypothesis testing at ART_a, using a mechanism called *match tracking* [5]. Match tracking sacrifices the minimum amount of generalization necessary to correct the predictive error. Speaking intuitively,

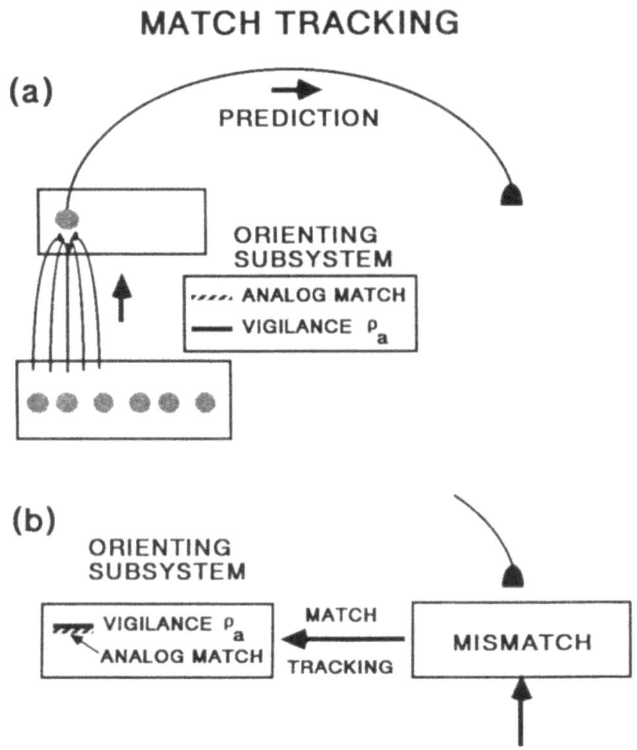

Figure 10. Match tracking: (a) A prediction is made by ART_a when the baseline vigilance ρ_a is less than the analog match value. (b) A predictive error at ART_b increases the baseline vigilance value of ART_a until it just exceeds the analog match value, and thereby triggers hypothesis testing that searches for a more predictive bundle of features to which to attend.

match tracking operationalizes the idea that the system must have accepted hypotheses with too little confidence to satisfy the demands of a particular environment. Match tracking increases the criterion confidence just enough to trigger hypothesis testing. Hypothesis testing leads to the selection of a new ART_a category, which focuses attention on a new cluster of $\mathbf{a}^{(p)}$ input features that is better able to predict $\mathbf{b}^{(p)}$. Due to the combination of match tracking and fast learning, a single ARTMAP system can learn a different prediction for a rare event than for a cloud of similar frequent events in which it is embedded. The equations for fuzzy ART and fuzzy ARTMAP are given in the Appendix in algorithmic form.

7 A Benchmark Study: Letter Recognition by Genetic Algorithms and Fuzzy ARTMAP

As summarized in Table 2, fuzzy ARTMAP has been benchmarked against a variety of machine learning, neural network, and genetic algorithms with considerable success. An illustrative study used a benchmark machine learning task that Frey and Slate [34] developed and described as a "difficult categorization problem" (p. 161). The task requires a system to identify an input exemplar as one of 26 capital letters A–Z. The database was derived from 20,000 unique black-and-white pixel images. The difficulty of the task is due to the wide variety of letter types represented: the twenty "fonts represent five different stroke styles (simplex, duplex, complex, and Gothic) and six different letter styles (block, script, italic, English, Italian, and German)" (p. 162). In addition each image was randomly distorted, leaving many of the characters misshapen. Sixteen numerical feature attributes were then obtained from each character image, and each attribute value was scaled to a range of 0 to 15. The resulting Letter Image Recognition file is archived in the UCI Repository of Machine Learning Databases and Domain Theories, maintained by David Aha and Patrick Murphy (ml_repository@ics.uci.edu).

Frey and Slate used this database to test performance of a family of classifiers based on Holland's genetic algorithms [35]. The training set consisted of 16,000 exemplars, with the remaining 4,000 exemplars used for testing. Genetic algorithm classifiers having different input representations, weight update and rule creation schemes, and system parameters were systematically compared. Training was carried out for 5 epochs, plus a sixth "verification" pass during which no new rules were created but a large number of unsatisfactory rules were discarded. In Frey and Slate's comparative study, these systems had correct prediction rates that ranged from 24.5% to 80.8% on the 4,000-item test set. The best performance (80.8%) was obtained using an integer input representation, a reward sharing weight update, an exemplar method of rule creation, and a parameter setting that allowed an unused or erroneous rule to stay in the system for a long time before being discarded. After training, the optimal case, that had 80.8% performance rate, ended with 1,302 rules and 8 attributes per rule, plus over 35,000 more rules that were discarded during verification. (For purposes of comparison, a rule is somewhat analogous to an ART_a category in ARTMAP, and the number of attributes per rule is analogous to the size $|\mathbf{w}_j^a|$ of ART_a category weight vectors.) Building on the results of their comparative study, Frey and Slate investigated two types of alternative algorithms, namely an accuracy-utility bidding system, that had slightly improved performance (81.6%) in the best case; and an exemplar/hybrid rule creation scheme that further improved performance, to a maximum of 82.7%, but that required the creation of over 100,000 rules prior to the verification step.

Fuzzy ARTMAP had an error rate on the letter recognition task that was consistently less than one third that of the three best Frey-Slate genetic algorithm classifiers described above. In particular, after 1 to 5 epochs, individual fuzzy ARTMAP systems had a robust prediction rate of 90% to 94% on the 4,000-item test set. A *voting strategy* consistently improved this performance. This voting strategy is based on the observation that ARTMAP fast learning typically leads to different adaptive weights and recognition categories for different orderings of a given training set, even when overall predictive accuracy of all simulations is similar. The different category structures cause the set of test items where errors occur to vary from one simulation to the next. The voting strategy uses an ARTMAP system that is trained several times on input sets with different orderings. The final prediction for a given test set item is the one made by the largest number of simulations. Since the set of items making erroneous predictions varies from one simulation to the next, voting cancels many of the errors. Such a voting strategy can also be used to assign confidence estimates to competing predictions given small, noisy, or incomplete training sets. Voting consistently eliminated 25% – 43% of the errors, giving a robust prediction rate of 92% – 96%. Moreover fuzzy ARTMAP simulations each created fewer than 1,070 ART_a categories, compared to the 1,040–1,302 final rules of the three genetic classifiers with the best performance rates. Most fuzzy ARTMAP learning occurred on the first epoch, with test set performance on systems trained for one epoch typically over 97% that of systems exposed to inputs for five epochs.

8 Concluding Remarks

Fuzzy ARTMAP is one of a rapidly growing family of attentive self-organizing learning hypothesis testing, and prediction systems that have evolved from the biological theory of cognitive information processing of which ART forms an important part [16, 23–26]. At the present time, unsupervised ART modules have found their way into such diverse applications as the control of mobile robots, learning and search of airplane part inventories, medical diagnosis, 3-D visual object recognition, automatic analysis of electrocardiogram traces, music recognition, diagnostic monitoring of nuclear plants, seismic recognition, prediction of protein secondary structure, sonar recognition, and laser radar recognition; e.g., [36–43]. All of these applications exploit the ability of ART systems to rapidly learn to classify large data bases in a stable fashion, to calibrate their confidence in a classification, and to focus attention upon those featural groupings that they deem to be important based upon their past experience. We anticipate that the growing family of supervised ARTMAP systems will find an even broader range of applications due to their ability to adapt the number, shape, and scale of their category boundaries to meet the on-line demands of large nonstationary data bases.

Appendix

Summary of the Fuzzy ART Algorithm

ART field activity vectors: Each ART system includes a field F_0 of nodes that represent a current input vector; a field F_1 that receives both bottom-up input from F_0 and top-down input from a field F_2 that represents the active code, or category. The F_0 activity vector is denoted $\mathbf{I} = (I_1, \ldots, I_M)$, with each component I_i in the interval [0,1], $i = 1, \ldots, M$. The F_1 activity vector is denoted $\mathbf{x} = (x_1, \ldots, x_M)$ and the F_2 activity vector is denoted $\mathbf{y} = (y_1, \ldots, y_N)$. The number of nodes in each field is arbitrary.

Weight vector: Associated with each F_2 category node $j (j = 1, \ldots, N)$ is a vector $\mathbf{w}_j \equiv (w_{j1}, \ldots, w_{jM})$ of adaptive weights, or LTM traces. Initially

$$w_{j1}(0) = \ldots = w_{jM}(0) = 1; \tag{1}$$

then each category is said to be *uncommitted*. After a category is selected for coding it becomes *committed*. As shown below, each LTM trace w_{ji} is monotone nonincreasing through time and hence converges to a limit. The fuzzy ART weight vector $\mathbf{w}_j$ subsumes both the bottom-up and top-down weight vectors of ART 1.

Parameters: Fuzzy ART dynamics are determined by a choice parameter $\alpha > 0$; a learning rate parameter $\beta \in [0, 1]$; and a vigilance parameter $\rho \in [0, 1]$.

Category choice: For each input **I** and F_2 node j, the *choice function* T_j is defined by

$$T_j(\mathbf{I}) = \frac{|\mathbf{I} \wedge \mathbf{w}_j|}{\alpha + |\mathbf{w}_j|}, \tag{2}$$

where the fuzzy AND [33] operator $\wedge$ is defined by

$$(\mathbf{p} \wedge \mathbf{q})_i \equiv \min(p_i, q_i) \tag{3}$$

and where the norm $| \cdot |$ is defined by

$$|\mathbf{p}| \equiv \sum_{i=1}^{M} |p_i|. \tag{4}$$

for any M-dimensional vectors **p** and **q**. For notational simplicity, $T_j(\mathbf{I})$ in (2) is often written as T_j when the input **I** is fixed.

The system is said to make a *category choice* when at most one F_2 node can become active at a given time. The category choice is indexed by J, where

$$T_J = \max\{T_j : j = 1 \ldots N\}. \tag{5}$$

If more than one T_j is maximal, the category j with the smallest index is chosen. In particular, nodes become committed in order $j = 1, 2, 3, \ldots$.

When the Jth category is chosen, $y_J = 1$; and $y_j = 0$ for $j \neq J$. In a choice system, the F_1 activity vector $\mathbf{x}$ obeys the equation

$$\mathbf{x} = \begin{cases} \mathbf{I} & \text{if } F_2 \text{ is inactive} \\ \mathbf{I} \wedge \mathbf{w}_J & \text{if the } J^{th}\ F_2 \text{node is chosen.} \end{cases} \tag{6}$$

Resonance or reset: *Resonance* occurs if the *match function* $|\mathbf{I} \wedge \mathbf{w}_J|/|\mathbf{I}|$ of the chosen category meets the vigilance criterion:

$$\frac{|\mathbf{I} \wedge \mathbf{w}_J|}{|\mathbf{I}|} \geq \rho; \tag{7}$$

that is, by (6), when the Jth category is chosen, resonance occurs if

$$|\mathbf{x}| = |\mathbf{I} \wedge \mathbf{w}_J| \geq \rho|\mathbf{I}|. \tag{8}$$

Learning then ensues, as defined below. *Mismatch reset* occurs if

$$\frac{|\mathbf{I} \wedge \mathbf{w}_J|}{|\mathbf{I}|} < \rho; \tag{9}$$

that is, if

$$|\mathbf{x}| = |\mathbf{I} \wedge \mathbf{w}_J| < \rho|\mathbf{I}|. \tag{10}$$

Then the value of the choice function T_J is set to 0 for the duration of the input presentation to prevent the persistent selection of the same category during search. A new index J is then chosen, by (5). The search process continues until the chosen J satisfies (7).

Learning: Once search ends, the weight vector $\mathbf{w}_J$ is updated according to the equation

$$\mathbf{w}_J^{(\text{new})} = \beta(\mathbf{I} \wedge \mathbf{w}_J^{(\text{old})}) + (1-\beta)\mathbf{w}_J^{(\text{old})}. \tag{11}$$

Fast learning corresponds to setting $\beta = 1$. The learning law used in the EACH system of Salzberg [44] is equivalent to equation (11) in the fast-learn limit with the complement coding option described below.

Fast-commit slow-recode option: For efficient coding of noisy input sets, it is useful to set $\beta = 1$ when J is an uncommitted node, and then to take $\beta < 1$ after the category is committed. Then $\mathbf{w}_J^{(\text{new})} = \mathbf{I}$ the first time category J becomes active. Moore [45] introduced the learning law (11), with fast commitment and slow recoding, to investigate a variety of generalized ART 1 models. Some of these models are similar to fuzzy ART, but none includes the complement coding option. Moore described a category proliferation problem that can occur in some analog ART systems when a large number of inputs erode the norm of weight vectors. Complement coding solves this problem.

Input normalization/complement coding option: Proliferation of categories is avoided in fuzzy ART if inputs are normalized. *Complement coding* is a normalization rule that preserves amplitude information. Complement coding represents both the on-response and the off-response to an input vector $\mathbf{a}$ (Figure 7). To define this operation in its simplest form, let $\mathbf{a}$ itself represent the on-response. The complement of $\mathbf{a}$, denoted by $\mathbf{a}^c$, represents the off-response, where

$$a_i^c \equiv 1 - a_i. \tag{12}$$

The complement coded input $\mathbf{I}$ to the field F_1 is the 2M-dimensional vector

$$\mathbf{I} = (\mathbf{a}, \mathbf{a}^c) \equiv (a_1, \ldots, a_M, a_1^c, \ldots, a_M^c). \tag{13}$$

Note that

$$\begin{aligned} |\mathbf{I}| &= |(\mathbf{a}, \mathbf{a}^c)| \\ &= \sum_{i=1}^{M} a_i + (M - \sum_{i=1}^{M} a_i) \\ &= M, \end{aligned} \tag{14}$$

so inputs preprocessed into complement coding form are automatically normalized. Where complement coding is used, the initial condition (1) is replaced by

$$w_{j1}(0) = \ldots = w_{j,2M}(0) = 1. \tag{15}$$

Fuzzy ARTMAP Algorithm

The fuzzy ARTMAP system incorporates two fuzzy ART modules ART$_a$ and ART$_b$ that are linked together via an inter-ART module F^{ab} called a *map field*. The map field is used to form predictive associations between categories and to realize the *match tracking rule* whereby the vigilance parameter of ART$_a$ increases in response to a predictive mismatch at ART$_b$. The interactions mediated by the map field F^{ab} may be operationally characterized as follows.

ART$_a$ and ART$_b$

Inputs to ART$_a$ and ART$_b$ are in the complement code form: for ART$_a$, $\mathbf{I} = \mathbf{A} = (\mathbf{a}, \mathbf{a}^c)$; for ART$_b$, $\mathbf{I} = \mathbf{B} = (\mathbf{b}, \mathbf{b}^c)$ (Figure 9). Variables in ART$_a$ or ART$_b$ are designated by subscripts or superscripts "a" or "b". For ART$_a$, let $\mathbf{x}^a \equiv (x_1^a \ldots x_{2M_a}^a)$ denote the F_1^a output vector; let $\mathbf{y}^a \equiv (y_1^a \ldots y_{N_a}^a)$ denote the F_2^a output vector; and let $\mathbf{w}_j^a \equiv (w_{j1}^a, w_{j2}^a, \ldots, w_{j,2M_a})$ denote the jth ART$_a$ weight vector. For ART$_b$, let $\mathbf{x}^b \equiv (x_1^b \ldots x_{2M_b}^b)$ denote the F_1^b output vector; let $\mathbf{y}^b \equiv (y_1^b \ldots y_{N_b}^b)$ denote the F_2^b output vector; and let $\mathbf{w}_k^b \equiv (w_{k1}^b, w_{k2}^b, \ldots, w_{k,2M_b}^b)$ denote the kth ART$_b$ weight vector. For the map field, let $\mathbf{x}^{ab} \equiv (x_1^{ab}, \ldots, x_{N_b}^{ab})$ denote the F^{ab} output vector, and let $\mathbf{w}_j^{ab} \equiv (w_{j1}^{ab}, \ldots, w_{JN_b}^{ab})$ denote the weight vector from the jth F_2^a node to F^{ab}. Vectors $\mathbf{x}^a, \mathbf{y}^a, \mathbf{x}^b, \mathbf{y}^b$, and $\mathbf{x}^{ab}$ are set to $\mathbf{0}$ between input presentations.

Map field activation

The map field F^{ab} is activated whenever one of the ART_a or ART_b categories is active. If node J of F_2^a is chosen, then its weights $\mathbf{w}_J^{ab}$ activate F^{ab}. If node K in F_2^b is active, then the node K in F^{ab} is activated by 1–to–1 pathways between F_2^b and F^{ab}. If both ART_a and ART_b are active, then F^{ab} becomes active only if ART_a predicts the same category as ART_b via the weights $\mathbf{w}_J^{ab}$. The F^{ab} output vector $\mathbf{x}^{ab}$ obeys

$$\mathbf{x}^{ab} = \begin{cases} \mathbf{y}^b \wedge \mathbf{w}_J^{ab} & \text{if the Jth } F_2^a \text{ node is active and } F_2^b \text{ is active} \\ \mathbf{w}_J^{ab} & \text{if the Jth } F_2^a \text{ node is active and } F_2^b \text{ is inactive} \\ \mathbf{y}^b & \text{if } F_2^a \text{ is inactive and } F_2^b \text{ is active} \\ \mathbf{0} & \text{if } F_2^a \text{ is inactive and } F_2^b \text{ is inactive.} \end{cases} \tag{16}$$

By (16), $\mathbf{x}^{ab} = \mathbf{0}$ if the prediction $\mathbf{w}_J^{ab}$ is disconfirmed by $\mathbf{y}^b$. Such a mismatch event triggers an ART_a search for a better category, as follows.

Match tracking

At the start of each input presentation the ART_a vigilance parameter ρ_a equals a baseline vigilance $\overline{\rho_a}$. The map field vigilance parameter is ρ_{ab}. If

$$|\mathbf{x}^{ab}| < \rho_{ab}|\mathbf{y}^b|, \tag{17}$$

then ρ_a is increased until it is slightly larger than $|\mathbf{A} \wedge \mathbf{w}_J^a||\mathbf{A}|^{-1}$, where $\mathbf{A}$ is the input to F_1^a, in complement coding form. Then

$$|\mathbf{x}^a| = |\mathbf{A} \wedge \mathbf{w}_J^a| < \rho_a|\mathbf{A}|, \tag{18}$$

where J is the index of the active F_2^a node, as in (10). When this occurs, ART_a search leads either to activation of another F_2^a node J with

$$|\mathbf{x}^a| = |\mathbf{A} \wedge \mathbf{w}_J^a| \geq \rho_a|\mathbf{A}| \tag{19}$$

and

$$|\mathbf{x}^{ab}| = |\mathbf{y}^b \wedge \mathbf{w}_J^{ab}| \geq \rho_{ab}|\mathbf{y}^b|; \tag{20}$$

or, if no such node exists, to the shut-down of F_2^a for the remainder of the input presentation.

Map field learning

Learning rules determine how the map field weights w_{jk}^{ab} change through time, as follows. Weights w_{jk}^{ab} in $F_2^a \to F^{ab}$ paths initially satisfy

$$w_{jk}^{ab}(0) = 1. \tag{21}$$

During resonance with the ART_a category J active, $\mathbf{w}_J^{ab}$ approaches the map field vector $\mathbf{x}^{ab}$. With fast learning, once J learns to predict the ART_b category K, that association is permanent; i.e., $w_{JK}^{ab} = 1$ for all time.

Acknowledgements: This research was supported in part by ARPA (ONR N00014-92-J-4015), the National Science Foundation (NSF IRI 90-00530), and the Office of Naval Research (ONR N00014-91-J-4100). The authors wish to thank Cynthia Bradford and Diana Meyers for their valuable assistance in the preparation of the manuscript.

References

1. Parker, D.B.: Learning-logic. Invention Report, 581-64, File 1, Office of Technology Licensing. Stanford University, October, 1982.
2. Rumelhart, D.E., Hinton, G., and Williams, R.: Learning internal representations by error propagation. In D.E. Rumelhart and J.L. McClelland (Eds.), Parallel distributed processing. Cambridge, MA: MIT Press, 1986.
3. Werbos, P.: Beyond regression: New tools for prediction and analysis in the behavioral sciences. PhD Thesis, Harvard University, Cambridge, MA, 1974.
4. Ratcliff, R.: Connectionist models of recognition memory: Constraints imposed by learning and forgetting functions. Psych. Rev. 97, 285–308 (1990).
5. Carpenter, G.A., Grossberg, S., and Reynolds, J.H.: ARTMAP: Supervised real-time learning and classification of nonstationary data by a self-organizing neural network. Neural Networks 4, 565–588 (1991).
6. Carpenter, G.A., Grossberg, S., Markuzon, N., Reynolds, J.H., and Rosen, D.B.: Fuzzy ARTMAP: A neural network architecture for incremental supervised learning of analog multidimensional maps. IEEE Trans. Neural Networks 3 698–713 (1992).
7. Grossberg, S.: Adaptive pattern classification and universal recoding, II: Feedback, expectation, olfaction, and illusions. Biol. Cybern. 23, 187–202 (1976).
8. Grossberg, S.: How does a brain build a cognitive code? Psych. Rev. 1, 1–51 (1980).
9. Carpenter, G.A. and Grossberg, S.: A massively parallel architecture for a self-organizing neural pattern recognition machine. Comp. Vis. Graph. Image Proc. 37, 54–115 (1987).
10. Carpenter, G.A. and Grossberg, S.: ART 2: Stable self-organization of pattern recognition codes for analog input patterns. Appl. Opt. 26, 4919–4930 (1987).
11. Carpenter, G.A. and Grossberg, S.: ART 3: Hierarchical search using chemical transmitters in self-organizing pattern recognition architectures. Neural Networks 3, 129–152 (1990).
12. Grossberg, S.: Neural expectation: Cerebellar and retinal analogs of cells fired by learnable or unlearned pattern classes. Kybernetik 10, 49–57 (1972).
13. Grossberg, S.: On the development of feature detectors in the visual cortex with applications to learning and reaction-diffusion systems. Biol. Cybern. 21, 145–159 (1976).

14. Grossberg, S.: Adaptive pattern classification and universal recoding, I: Parallel development and coding of neural feature detectors. Biol. Cybern. 23, 121–134 (1976).
15. Grossberg, S.: A theory of human memory: Self-organization and performance of sensory-motor codes, maps, and plan. In R. Rosen and F. Snell (Eds.), Progress in theoretical biology, Vol. 5. New York: Academic Press, 1978. [Reprinted in S. Grossberg, Studies of mind and brain: Neural principles of learning, perception, development, cognition, and motor control. Boston: Reidel Press, 1982].
16. Grossberg, S.: Studies of mind and brain: Neural principles of learning, perception, development, cognition, and motor control. Boston: Reidel Press, 1982.
17. von der Malsburg, C.: Self-organization of orientation sensitive cells in the striate cortex. Kybernetik 14, 85–100 (1973).
18. Willshaw, D.J. and von der Malsburg, C.: How patterned neural connections can be set up by self-organization. Proc. Roy. Soc. London (B) 194, 431–445 (1976).
19. Cohen M.A. and Grossberg, S.: Neural dynamics of speech and language coding: Developmental programs, perceptual grouping, and competition for short term memory. Human Neurobiol. 5, 1–22 (1986).
20. Cohen, M.A. and Grossberg, S.: Masking fields: A massively parallel architecture for learning, recognizing, and predicting multiple groupings of patterned data. Appl. Opt. 26, 1866–1891 (1987).
21. Grossberg, S. and Kuperstein, M.: Neural dynamics of adaptive sensory-motor control: Ballistic eye movements. Amsterdam: Elsevier/North Holland, 1986. Grossberg, S. and Kuperstein, M.: Neural dynamics of adaptive sensory-motor control: Expanded edition. Elmsford, NY: Pergamon Press, 1989.
22. Kohonen, T.: Self-organization and associative memory. New York: Springer-Verlag, 1988.
23. Carpenter, G.A. and Grossberg, S. (Eds.): Pattern recognition by self-organizing neural networks. Cambridge, MA: MIT Press, 1991.
24. Grossberg, S. (Ed.): The adaptive brain, I: Cognition, learning, reinforcement, and rhythm. Amsterdam: Elsevier/North-Holland, 1987.
25. Grossberg, S. (Ed.): The adaptive brain, II: Vision, speech, language, and motor control. Amsterdam: Elsevier/North-Holland, 1987.
26. Grossberg, S. (Ed.): Neural networks and natural intelligence. Cambridge, MA: MIT Press, 1988.
27. Carpenter, G.A. and Grossberg, S.: Neural dynamics of category learning and recognition: Attention, memory consolidation, and amnesia. In S. Grossberg (Ed.), The adaptive brain, I: Cognition, learning, reinforcement, and rhythm. Amsterdam: Elsevier/North Holland, pp. 238–286, 1987.

28. Grossberg, S. and Merrill, J.W.L.: A neural network model of adaptively timed reinforcement learning and hippocampal dynamics. Cog. Brain Res. 1, 3–38 (1992).
29. Desimone, R.: Neural circuits for visual attention in the primate brain. In G.A. Carpenter and S. Grossberg (Eds.), Neural networks for vision and image processing. Cambridge, MA: MIT Press, pp. 343–364, 1992.
30. Laird, J.E., Newell, A., and Rosenbloom, P.S.: SOAR: An architecture for general intelligence. Artificial Intell. 33, 1–64 (1987).
31. Carpenter, G.A., Grossberg, S., and Rosen, D.B.: Fuzzy ART: Fast stable learning and categorization of analog patterns by an adaptive resonance system. Neural Networks 4, 759–771 (1991).
32. Kosko, B.: Fuzzy entropy and conditioning. Info. Sci. 40, 165–174 (1986).
33. Zadeh, L.: Fuzzy sets. Info. Control 8, 338–353 (1965).
34. Frey, P.W. and Slate, D.J.: Letter recognition using Holland-style adaptive classifiers. Mach. Learn. 6, 161–182 (1991).
35. Holland, J.H.: Adaptive algorithms for discovering and using general patterns in growing knowledge bases. Int. J. Pol. Anal. Info. Sys. 4, 217–240 (1980).
36. Baloch, A.J. and Waxman, A.M.: Visual learning, adaptive expectations, and learning behavioral conditioning of the mobil robot MAVIN. Neural Networks 4, 271–302 (1991).
37. Caudell, T., Smith, S., Johnson, C., Wunsch, D., and Escobedo, R.: An industrial application of neural networks to reusable design. Adaptive neural systems, Technical Report BCS-CS-ACS-91-001, Seattle, WA: The Boeing Company, pp. 185–190, 1991.
38. Gjerdingen, R.O.: Categorization of musical patterns by self-organizing neuronlike networks. Music Percep. 7, 339–370 (1990).
39. Goodman, P., Kaburlasos, V., Egbert, D., Carpenter, G.A., Grossberg, S., Reynolds, J.H., Hammermeister, K., Marshall, G., and Grover, F.: Fuzzy ARTMAP neural network prediction of heart surgery mortality. Proceedings of the Wang Institute research conference: Neural networks for learning, recognition, and control. Boston, MA: Boston University, p. 48, 1992.
40. Ham, F.M. and Han, S.W.: Quantitative study of the QRS complex using fuzzy ARTMAP and MIT/BIH arrythmia database. Proceedings of the World Congress on Neural Networks (WCNN'93) I, 207–211 (1993).
41. Keyvan, S., Durg, A., and Rabelo, L.C.: Application of artificial neural networks for development of diagnostic monitoring system in nuclear plants. Trans. Amer. Nuclear Soc. 1, 515–522 (1993).
42. Mehta, B.V., Vij, L., and Rabelo, L.C.: Prediction of secondary structures of proteins using fuzzy ARTMAP. Proceedings of the World Congress on Neural Networks (WCNN'93) I, 228–232 (1993).

43. Seibert, M. and Waxman, A.M.: Learning and recognizing 3D objects from multiple views in a neural system. In H. Wechsler (Ed.) Neural networks for perception, Vol. 1. New York: Academic Press, 1991.
44. Salzberg, S.L.: Learning with nested generalized exemplars. Boston: Kluwer Academic Publishers, 1990.
45. Moore, B.: ART 1 and pattern clustering. In D. Touretzky, G. Hinton, and T. Sejnowski (Eds.), Proceedings of the 1988 connectionist models summer school. San Mateo, CA: Morgan Kaufmann, pp. 174–185, 1989.

Recognition of 3-D Objects from Multiple 2-D Views by a Self-Organizing Neural Architecture

Gary Bradski and Stephen Grossberg

Center for Adaptive Systems and
Department of Cognitive and Neural Systems,
Boston University, 111 Cummington Street,
Boston, Massachusetts 02215 USA

Abstract

The recognition of 3-D objects from sequences of their 2-D views is modeled by a neural architecture, called VIEWNET, that uses View Information Encoded With NETworks. VIEWNET illustrates how several types of noise and variability in image data can be progressively removed while incomplete image features are restored and invariant features are discovered using an appropriately designed cascade of processing stages. VIEWNET first processes 2-D views of 3-D objects using the CORT-X 2 filter, which discounts the illuminant, regularizes and completes figural boundaries, and removes noise from the images. Boundary regularization and completion are achieved by the same mechanisms that suppress image noise. A log-polar transform is taken with respect to the centroid of the resulting figure and then re-centered to achieve 2-D scale and rotation invariance. The invariant images are coarse coded to further reduce noise, reduce foreshortening effects, and increase generalization. These compressed codes are input into a supervised learning system based on the fuzzy ARTMAP algorithm. Recognition categories of 2-D views are learned before evidence from sequences of 2-D view categories is accumulated to improve object recognition. Recognition is studied with noisy and clean images using slow and fast learning. VIEWNET is demonstrated on an MIT Lincoln Laboratory database of 2-D views of jet aircraft with and without additive noise. A recognition rate of 90% is achieved with one 2-D view category and of 98.5% correct with three 2-D view categories.

1 Introduction

This article describes a neural architecture that is capable of learning to recognize 3-D objects in a self-organizing manner. Much prior research on 3-D visual object recognition relies on appearance based approaches. Appearance based approaches use input imagery to construct 3-D object models. Koenderink and van Doorn (1979) created *Aspect Graphs* consisting of 2-D views of a 3-D object along the nodes of the graph, with legal view transitions indicated by the arcs among nodes. In their approach, 2-D views and view transitions are equally important for recognizing the object. Gigus and Malik (1988, 1990) and Plantinga and Dyer (1990) have attempted to automatically construct aspect graphs from objects in a CAD database using convex polyhedra. Other efforts for automatically generating perspective projection aspect graphs from a CAD database using curved objects and non-convex polyhedra have been pursued by Bowyer, Eggert, Stewman, and Stark (1989), Sripradisvarakul and Jain (1989), Ponce and Kriegman (1990), Rieger (1990), Stewman and Bowyer (1990), Chang and Huang (1992), and Eggert and Bowyer (1993). Hidden Markov models have also been applied to learning an aspect graph from a view sequence by Rimey and Brown (1991).

Seibert and Waxman (1992) have developed a neural network architecture that self-organizes aspect graph representations of 3-D objects from 2-D view sequences. Images of rotating jets were binarized and points of high curvature and the object centroid were found using a reaction-diffusion process. A log-polar transform around the object centroid was used to remove 2-D rotation and scale variations. The result was coarse coded (compressed to 5x5 pixels from 128x128) using Gaussian filters. The coarse codes (25 data points) were fed into an ART 2 (Carpenter and Grossberg 1987) network for clustering and categorization. These "categorical" 2-D views were then fed into a series of cross-correlation matrices, or view graphs, one for each possible 3-D object, so that views and view transitions could be learned by a 3-D object categorization layer. The 3-D categorization layer incorporated "evidence accumulation" nodes which integrate activations that they receive from learned connections to the correlation matrix. The node receiving maximal evidence in the 3-D layer is chosen as the network's recognition of the 3-D object being viewed.

In the Seibert and Waxman model, given N 2-D views and M objects, the architecture must have the potential to encode on order of $M \times N^2$ 2-D view transitions. As reported in Seibert and Waxman (1992), 75% of the 2-D jet images were ambiguous to some degree. That is, 75% of the 2-D view categories formed by ART 2 gave evidence for more than one type of jet. Even if several views are ambiguous, the transitions between them may unambiguously identify a particular 3-D object. Thus, view transitions are critically important in the Seibert and Waxman architecture, which may then incur the cost of needing up to $M \times N^2$ view transitions.

Bradski, Carpenter, and Grossberg (1991) described an alternative architecture that potentially overcomes the problem of proliferating view transitions. It learns to code 2-D views in recognition categories, as do Seibert and Waxman, but stores these categories in a working memory, called a STORE network, whose activity pattern implicitly represents the order in which the 2-D views occurred, as well as the views themselves. An ART module then learns to categorize the stored combination of 2-D views and (implicitly coded) view transitions into a 3-D object category. Such an algorithm needs no more than N+M nodes to code N 2-D views in working memory for M 3-D objects.

This paper further develops the perspective that, although multiple views may facilitate recognition, view transitions, as such, may not be needed to achieve high recognition accuracy from one or more views. A neural network architecture, called **VIEWNET**, for **V**iew **I**nformation **E**ncoded **W**ith **NET**works is proposed that can categorize individual views with high accuracy, in accord with the human experience that many objects can be identified with a single view, except when they are observed from an unfamiliar perspective or from a perspective that reduces the objects apparent dimension. Single view recognition accuracy of up to 90% is achieved by this architecture on the Seibert and Waxman database.

As diagramed in Figure 1, the architecture consists of three parts: an image preprocessor, a supervised self-organizing recognition network, and a network to accumulate evidence over multiple views. It is assumed that the figure to be recognized is separated from its background. Neural networks for figure-ground separation that use computations consistent with those in the preprocessors are described in Grossberg (1993) and Grossberg and Wyse (1992). The image figure is then processed by a feedforward network, called the CORT-X 2 filter (Carpenter, Grossberg, and Mehanian, 1989; Grossberg and Wyse, 1991, 1992) that suppresses image noise while it completes and regularizes a boundary segmentation of the figure. The noise-suppressed boundary segmentation is made invariant under 2-D rotation, translation, and scale invariance by a centering, log-polar, centering operation (Schwartz, 1977). The resulting spectra are coarse coded to gain some insensitivity to 3-D deformation effects and to reduce memory requirements. This coarse-coded, invariant spectrum of a noise-suppressed boundary segmentation defines the input vectors to the self-organizing neural network classifier.

Fuzzy ARTMAP (Carpenter, Grossberg, Markuzon, Reynolds and Rosen, 1992) was used to categorize the output spectra. This architecture is capable of fast, stable learning of recognition categories in response to nonstationary multidimensional data, and of learning to generate many-to-one output predictions from recognition categories to output labels. Erroneous predictions trigger hypothesis testing, or memory search, in the input classifier. Memory search discovers and learns recognition categories that conjointly maximize code compression and minimize predictive error using a mechanism that is called *match tracking*. Fuzzy ARTMAP can hereby use supervised learning to rapidly fit the number, size, and shape of input categories to the statistical demands of the environment. Each category codes a range of target views.

Evidence accumulation stores several learned categories in working memory, and derives decisions from a voting procedure. On the test set, a single view category leads to up to 90% recognition accuracy, voting with two view categories achieves up to 94%, and voting with three view categories up to 98.5%.

2 Data

The image database used to test the architecture described below consists of multiple 2-D images images of three jets [1]. Video images were taken of

[1] Special thanks to Michael Seibert, Alan Waxman and MIT Lincoln Laboratory for their assistance and use of their data.

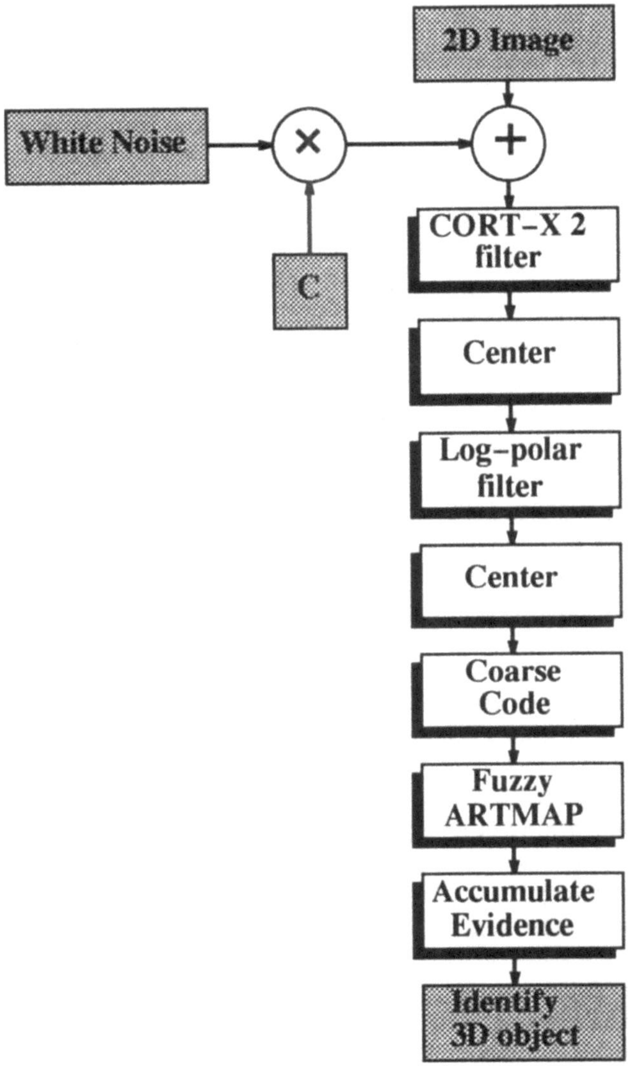

Figure 1: The image processing flow chart of the VIEWNET system from presenting a 2-D image in the image database till the read out of the predicted 3-D object.

3 jet models: an F-16, an F-18, and an HK-1. Each jet was painted black and suspended by string against a light background to facilitate figure-ground separation. The camera was mounted anywhere in an arc around the jets that started at 0.0 degrees above horizontal and went in increments of 4.5 degrees to a maximum of 72.0 degrees above horizontal. For each camera angle, the jets were spun and frames covering one full revolution (an average of 88 frames) were retained resulting in 1200 to 1400 images per object. The images themselves were 128x128 pixel gray scale. The images were then thresholded and binarized into a SUN raster format to form the "raw" database. Data were converted into a floating point format scaled between 0.0 and 1.0 and an additive noise process was introduced. The noise consisted of a 128×128 pixel images with each pixel taken from a uniform distribution between 0.0 and 1.0 scaled by a constant $C \geq 0.0$. These scaled, 128×128 noise images were then added to the 128×128 jet images prior to preprocessing. Thus, both noise-free and noisy 2-D views covering a half-sphere surrounding the 3-D object were collected, keeping their spatial relationships intact.

Even numbered rotation images from each camera angle were taken as the training set with the odd numbered images forming the test set. The system was trained using random walks over the half-sphere of training images. Testing was done using random walks over the half-sphere of test images so that the paths taken and views seen were never the same between the training and test sets.

3 CORT-X 2 filter

The CORT-X 2 filter (Grossberg and Wyse, 1991, 1992) discounts the illuminant and normalizes image contrasts, regularizes and completes figural boundaries, and suppresses image noise. See CORT-X 2 stages in Figure 2(a), filter kernels in Figure 2(b), and equations in the Appendix.

Step 1. Discount the illuminant. A shunting on-center/off-surround network ("ON-C") and an off-center/on-surround network ("OFF-C") operating on the image in parallel are used to discount variable illumination in the image. The ON-C network has a zero baseline activity and the OFF-C network has a positive baseline activity. The OFF-C filter performs an image inversion. Figure 3 shows a noise-free image as well as the ON-C and OFF-C outputs.

Along straight contrast boundaries in an image, both the ON-C and OFF-C networks enhance the contrast. The ON-C network has a stronger response to concave corners of activity in an image than the OFF-C network, while the converse is true at convex corners (Grossberg and Todorović 1988). These complementary responses are used to build better boundary segmentations, as illustrated below.

Step 2. Boundary Segmentation. Two sets of convolution kernels at two different scales are combined to produce a segmentation that takes advantage of another complementary processing property: larger scales achieve better noise reduction and smaller scales achieve better positional localiza-

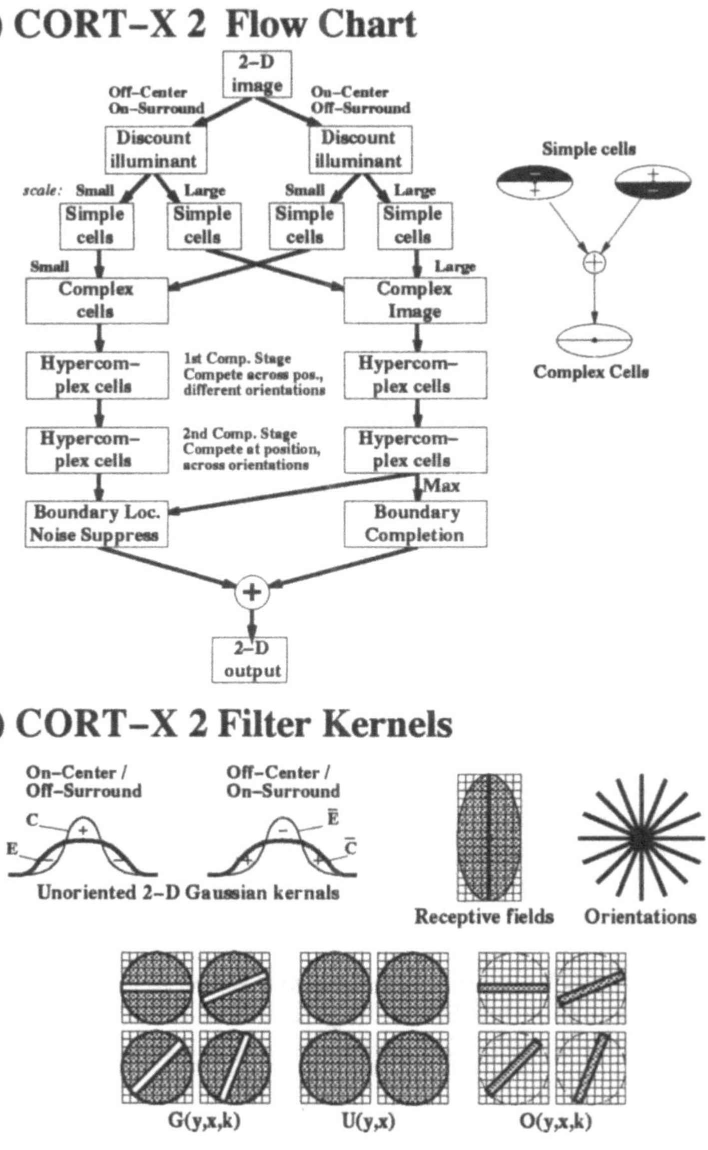

Figure 2: CORT-X 2 flow chart and filter kernels. The image is processed in parallel with small and large scale filters. Grey areas in the kernels are the active regions. All kernels are normalized to have an area equal to one.

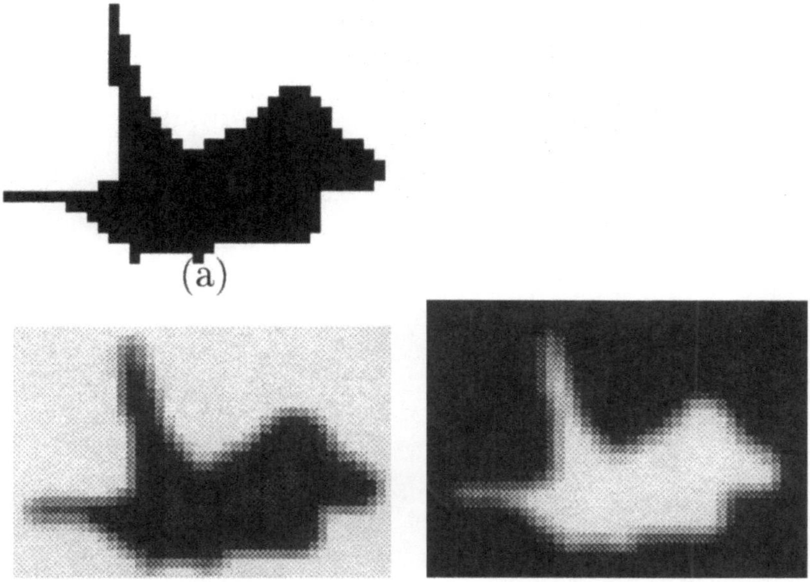

(a) (b) (c)

Figure 3: (a) The original F16 image. (b) CORT-X 2 ON-C output. (c) CORT-X 2 OFF-C output.

tion. The ON-OFF and large-small complementary properties are both exploited in the filter. The first stage, called the simple cell layer, consists of oriented contrast detectors that are sensitive to the orientation, amount, direction, and spatial scale of image contrast at a given image location. The orientation sensitivity results from an elliptically shaped kernel, or input field, one for each of eight orientations spaced 45° apart that operate in parallel at each position in the image. Sensitivity to direction-of-contrast results from a kernel in which one half is excitatory and the other half inhibitory. At each orientation, a pair of detectors sensitive to opposite directions-of-contrast processes the image. The net activity of each detector is rectified, giving rise to a half-wave rectified output signal. Figure 4(a) illustrates processing the ON-C and Figure 4(b) the OFF-C image with the small spatial scale (6x3 pixels) simple cell layer. The same thing is done using the larger spatial scale (10x5 pixels) simple cell layer. Lines in the figure indicate the magnitude of the simple cell response at each orientation at each position.

The complex cell layer combines outputs from the simple cells at each position. Complex cells sum up the half-wave rectified outputs of like-oriented simple cells of both directions-of-contrast at each position from the ON-C and

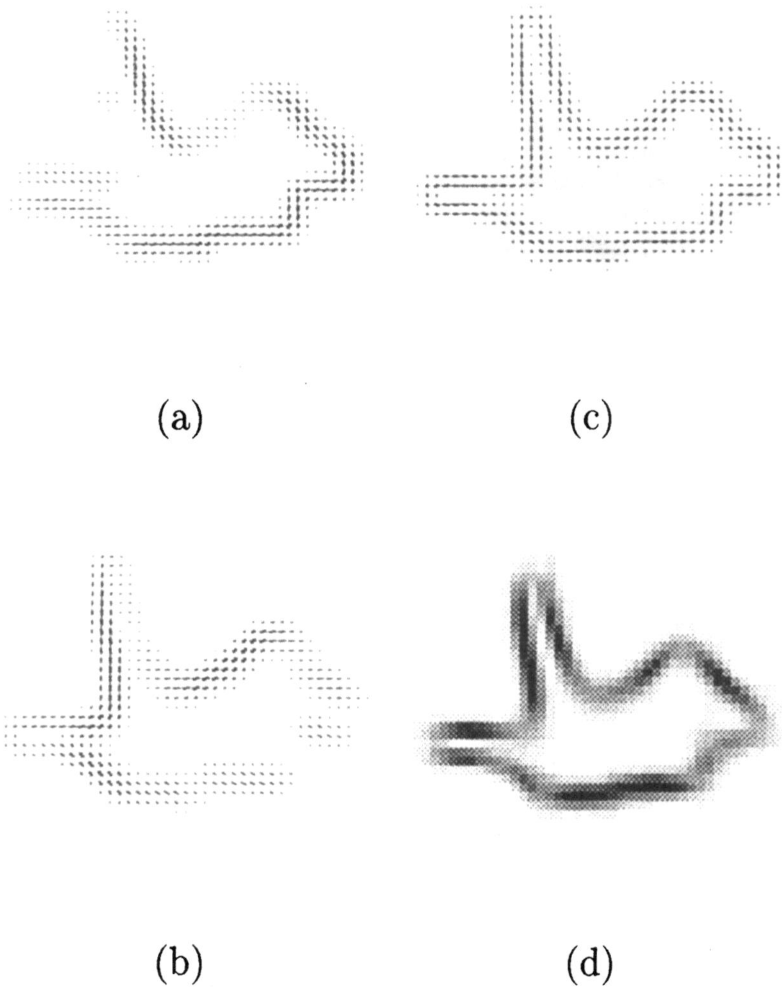

Figure 4: CORT-X 2 processing. (a) Output resulting from the ON-C network, using left sided elliptical filters (simple cell output). A "left sided" filter refers to filters that respond to a vertical left-to-right, high-to-low contrast transition area in the image when the filter is in vertical orientation. A "right sided" filter is the opposite. Lines in the figure are proportional to the magnitude of the response at each orientation at each position. (b) Output from the OFF-C network using left sided elliptical filters. (c) Hypercomplex cell output for the small scale. (d) The final CORT-X 2 output.

OFF-C networks to achieve sensitivity to the orientation, amount, and spatial scale of the contrast in the image, but not to its direction-of-contrast. The complementary deficiencies of the ON-C and OFF-C responses in Figure 4a and 4b are hereby overcome.

Complex cells excite hypercomplex cells in the next layer at their position and orientation while inhibiting hypercomplex cells at nearby locations that are not co-linear with the complex cell's orientation. This interaction is called the first competitive stage. Figure 4(c) shows the output of the hypercomplex cells for the small scale. The next layer, called the second competitive stage, chooses the hypercomplex cell whose orientation is maximally activated to represent the activity at each position.

The final stages of CORT-X 2 involve cooperative interactions between the large and small scale filters. Larger scale filters are better able to complete gaps in image boundaries and to suppress noise, but do a worse job of boundary localization than smaller scale filters. The final CORT-X 2 operations include cooperative interactions between both filter scales that enhance their desirable properties.

Boundary gaps become more likely as the noise in the image increases. To overcome this problem, cooperative interactions among the hypercomplex cells activate an inactive cell if enough cells that share the inactive cell's orientation are active on both sides of its oriented axis. Large and small scales are combined in such a way that the better localization properties of the smaller scale filters have an effect only within regions where the larger scales have located a boundary. Figure 4(d) shows the final CORT-X 2 output consisting of the sum of output of the cooperative and multiple scale interactions. Figure 5 shows the results of processing images with two levels of additive noise: C = 0.5 or 50% noise (a), and C= 1.0 or 100% noise (b).

4 Translation, rotation and scale invariance

The 2-D boundary segmentation is centered by dividing its 1st moments by its 0th moment to find the figure centroid, subtracting off the center of the image and then shifting the figure by this amount. A log-polar transform is then taken with respect to the center of the image. Each point (x, y) is represented as $re^{i\theta}$. Taking the logarithm yields coordinates of log radial magnitude and angle. As is well known (Schwartz, 1977), figural sizes and rotations are converted into figural shifts under log-polar transformation. Using these shift parameters to center the log-polar transformed image leads to a figural representation that is invariant under 2-D changes in position, size and rotation.

5 Coarse coding

Coarse coding reduces memory requirements while compensating for inaccuracies of figural alignment, 3-D viewpoint specific foreshortening, and self-occlusions. On the other hand, too much coarse coding can obscure critical input features and thereby harm recognition performance. The analysis below suggests how to balance these effects to maximize the benefits of coarse coding.

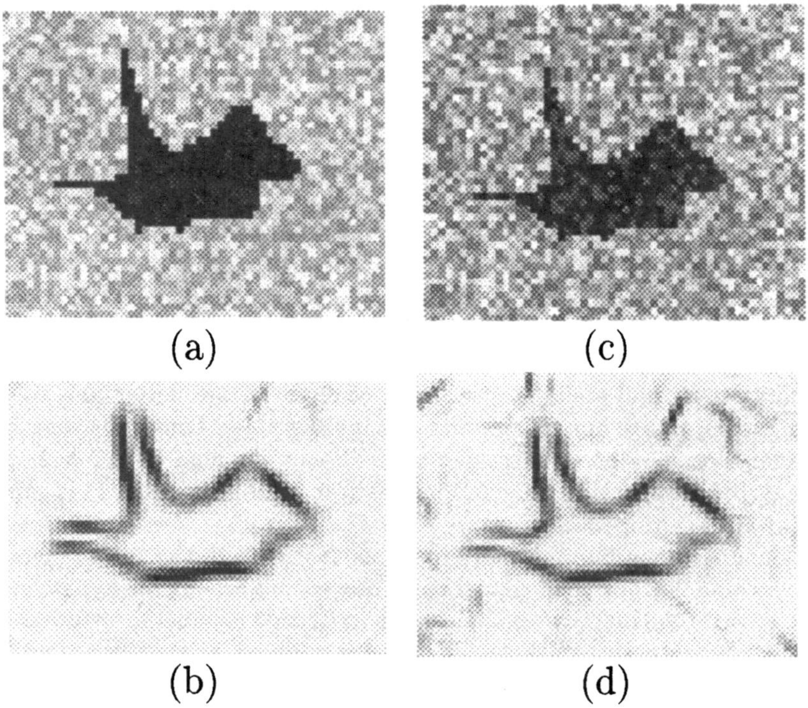

Figure 5: Results of processing noisy images with CORT-X 2. Uniform random noise was added to every pixel in the original image. The original image (left column) had pixels with activity levels between 0.0 and 1.0. Uniform random noise with pixel values ranging between 0.0 and 1.0 was scaled by C and added to the clean image prior to processing by CORT-X 2 with results shown in the right column. In (a,b), random noise between 0.0 and 0.5 ($C = 0.5$ or 50% noise) was added. In (c,d), noise between 0.0 and 1.0 ($C = 1.0$ or 100% noise) was added.

Coarse coding of the 2-D images used a spatial averaging method. Spatial averaging consists of convolving the original image I with a function Ψ and then sampling the resultant image with delta functions spaced every T pixels: $\delta(x - nT, y - kT)$. For simplicity, in 1-D this is

$$(I * \Psi) \cdot \sum_{n=-\infty}^{\infty} \delta(x - nT). \tag{1}$$

If the Fourier transform of I is $\hat{I}$, and that of Ψ is $\hat{\Psi}$, then the Fourier transform of equation (1) is

$$(\hat{I} \cdot \hat{\Psi}) * \frac{2\pi}{T} \sum_{k=-\infty}^{\infty} \delta(\Omega - k\Omega_s), \tag{2}$$

where $\Omega_s = 2\pi/T$, and T is the sampling period in pixels. If Ω_N is the highest frequency in the image, then for the image to be uniquely determined by its samples, we must have by the Nyquist sampling theorem that

$$\Omega_s = \frac{2\pi}{T} > 2\Omega_N. \tag{3}$$

Two simple spatial averaging functions Ψ are: (1) uniform averaging of the input image so that all pixels in a window of some width are summed and divided by the number of pixels in the window; (2) Gaussian averaging of the input image so that a normalized, Gaussian weighted sum of all pixels is taken over a window of some width. Both approaches were investigated in this paper.

Method (1) has the problem that uniform averaging is a rectangular filter in the space domain and a sinc function in the frequency domain which introduces high frequency aliasing ("ringing") in the resultant image. The Gaussian function of method (2) is a "smoother" low pass filter and so does not suffer from this problem. A Gaussian is also an eigenfunction of a Fourier transform, which simplifies calculation.

To best set the standard deviation σ of the Gaussians, we define two standard deviations away from the Gaussian midpoint to be essentially zero. The cutoff frequency of such a low pass filter is then $\pi/2\sigma$, which by equation (3) yields at equality:

$$\sigma = \frac{T}{2}. \tag{4}$$

Thus, the zero point of each Gaussian just touches the center of the next Gaussian. Figure 6 summarizes the preprocessing: 6(a) shows the output of CORT-X 2, 6(b) the centered log polar transform of (a), 6(c) depicts Gaussian coarse coding according to equation (4), and 6(d-f) show coarse coding down to 16×16, 8×8, and 4×4 pixels.

6 Recognition using Fuzzy ARTMAP

A simplified version of the Fuzzy ARTMAP network discussed in Carpenter *et al.* (1992) is used here consisting of a Fuzzy ART module (Carpenter, Grossberg, and Rosen 1991) ART_a and a field of output nodes F^b linked together by an associative memory F^{ab} that is called the *Map Field.* Figure 7 shows

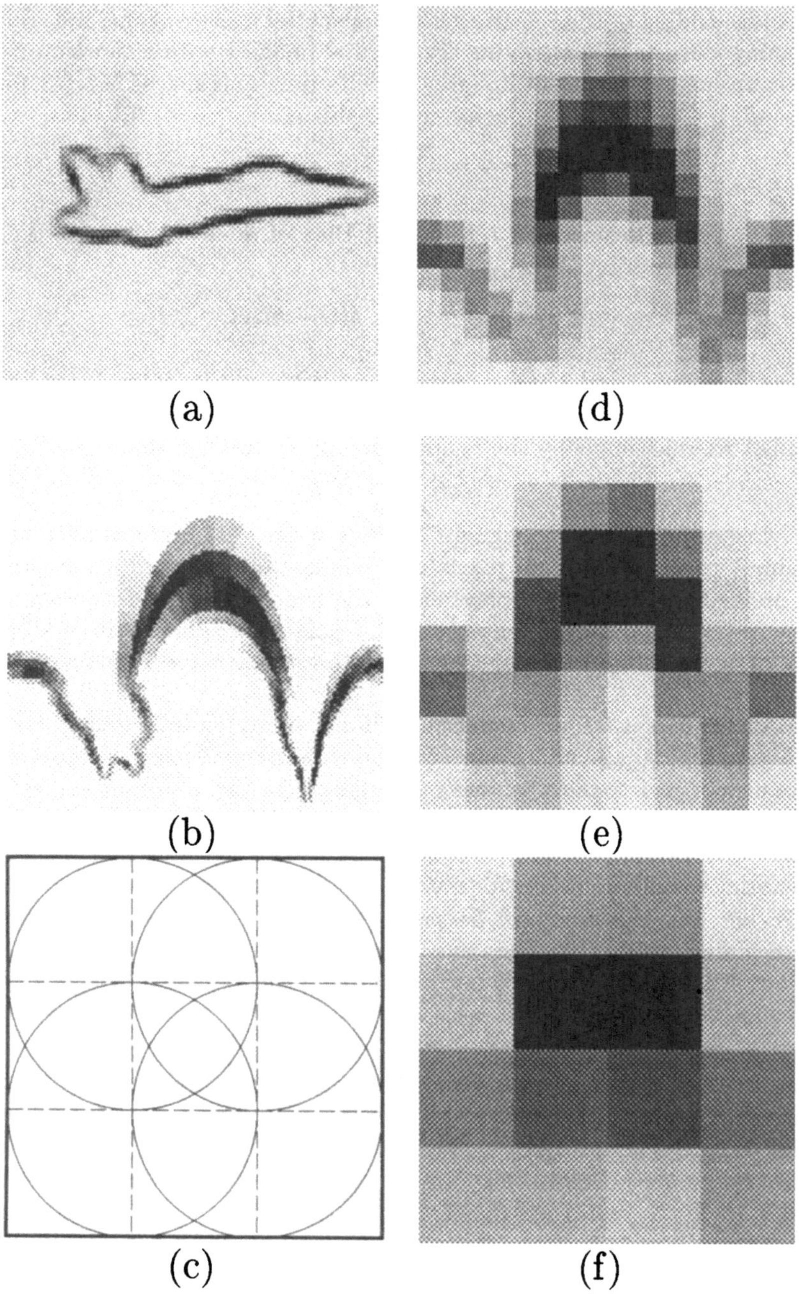

Figure 6: Preprocessing summary. (a) Output of CORT-X 2 preprocessing. (b) Centered log-polar image. (c) Gaussian coarse coding pattern. (d-f) Coarse coding reduction from 128 × 128 pixels down to 16 × 16, 8 × 8, and 4 × 4 pixels.

a block diagram of Fuzzy ARTMAP, and Figure 8 shows a flow chart with equations. In supervised learning mode, Fuzzy ARTMAP receives a sequence of input pairs $(\mathbf{a}_p, \mathbf{b}_p)$ where $\mathbf{b}_p$ is the correct output class given the analog input pattern $\mathbf{a}_p$. The ART_a module classifies analog input vectors $\mathbf{a}_p$ into categories and the Map Field makes associations from the ART_a categories to the outputs $\mathbf{b}_p$ in F^b. If $\mathbf{a}_p$ is categorized into an ART_a category that predicts an incorrect $\mathbf{b}_p$, the mismatch between actual and predicted $\mathbf{b}_p$ causes a memory search within ART_a via a mechanism called *match tracking*. Match tracking raises the ART_a vigilance parameter ρ_a by the minimum amount that will trigger a memory search. Since low vigilance leads to learning of large, coarse categories and high vigilance leads to learning of small, fine categories, match tracking sacrifices the minimum amount of category compression needed to correct each predictive error. Memory search by match tracking continues until a pre-existing ART_a category that predicts the correct ART_b category is found, or a new ART_a category is chosen after which learning takes place. Between learning trials, vigilance relaxes to its baseline vigilance $\bar{\rho}_a$. In test mode, input vectors $\mathbf{a}_p$ are classified by ART_a and the chosen category reads out its prediction to the Map Field. The index of the maximally activated node in the Map Field is taken to represent the predicted output class. (See Carpenter and Grossberg (1994) for more details.)

Fuzzy ARTMAP was modified to allow for on-line slow learning from ART_a F_2^a to the Map Field nodes. A maximal ART_a vigilance level, $\bar{\rho}_{max}$ is introduced (see Figure 8) such that an error at the Map Field triggers match tracking only if match tracking leads to a vigilance $\rho_a \leq \bar{\rho}_{max}$. If $\rho_a > \bar{\rho}_{max}$, learning takes place instead of memory search. By setting the Map Field learning rate β_{ab}, baseline $(\bar{\rho})$ and maximal $(\bar{\rho}_{max})$ vigilance levels appropriately, weights from F_2^a nodes to the Map Field approximate the conditional probability of the true class given the selected F_2^a category. A related approach to slow probability learning is described in Carpenter, Grossberg, and Reynolds (1993).

7 Simulation results

A computer simulation on the jet airplane database was done using the CORT-X 2 parameters in Table 1. The database was processed twice by CORT-X 2 using a larger and a smaller pair of oriented filters in order to compare recognition results at different scales. Coarse coding was done with both simple spatial averaging and Gaussian averaging, reducing the image down to 16×16, 8×8, and 4×4 pixels from an original size of 128×128. Except where mentioned, the simulations were run with the parameters shown in Tables 1 and 2.

The data were presented to the network in two different ways: (1) 2-D views were presented in the "natural" order in which they would appear if viewing the actual object in motion; (2) 2-D views were presented in random order. This was done to test whether presenting views in natural order helps recognition scores. Training in natural order consisted of 160 runs of from 1

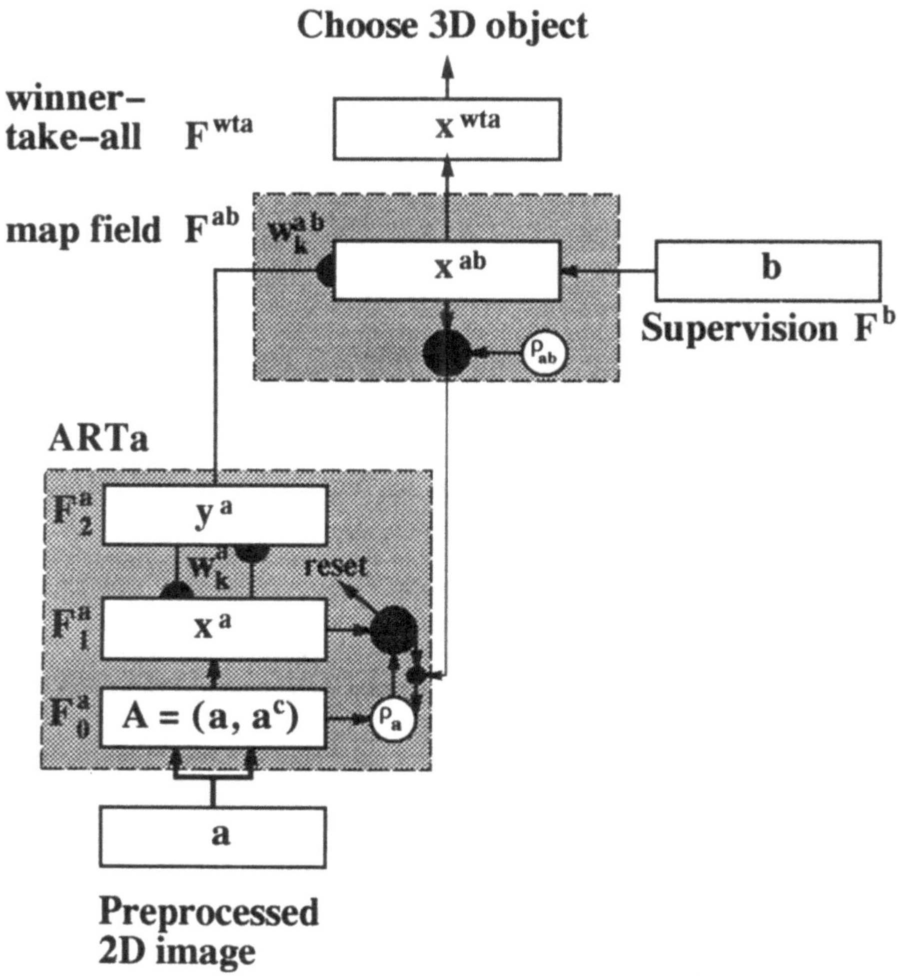

Figure 7: Fuzzy ARTMAP architecture. Each preprocessed 2-D input vector **a** is fed sequentially to the network as it becomes available. The inputs are complement coded which transforms the M-vector **a** into the $2M$-vector $\mathbf{A} = (\mathbf{a}, \mathbf{a}_j^c)$ at field F_0^a which is then fed into the input field F_1^a. A category node k is chosen at F_2^a which reads out its prediction to the Map Field via weights $\mathbf{w}_k^{ab}$. If the prediction is disconfirmed, a match tracking process is invoked in ART_a. Match tracking raises the ART_a vigilance ρ_a to just above the match ratio $|\mathbf{x}^a|/|\mathbf{A}|$. This triggers an ART_a search which activates either a different existing category, or a previously uncommitted category node at F_2^a. After the search process concludes, F^{wta} chooses the maximally activated node in F^{ab} as the 3-D object being viewed.

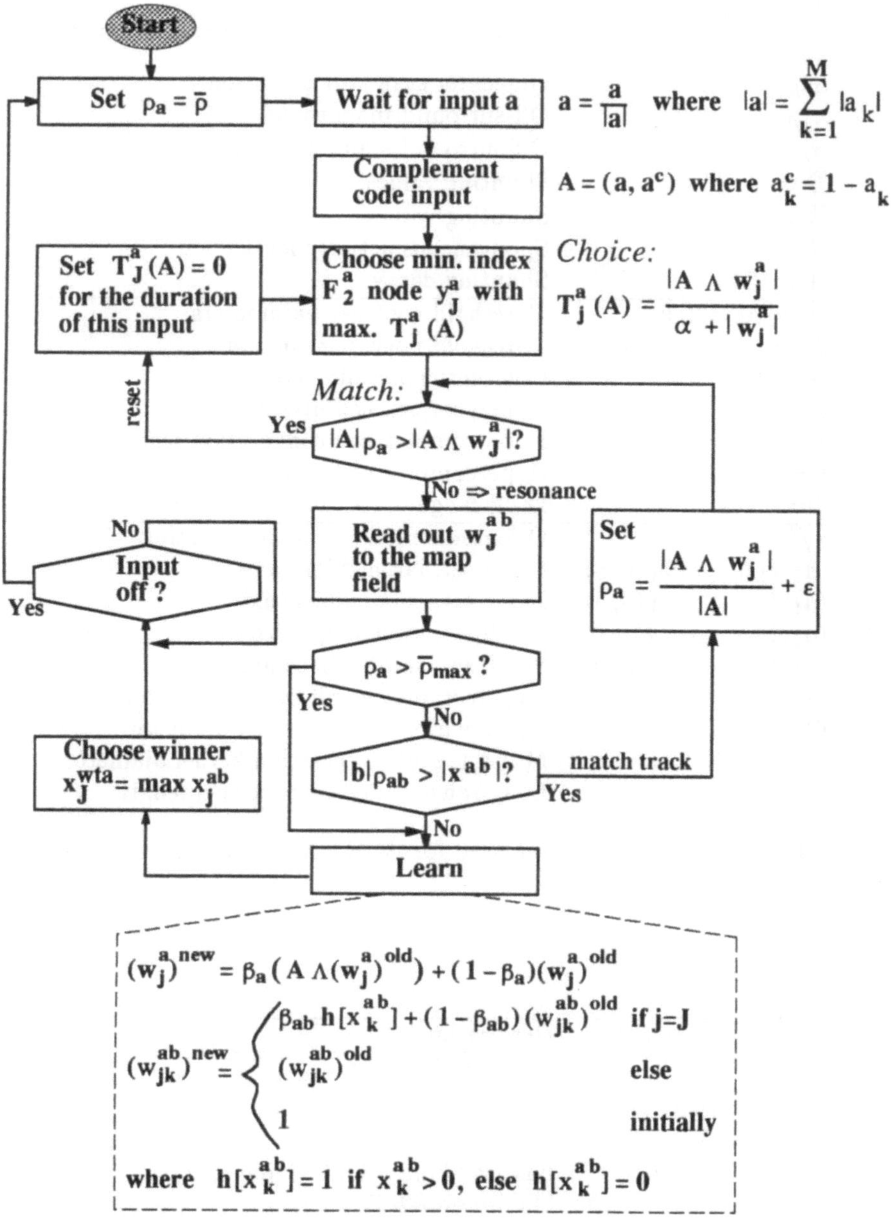

Figure 8: Fuzzy ARTMAP flow chart with reference to Figure 7. The operator $\wedge$ is defined as fuzzy AND (Zadeh, 1965) $(p \wedge q)_k \equiv \min(p_k, q_k)$.

Parameter	*Description*
$\kappa_{onC} = 7.0$	On-center magnitude
$\alpha_{onC} = 1.3$	On-center standard deviation
$\kappa_{offS} = 3.333$	Off-surround magnitude
$\alpha_{offS} = 1.875$	Off-surround standard deviation
$\overline{D} = B = 1.0$	Shunting values
$\overline{B} = D = 0.5$	Shunting values
$S = 0.2$	Spontaneous activity level
$A = 134$	Shunting decay
$\alpha_1 = \alpha_2 = 1.1$	Threshold contrast parameters
$\beta_1 = \beta_2 = \beta = .003$	Threshold noise parameters
$F = 0.5$	Complex cell scaling constant
$\epsilon = 0.1$	Hypercomplex cell divisive offset
$\mu = 5.0$	Hypercomplex cell convolution scaling
$\tau = 0.004$	Hypercomplex cell threshold
$\delta = 0.001$	Long range cooperation threshold
$\pi/8$	Oriented kernel orientation spacing
$(a_2, b_2)_{large} = (16, 8)$	Large set, large ellipse axis
$(a_1, b_1)_{large} = (10, 5)$	Large set, small ellipse axis
$(a_2, b_2)_{small} = (10, 5)$	Small set, large ellipse axis
$(a_1, b_1)_{small} = (6, 3)$	Small set, small ellipse axis
$G_1 = 2a_1/3$	Hypercomplex small kernel diameter
$G_2 = 2a_2/3$	Hypercomplex large kernel diameter
$U = 2a_2/5$	Multiple scale interaction kernel diameter
$O = 3a_2/5$	Long-range cooperation kernel length

Table 1: The parameter set used for CORT-X 2 in the simulations.

Parameter	*Description*
$\alpha = 0.6$	Fuzzy ART search order
$\beta_a = 1.0$	Fuzzy ART learning rate
$\beta_{ab} = 1.0$	Map Field learning rate
$\bar{\rho} = 0.1$	Baseline Fuzzy ART vigilance ρ_a
$\bar{\rho}_{max} = 1.0$	Maximum ART_a vigilance
$\rho_{ab} = 1.0$	Map Field vigilance

Table 2: The FuzzyARTMAP parameter set used for the simulations.

CORT-X 2 filter set	*Data presentation*	*Coarse code using spatial / Gaussian avg* 4x4	8x8	16x16
Small	Ordered	81.0/83.1	84.4/86.4	86.7/90.5
Small	Unordered	80.3/83.9	84.9/86.5	86.8/89.3
Large	Ordered	76.8/78.7	79.0/81.6	79.1/80.1
Large	Unordered	77.4/79.7	80.5/81.5	77.1/80.5

Table 3: Recognition results on a noise free database ($C = 0$). In the table, "Large" refers to the run with the larger set of CORT-X 2 oriented filters, "Small" refers to the run with the smaller set of filters. Views were presented either in natural order or in random order. Data was coarse coded from 128x128 down to 4x4, 8x8, or 16x16 using simple spatial averaging or Gaussian averaging. Recognition scores refer to the percent of 2-D views correctly associated with a 3-D object.

to 50 views over each object. Training in random order consisted of a series of 40 runs of 100 training set views over each object. Recognition scores are taken as an average of fifteen separate training-testing cycles.

7.1 Fast learning without noise

No clear advantage results from ordered presentation as compared to unordered presentation using noise-free data ($C = 0$) and fast learning, as shown by the results in Table 3. It can be seen that the smaller CORT-X 2 filter set resulted in better recognition performance overall and did better given more detail (less coarse coding).

7.2 Fast learning simulation with noise

The system was next tested with noisy data using additive white noise scaled by $C = 1.0$. Table 4 shows what percent of the additive noise survives processing by CORT-X 2 alone, and by CORT-X 2 and coarse coding together. The percent noise surviving these transformations was measured by the following formula:

$$\max_{\forall(x,y)} \left[\frac{\Psi(\mathbf{I}+\mathbf{N}) - \Psi(\mathbf{I})}{C} \right] \times 100, \tag{5}$$

where $\mathbf{I}$ is the image, $\mathbf{N}$ is the noise image, Ψ is the CORT-X 2 filter, $C > 0$ is the noise scaling parameter and (x, y) is the pixel index in the images. Table 4 represents the average results from ten measurements using equation (5). With such noise reduction, the recognition results shown in Table 5 were similar to those for the noise-free case in Table 3, except for some falling off of recognition scores at the lowest level of coarse coding (the 16×16 case).

Table 6 shows the number of nodes created by the network after training for the no noise (left entry) and noise (right entry) results reported above. Noise causes a small increase in the number of categories formed on average as the network attempts to correct a greater number of noise-induced errors during supervised training.

% noise surviving CORT-X 2 filtering and Coarse Coding:		
	Large CORT-X 2 filters (16x8, 10x5)	*Small CORT-X 2 filters (10x5, 6x3)*
	1.79	2.42
After Gaussian coarse coding from 128x128 down to:		
16x16	0.33	0.34
8x8	0.23	0.29
4x4	0.19	0.26
After spatial average coarse coding from 128x128 down to:		
16x16	0.40	0.40
8x8	0.28	0.30
4x4	0.21	0.28

Table 4: Percent of additive white noise surviving processing by CORT-X 2 and coarse coding.

CORT-X 2 filter set	*Data presentation*	*Coarse code using spatial / Gaussian avg* 4x4	8x8	16x16
Small	Ordered	80.1/83.3	84.5/85.9	84.2/89.1
Small	Unordered	79.4/83.2	83.9/86.4	84.3/88.0
Large	Ordered	76.6/79.4	79.3/80.8	75.8/79.3
Large	Unordered	76.0/79.7	78.4/80.7	75.5/79.0

Table 5: Recognition results on noisy data ($C = 1$) with fast learning ($\beta_{ab} = 1.0$). These results differ little from the noise-free results in Table 3 (no noise condition) with the exception of some consistent reduction in scores for the 16x16 coarse coding.

CORT-X 2 filter set	*Data presentation*	*Coarse code using spatial / Gaussian avg* 4x4	8x8	16x16
Small	Ordered	[172, 184]	[77, 73]	[34, 33]
		[165, 169]	[70, 73]	[33, 35]
Small	Unordered	[191, 198]	[76, 77]	[34, 35]
		[175, 179]	[73, 76]	[35, 36]
Large	Ordered	[168, 179]	[71, 68]	[31,33]
		[160, 162]	[67, 71]	[30, 31]
Large	Unordered	[183, 192]	[73, 75]	[32, 32]
		[169, 174]	[69, 72]	[33, 32]

Table 6: Average number of ART_a categories formed during training for the simulations of Table 3 (no noise) and Table 5 (noise). The format in the table is as follows: [spatial avg.]/[Gaussian avg.] = [No noise, Noise]/[No noise, Noise].

CORT-X 2 filter set	*Data presentation*	*Coarse code using spatial / Gaussian avg* 4x4	8x8	16x16
Small	Ordered	79.9/83.1	84.0/85.6	84.7/89.9
Small	Unordered	78.8/83.3	83.2/85.7	84.9/89.1
Large	Ordered	76.3/78.2	78.5/81.5	77.0/78.8
Large	Unordered	77.4/80.2	79.6/80.41	75.8/79.2

Table 7: Recognition results on noisy data ($C = 1$) with slow learning to the Map Field ($\beta_{ab} = 0.2$, $\bar{\rho}_{max} = 0.95$). Due to the low levels of noise surviving preprocessing, the recognition results here are not substantially different than those found using fast learning in noise in Table 5 except where noise was highest as in the 16x16 coarse coding. As noise increases, slow learning becomes more important for maintaining good recognition scores.

7.3 Slow learning simulation with noise

For the next set of computer simulations, the network was run on the noisy data using slow learning to the Map Field ($\beta_{ab} = 0.2$). Fast learning was still used within the ART_a module itself ($\beta_a = 1.0$). Note that for $\bar{\rho}_{max} = 1.0$, the results for slow learning and fast learning (Section 7.2) to the Map Field are equivalent. They are equivalent because with Map Field vigilance set to $\rho_{ab} = 1.0$ as in Table 2, the slightest mismatch at the Map Field will invoke match tracking and a new category will be created. To derive benefit from slow learning in the case $\rho_{ab} = 1.0$, we set $\bar{\rho}_{max} = 0.95$. Table 7 records the results using slow learning in large amplitude noise ($C = 1$). Where noise levels after preprocessing were very small, the results were approximately the same as in the fast learning case shown in Table 5. Slow learning begins to help when the noise level increases, as with the 16×16 coarse coding. Table 8 records the average number of categories formed for the noisy data case using fast learning and slow learning. Slow learning with $\bar{\rho}_{max} = 0.95$, caused approximately 10% fewer categories to be formed than with $\bar{\rho}_{max} = 1.0$, since noise-induced errors do not always cause the formation of a new category in the former case.

8 Voting versus view transitions

For the jet data set as processed by VIEWNET, it was found that the average overall length of an error sequence was 1.31 2-D views with a standard deviation of 0.57 views. Thus, when an error occurs, collecting evidence from (or voting over) two more views will usually be sufficient to correct the error. This can be done in VIEWNET by adding an integration field (F^{int}) between the Map Field (F^{ab}) and the winner-take-all field (F^{wta}) in Figure 7. The equation for the integrator field is stepped once each time ART_a chooses a category:

$$(x_k^{int})^{new} = \beta_{int} x_k^{ab} + (1 - \beta_{int})(x_k^{int})^{old}, \tag{6}$$

where x_k^{int} is an integrator node for the kth object, β_{int} is the integration rate each time the equation is stepped, and x_k^{ab} is the kth Map Field category. The

CORT-X 2 filter set	*Data presentation*	*Coarse code using spatial / Gaussian avg* 4x4	8x8	16x16
Small	Ordered	[184, 165] [169, 150]	[73, 67] [73, 66]	[33, 30] [35, 32]
Small	Unordered	[198, 180] [179, 163]	[77, 69] [76, 70]	[35, 32] [36, 33]
Large	Ordered	[179, 160] [162, 147]	[68, 61] [71, 66]	[33 , 30] [31, 29]
Large	Unordered	[192, 175] [174, 160]	[75, 69] [72, 67]	[32, 30] [32, 30]

Table 8: Average number of nodes formed during training for the simulations of Tables 5 (noise with fast learning) and 7 (noise with slow learning). The format in the table is as follows: [spatial avg.]/[Gaussian avg.] = [fast learning, slow learning]/[fast learning, slow learning]. It can be seen that slow learning reduced the number of nodes formed by approximately 10%.

maximal integration node is chosen by the winner-take-all field (F^{wta}) as the network's identification of the 3-D object.

Figure 9 shows the average recognition scores for voting with $\beta_{int} = 0.2$ over one, two, and three views under CORT-X 2 preprocessing with large and small scale filter sets and coarse coding to 4×4, 8×8 and 16×16 pixels using both Gaussian and spatial averaging. Voting over 3 frames improves recognition results by an average of ten percent with the best results being 98.5% correct for small scale filtered 16×16 Gaussian coarse coded data.

The advantage of voting over using 2-D view transitions is that given N 2-D views, the $O(N^2)$ cost for learning view transitions is avoided. To compare how well voting over view sequences does to using view transitions, the architecture described in Bradski, Carpenter, and Grossberg (1991) (Section 1) that incorporates 2-D views and 2-D view transitions for recognition was simulated.

In Figure 9, the black circles and squares represent the recognition scores using view transitions for preprocessing with the large and small scale CORT-X 2 filters respectively. Recognition scores from view transitions and from evidence accumulation are similar. Since evidence accumulation does not require the $O(N^2)$ nodes needed for learning 2-D view transitions, evidence accumulation over view transitions seems sufficient for this application.

9 Concluding Remarks

Using the smaller set of CORT-X 2 filters, a 3-D object recognition rate of approximately 90% may be achieved from single 2-D views alone without recourse to more elaborate methods of generating aspect graph models of the 3-D objects. When evidence integration or voting over a sequence of views is added, recognition rates reach 98.5% within three views. Voting over two views did as well as using view transitions on this database, but

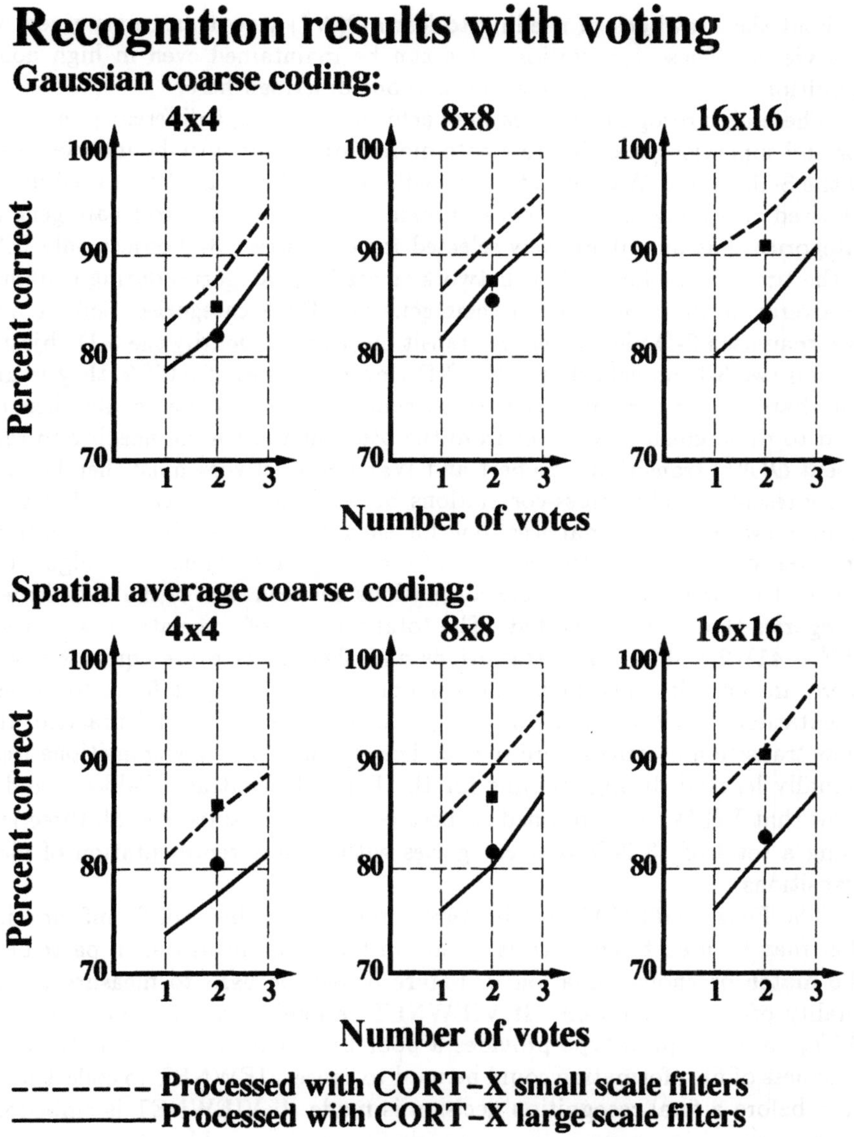

Figure 9: Recognition results for voting with an integration rate of $\beta_{int} = 0.2$. The graphs show the recognition results after gathering evidence over one, two and three 2-D views for data preprocessed using large (solid line) and small (dotted line) scale CORT-X 2 filters. Results from both Gaussian and spatial averaging coarse coding methods are shown where the images were reduced from 128×128 down to 4×4, 8×8 and 16×16 pixels. The circles and squares represent recognition scores resulting from using view transitions as discussed in Section 8.

without the drawback of needing to learn $O(N^2)$ view transitions given N, 2-D views. These recognition rates can be maintained even in high noise conditions using the preprocessing methods described here.

These high recognition rates were achieved by using a different preprocessor and supervised learning to create more optimal category boundaries than in the Seibert and Waxman studies. Seibert and Waxman (1992) used unsupervised clustering of coarse coded maximal curvature data to create general categories that unambiguously selected for the correct 3-D object only 25% of the time. In so doing, their network created 41 categories during training. To overcome the ambiguity of their general ART 2 categories, Seibert and Waxman used 2-D view category transitions to help identify the 3-D objects. Even if two 3-D objects shared the 2-D view categories of ART 2, they might not share the particular 2-D view category transitions that could then be used to distinguish one object from the other at the cost of needing to represent $O(N^2)$ transitions. Seibert and Waxman's network must then be able to represent possible cross-correlations between every categorical 2-D view in its view transition matrices, one for each object, even if no correlations are eventually found between some of the categories. Thus, their algorithm needed to represent the possible correlations between each of the 41 2-D view categories that were generated. The total number of correlations were then $(41^2 - 41)/2 = 820$, since transitions and their reverse are equivalent and there are no self-transitions. This is done for each object for a total representation of $820 \times 3 = 2460$ possible correlations. In actual practice, the view transition matrices were sparse. For example, 70 view transitions were actually learned during training for the F-16. In contrast, Tables 3 and 6 show that VIEWNET obtained its best recognition results over all three jets using a total of 33 2-D view categories without any representation of view transitions.

The Fuzzy ARTMAP architecture computes goodness of fit information that may be used to enhance its power in future applications. In particular, the match or choice equation in Figure 8 may be used to measure to the quality of the recognition. If VIEWNET recognizes a 3-D object, but its ART_a category prototype provides a poor fit to the input vector, then the goodness of fit information could be used to cause VIEWNET to collect more data before a final recognition decision is made. If VIEWNET is embedded in an active vision system, then a poorly fitting view could be used to trigger the system to move to get a better perspective.

A Appendix: CORT-X 2 equations

The equations for the CORT-X 2 filter as described in Section 3 are discussed below. Figure 2 shows the flow chart and filter kernels. Table 1 summarizes the parameters used in the simulations. Filter kernels G, U, and O are normalized to have area equal to one.

A.1 Step 1. Discounting the Illuminant

ON-C and OFF-C Network: The activation x_{ij} at node v_{ij} at position (i,j) obeys the shunting on-center off-surround equation:

$$\frac{d}{dt}x_{ij} = -Ax_{ij} + (B - x_{ij})C_{ij} - (x_{ij} + D)E_{ij}, \tag{7}$$

and $\bar{x}_{ij}$ obeys the off-center, on-surround equation:

$$\frac{d}{dt}\bar{x}_{ij} = -A(\bar{x}_{ij} - S) + (\overline{B} - \bar{x}_{ij})\overline{C}_{ij} - (\bar{x}_{ij} + \overline{D})\overline{E}_{ij} \tag{8}$$

where C_{ij}, $\overline{C}_{ij}$, E_{ij}, $\overline{E}_{ij}$ are discrete convolutions of the input with gaussian kernels of the form:
$K_{ij} = \sum_{p,q} I_{pq}K_{pqij}$ with $K_{pqij} = \kappa \exp\left\{-\alpha^{-2}\log 2[(p-i)^2 + (q-j)^2]\right\}$.

The on-center kernel of $\bar{x}_{ij}$ is the off-surround kernel of x_{ij}, and the off-surround kernel of $\bar{x}_{ij}$ is the on-center kernel of x_{ij}. Then $\overline{C}_{ij} = E_{ij}$, $\overline{E}_{ij} = C_{ij}$. Also in equations (7) and (8), $\overline{B} = D$ and $\overline{D} = B$. At equilibrium in the ON-C network,

$$x_{ij} = \frac{\sum_{(p,q)}(BC_{pqij} - DE_{pqij})I_{pq}}{A + \sum_{(p,q)}(C_{pqij} + E_{pqij})I_{pq}}, \tag{9}$$

and in the OFF-C network,

$$\overline{x}_{ij} = \frac{AS + \sum_{(p,q)}(DE_{pqij} - BC_{pqij})I_{pq}}{A + \sum_{(p,q)}(C_{pqij} + E_{pqij})I_{pq}}. \tag{10}$$

A.2 Step 2. CORT-X 2 Filter

Oriented receptive fields are elliptical with $y^2/a_s^2 + x^2/b_s^2 = 1$, where a_s is the major axis and b_s is the minor axis with $a_s \geq b_s$. Two sizes of receptive fields were used, indexed by the subscript s with 1 = small scale and 2 = large scale. Orientations are indexed below by subscript k.

Simple Cells: Simple cells of scale s with activation variable $x = x_{ij}$ and receptive field orientation k have outputs

$$S_{sL}(i,j,k) = \max[L_s(x,k) - \alpha_s R_s(x,k) - \beta_s, 0] \tag{11}$$

$$S_{sR}(i,j,k) = \max[R_s(x,k) - \alpha_s L_s(x,k) - \beta_s, 0] \tag{12}$$

where $L_s(x,k)$ and $R_s(x,k)$ are the left or right oriented receptive field inputs

$$L_s(x,k) = \frac{\sum_{(p,q)\in l_s(i,j,k)} x_{pq}w_{pq}}{\sum_{(p,q)\in l_s(i,j,k)} w_{pq}} \tag{13}$$

and

$$R_s(x,k) = \frac{\sum_{(p,q)\in r_s(i,j,k)} x_{pq}w_{pq}}{\sum_{(p,q)\in r_s(i,j,k)} w_{pq}}, \tag{14}$$

where w_{pq} is a weighting factor proportional to the area of a cell covered by the receptive field. L and R in S_{sL} and S_{sR} indicate that each receptive field is sensitive to the opposite direction-of-contrast from its companion. The ON and OFF networks have separate sets of simple cells with the ON simple cells denoted by S_{sL}^+ and S_{sR}^+, and the OFF simple cells denoted by S_{sL}^- and S_{sR}^-.

Complex Cells: The complex cell output $C_s(x,k)$ is defined by

$$C_s(i,j,k) = F[S_{sL}^+(i,j,k) + S_{sR}^+(i,j,k) + S_{sL}^-(i,j,k) + S_{sR}^-(i,j,k)]. \tag{15}$$

Hypercomplex Cells (First Competitive Stage): The hypercomplex cells $D_s(i,j,k)$ receive input from the spatial competition among the complex cells:

$$D_s(i,j,k) = \max\left[\frac{C_s(i,j,k)}{\epsilon + \mu \sum_m \sum_y C_s(p,q,m)G_s(p,q,i,j,k)} - \tau, 0\right]. \quad (16)$$

Hypercomplex Cells (Second Competitive Stage): Hypercomplex cells $D_s(i,j)$ compute the competition among oriented activities $D_s(i,j,k)$ at each position. This process is simplified as a winner-take-all process

$$D_s(i,j) = D_2(i,j,K) = \max_k D_s(i,j,k), \quad (17)$$

where K denotes the orientation of the maximally activated cell.

Multiple Scale Interaction: The interaction between the small and large scales is defined by

$$B_{12}(i,j) = D_1(i,j)\sum_{p,q} D_2(p,q)U(p,q,i,j). \quad (18)$$

Long-Range Cooperation: The large detectors $D_2(i,j)$, are capable of responding across locations where pixel signal strength has been reduced by noise. Such boundary signals may, however, be poorly localized. To overcome this tradeoff between boundary completion and localization, large-scale cells interact cooperatively as

$$B_2(i,j) = D_2(i,j)\max\left[\sum_{p,q} D_2(p,q,K)O(p,q,i,j,K) - \delta, 0\right]. \quad (19)$$

CORT-X 2 Output: The final output of the CORT-X 2 filter is the sum of the multiple scale interaction and the cooperative process:

$$B(i,j) = B_{12}(i,j) + B_2(i,j). \quad (20)$$

Acknowledgements

Gary Bradski was supported in part by the National Science Foundation (NSF IRI 90-24877) and the Office of Naval Research (ONR N00014-92-J-1309).

Steve Grossberg was supported in part by the Air Force Office of Scientific Research (AFOSR F49620-92-J-0499), ARPA (AFOSR 90-0083 and ONR N00014-92-J-4015) and the Office of Naval Research (ONR N00014-91-J-4100).

References

Bowyer, K., Eggert, D., Stewman, J., & Stark, L. (1989). Developing the aspect graph representation for use in image understanding. In *Proc. 1989 Image Understanding Workshop*, pp. 831–849.

Bradski, G., Carpenter, G., & Grossberg, S. (1991). Working memory networks for learning multiple groupings of temporally ordered events: Application to 3-D visual object recognition. In *Proceedings of the IJCNN-91, Seattle, WA.*, Vol. 1, pp. 723–728. Piscataway, NJ: IEEE Service Center.

Carpenter, G., & Grossberg, S. (1987). ART 2: Self-organization of stable category recognition codes for analog input patterns. *Applied Optics*, *26*, 4919–4930.

Carpenter, G., & Grossberg, S. (1994). Self-organizing neural networks for supervised and unsupervised learning and prediction.. In Cherkassky, V., Friedman, J., & Wechsler, H. (Eds.), *From Statistics to Neural Networks. Theory and Pattern Recognition Applications.* New York, NY: Springer-Verlag.

Carpenter, G., Grossberg, S., Markuzon, N., Reynolds, J., & Rosen, D. (1992). Fuzzy ARTMAP: A neural network architecture for incremental supervised learning of analog multidimensional maps. *IEEE Transactions on Neural Networks*, *3*, 698–713.

Carpenter, G., Grossberg, S., & Mehanian, C. (1989). Invariant recognition of cluttered scenes by a self-organizing ART architecture: CORT-X boundary segmentation. *Neural Networks*, *2*, 169–181.

Carpenter, G., Grossberg, S., & Reynolds, J. (1993). Fuzzy ARTMAP, slow learning and probability estimation. Tech. rep. CAS/CNS-TR-93-014, Boston University, Boston, MA: Boston University.

Carpenter, G., Grossberg, S., & Rosen, D. (1991). Fuzzy ART: Fast stable learning and categorization of analog patterns by an adaptive resonance system. *Neural Networks*, *4*.

Carpenter, G., & Ross, W. (1993). ART-EMAP: A neural network architecture for learning and prediction by evidence accumulation. In *Proceedings of the World Congress on Neural Networks, (WCNN-93).*, Vol. III, pp. 649–656.

Chang, I., & Huang, C. (1992). Aspect graph generation for non-convex polyhedra from perspective projection view. *Pattern Recognition*, *25*(10), 1075.

Eggert, D., & Bowyer, K. (1993). Computing the perspective projection aspect graph of solids of revolution. *IEEE Trans. on Pattern Analysis and Machine Intelligence*, *15*(2), 109.

Gigus, Z., & Malik, J. (1988). Computing the aspect graph for line drawings of polyhedral objects. In *Proc. IEEE Conf. Comput. Vision Pattern Recognition*, pp. 654–661.

Gigus, Z., & Malik, J. (1990). Computing the aspect graph for line drawings of polyhedral objects. *IEEE transactions on pattern analysis and machine vision*, *12*(2), 113.

Grossberg, S. (1993). 3-D vision and figure-ground separation by visual cortex. Tech. rep. CAS/CNS-TR-92-019, Boston University, Perception and Psychophysics, in press.

Grossberg, S., & Todorovic, D. (1988). Neural dynamics of 1-D and 2-D brightness perception: A unified model of classical and recent phenomena. *Perception and Psychophysics*, *43*, 241–277.

Grossberg, S., & Wyse, L. (1991). A neural network architecture for figure-ground separation of connected scenic figures. *Neural Networks*, *4*, 723–742.

Grossberg, S., & Wyse, L. (1992). A neural network architecture for figure-ground separation of connected scenic figures. In Pinter, R., & Nabet, B. (Eds.), *Nonlinear Vision: Determination of Neural Receptive Fields, Function, and Networks* (1 edition)., chap. 21, pp. 516–543. CRC Press, Inc.

Koenderink, J., & van Doorn, A. (1979). The internal representation of solid shape with respect to vision. *Biological Cybernetics.*, *32*, 211–216.

Plantinga, H., & Dyer, C. (1990). Visibility, occlusion, and the aspect graph. *Int. J. Comput. Vision*, *5*(2), 137–160.

Ponce, J., & Kriegman, D. (1990). Computing exact aspect graphs of curved objects: Parametric surfaces. In *Proc. 8th National Conf. on Artificial Intell.*, pp. 1074–1079.

Rieger, J. (1990). The geometry of view space opaque objects bounded by smooth surfaces. *Artificial Intell.*, *44*, 1–40.

Rimey, R., & Brown, C. (1991). Hmms and vision: Representing structure and sequences for active vision using hidden markov models. Tech. rep., University of Rochester Computer Science Department TR No. 366.

Schwartz, E. (1977). Spatial mapping in primate sensory projection: analytic structure and relevance to perception. *Biological Cybernetics*, *25*, 181–194.

Seibert, M., & Waxman, A. (1992). Adaptive 3-D-object recognition from multiple views. *IEEE Transactions on Pattern Analysis and Machine Intelligence*, *11*, 107–124.

Sripradisvarakul, T., & Jain, R. (1989). Generating aspect graphs for curved objects. In *Proc. IEEE Workshop Interpretation of 3-D Scenes*, pp. 109–115.

Stewmen, J., & Bowyer, K. (1990). Direct construction of the perspective projection aspect graph of convex polyhedra. *Computer vision, graphics, and image processing*, *51*(1), 20.

Zadeh, L. (1965). Fuzzy sets. *Information Control*, *8*, 338–353.

Chaotic Dynamics in Neural Pattern Recognition

Walter J Freeman

Division of Neurobiology
Department of Molecular & Cell Biology
University of California at Berkeley CA 94720 USA

Abstract. The use of impulse inputs for characterizing neural "signals" that are embedded in electroencephalographic EEG "noise" is reviewed in the context of linear systems analysis. Examples are given of the use of linear and nearly linear basis functions with statistics for measurement of neural activity patterns of single cells and populations, with emphasis on the relations between microscopic and macroscopic activity, including measurement of local mean fields and description of the transfer of microscopic sensory information to the macroscopic level of perception and then back to microscopic cortical output by action potentials. Some elements of nonlinear dynamics are introduced that are needed to understand the emergence of low-dimensional aperiodic activity in sensory cortex, and its possible uses for the operation of Hebbian synapses during the learning of new generalization gradients.

1 Introduction

Biological neural networks even in simpler animals are adept at pattern recognition, including goal-directed management of figure-ground relations, feature definition and extraction, generalization on classes of examples during reinforcement learning, the exclusion of irrelevant and ambiguous inputs by habituation, and adaptation to rapid and/or long term evolutionary changes in both target stimuli and background clutter.

These operations are performed by masses of nerve cells forming two dimensional sheets in serial layers, with multiple distributed feedback connections among the cells both within and between the layers. The characteristic relaxation rates and point spread functions of the component cells are the determinants of the time and distance metrics of the continuous time dynamics of the populations (Freeman, 1975; Basar, 1980).

The dynamics of each population of neurons can be modeled with networks of coupled ordinary differential equations. The solutions sets of such systems contain point, limit cycle and chaotic attractors with their attendant basins of attraction delimited in state space. During normal operations of sensation and perception each sensory cortex maintains a global chaotic attractor, which has multiple wings, each of which has been formed during a prior learning experience with a class of stimuli. An act of recognition takes place through the confinement of the cortex into an appropriate wing by the bias that is imposed by an expected stimulus. Generalization occurs by the basin of attraction for the wing. Adaptation occurs by update of the attractor through continuing learning (Basar, 1990; Freeman, 1992).

This review is in three parts. First, the elements of signal detection theory for linear systems is reviewed. Second, the uses of statistics for measurement of neural activity patterns of single cells and populations are discussed, with emphasis on the relations between microscopic and macroscopic activity, including derivation and measurement of local mean fields, and description of the transfer of microscopic sensory information to the macroscopic level of perception and then back to output by action potentials. The microscopic activity of single neurons is patterned by the macroscopic population activity acting as an order parameter (Haken and Stadler, 1990). Third, elements of nonlinear dynamics are introduced that are needed to understand the emergence of low-dimensional aperiodic activity in sensory cortex, and its possible uses for the operation of Hebbian synapses during the learning of new generalization gradients. Attention is given to the goal-oriented and self-organizing properties of biological systems, which are not at present sufficiently used in artificial neural networks, and which may provide challenges as well as opportunities in the future embodiments of the principles of neurodynamics into systems designed for artificial intelligence.

2. Characterizing neural activity as "signal" vs. "noise"

The description of a neural operation requires measurement of inputs and outputs in pairs, from which a transformation is derived that maps the one into the other. For study of these operations in early stages of the olfactory system, pulses are elicited in the sensory axons by electrical stimulation, and the pulses and dendritic currents formed by the neurons in response to the stimuli are measured. Paired shock testing in conjunction with the superposition principle shows that a small-signal near-linear range exists for input-output pairs. Measurement is done by fitting the sums of linear basis functions (exponential and damped cosine basis functions) to the time-averaged impulse responses, and the dynamics is modeled with nonlinear ordinary differential equations linearized at point attractors far from equilibrium (Freeman, 1975, 1987b; Basar, 1980).

In this paradigm the stimulus is used to elicit a "signal" in the brain, the impulse response, and the persisting background activity is treated as "noise" to be removed by averaging and by filtering. The basal neural activity of the brain, as manifested in recordings of "spontaneous" unit and EEG potentials, is assumed to be stochastic in order to design filters so to extract the "signal" from "noise". The neurons are conceived to be unreliable elements for processing information, and the reason for having so many of them connected in parallel is to achieve reliability through redundancy of the noisy processors. Models of brain function are made from reliable components that simulate the neurons in parallel, and noise is introduced into the models by use of random number generators or thermal white noise, when the need for it arises. Noise is regarded as a nuisance that is needed to simulate biological processes, or it is introduced as an adjuvant for data processing, as in its use for simulated annealing or as a means for inducing state changes by arbitrary fluctuations.

The discovery independently by several investigators that the EEG is not a purely stochastic variable (e.g. Babloyantz and Destexhe, 1986) came with new mathematical tools for the analysis of the behavior of deterministic systems, whose activity patterns are aperiodic and unpredictable (e.g., Thompson and Stewart, 1986). These tools were designed for study of turbulence in physical and chemical systems and of pseudorandomness in computer programs, but they found immediate use in the measurement of the correlation dimensions of neural systems that generate electrical activity. Although the numerical values and even the meaning of the concept of "dimension" in this context are controversial, the basic idea is now clear and incontrovertible, that at some levels the activity of brains is chaotic and not stochastic (Skarda and Freeman, 1987).

This discovery has caused profound shifts in the way in which we think about and understand brain function. At the experimental level we now place less reliance on Fourier analysis and its underlying assumptions of linearity and periodicity. We entertain the hypothesis that the "noise" in brain function is the "signal". Already this has born fruit in the discovery that EEG patterns in several sensory systems merely appear to be random time series, but carry information that is behaviorally significant for animals.

In our new models we have re-evaluated our networks of nonlinear ordinary differential equations with parameter values that yield chaotic solutions, that is, solutions that are neither steady state, limit cycle, or quasiperiodic (decomposable into finite sets of Fourier terms). Our dynamical models, backed by new experimental results that were predicted from them, have shown that time series can be generated from deterministic equations, which are structured in respect to the known anatomy and physiology of the olfactory system. The time series and their spatial patterns of amplitude and phase closely resemble forms of EEGs under normal and abnormal conditions Freeman, 1987a,b, 1992).

3. Experimental observations on the olfactory system

The olfactory system is the simplest and phylogenetically oldest sensory system, and it is the most important of the senses for cats, rabbits and rats, so it is optimal for the study of brain mechanisms of perception in animals. The basic approach to it as a dynamic system is to measure its input and output in pairs on repeated trials and describe the operations by which the input is transformed to the output. That description has the form of a network of nonlinear ordinary differential equations, and the test of the model is to fit the solutions of the equations to measurements of the electrical activity of the olfactory system during the perceptual discriminations.

The crucial experiments were simple in conception. Rabbits were implanted with arrays of 64 electrodes in an 8 x 8 grid placed onto the surface of the olfactory bulb. They were trained to respond by licking to one odorant, such as amyl acetate that was accompanied by a reward (water), and merely to sniff in response to another odorant (such as butyric acid) as an unrewarded stimulus. On each trial a set of 64 EEG traces was recorded for 6 sec, that included a control period and a test period (Figure 1). Brief EEG segments lasting 0.1 msec were selected during the times of inhalation of the background air as a control (C) or either of the two odors presented as conditioned stimuli (CS) on randomly interspersed trials, one with the reinforcement (CS+) and the other without (CS-). Sets of several hundred of these EEG segments were analyzed for each animal. We knew which of the three states each segment came from. The operational question was, what aspect or aspects of the segments would enable us to classify the segments correctly in respect to the odorant conditions?

The hypotheses were that, between the time of inhalation and the performance of a correct response, odorant information existed in the bulb as a pattern of neural activity, on the basis of which the animal made the discrimination, and that this information would be

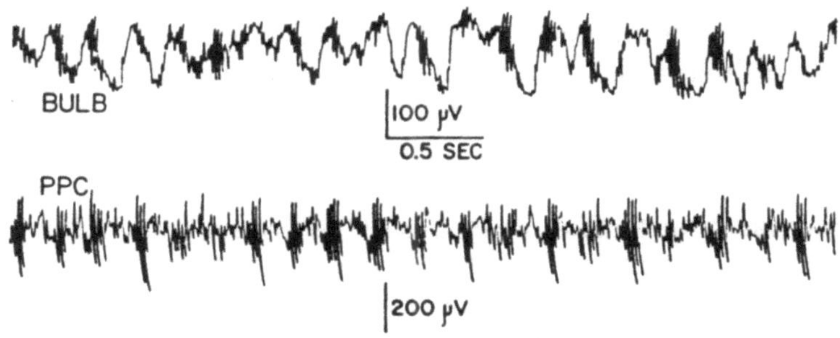

Figure 1. An example is shown of single EEG traces recorded from the olfactory bulb and prepyriform cortex (PPC) of a cat together with an electromyogram of the leg during stimulation with an odorant without reinforcement (CS-) ("safe" odor) with no conditioned response (CR). The low frequency wave manifests respiratory forcing function, and the high frequency oscillations are the "bursts" that manifest the state transition from the basal state to a perceptual state.

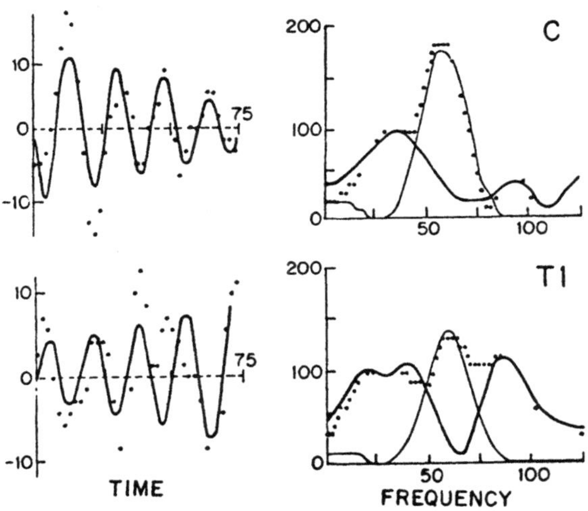

Figure 2. Examples are shown on the left of the spatial ensemble averages of three bursts (dots) from the control (C) and odorant states (T1). Time is in msec and amplitude is in arbitrary units. The Fourier transforms are shown on the right as the dots. The nonlinear basis function fitted to the dots by nonlinear regression for the dominant component $S_m(t)$ is shown by the heavy curve, and its Fourier transform is shown at the right by the light curve. The dark curve on the right shows the residual spectrum after subtracting the light curve from the dots. The frequency and phase at its maximum of power provide the initial guesses for determining the largest component of the clutter $C_{m,2}(t)$.

detectable in some as yet to be determined properties of the EEGs. We collected 60 samples of bursts, 20 from each of 3 classes: C, CS+ and CS-. Visual inspection of the 60 bursts showed that there was a common wave form of oscillation on all 64 of the records for each burst, which varied in amplitude and phase over the channels to form patterns of amplitude and phase modulation of the wave form seen as a "carrier" wave, but obscured by noise. On the basis of the near-linear performance of the system as tested by superposition with electrical stimuli, the signal was conceived as a linear basis function embedded in two kinds of noise. One kind was white noise that was spectrally colored by the pass band of the filters used to preprocess the EEG data (10 Hz and 160 Hz). The other kind was non-white noise designated as "clutter", a sum of linear basis functions. The form of the equation was

$$V_m(x, y, t) = A_{m,1}(x, y)\, S_m(t) \qquad \text{signal}$$

$$+ \sum_{i=2}^{k} A_{m,i}(x, y)\, C_{m,i}(t) \qquad \text{clutter}$$

$$+ e_{m,i}(x, y, t) \qquad \text{noise}$$

Here $V_m(8,8,40)$ is the EEG on one sniff for 64 channels and 40 time points spaced at 2 msec (80 msec); $S_m(40)$ is the carrier signal as a function of time; $C_{m,i}(40)$ is the set of k - 1 basis functions for the clutter; $A_{m,1}(8x8)$ and $A_{m,i}(8x8)$, i = 2, ... ,k are 64x1 column vectors each representing the spatial amplitude modulation of a temporal basis function; and $e_{m,i}(8,8,40)$ is noise that is normally distributed, spatially and spectrally uniform, and time invariant.

The search for the common wave form was facilitated by forming the spatial ensemble average for each EEG segment, m, and fitting basis functions to this average with nonlinear regression, so as to use the resulting optimized coefficients as starting guesses for each of the 64 traces:

$$\bar{V}_m(t) = \sum_{x=1}^{8} \sum_{y=1}^{8} V_m(x, y, t)$$

Our initial choice of analytic basis functions was a set of cosines, based on the assumption that the EEG segments could be decomposed numerically by the Fast Fourier Transform. We quickly found that the data were inappropriate for this set of basis functions, owing to the temporal modulation of the bursts in both amplitude and frequency. By visual inspection we determined that the temporal AM and FM could be approximated by linear functions of amplitude and frequency with time during each burst (Figure 2). The modified analytic basis functions were given the form:

$$V_m(t) = \sum_{i=1}^{5} A_{m,i}\,[1+a_{m,i}(t - t_o)]\,\cos[2pt(f_{m,i}+ b_{m,i}\,(t - t_o)) + F_{m,i})]$$

$a_{m,i}(t)$ = coefficient for linear function in temporal AM

$b_{m,i}(t)$ = coefficient for linear function in temporal FM

t_o = center time of each segment

Here $f_{m,i}$ is the center frequency of each component, $b_{m,i}(t - t_o)$ is the linear ramp of FM, $A_{m,i}$ is the initial amplitude, $a_{m,i}(t - t_o)$ is the linear ramp of AM, and $F_{m,i}$ is the phase of each component. The number $k = 5$ was selected on the basis of visual inspection of the residuals to test for conformance in regard to the assumptions about the noise.

This function was fitted serially to the spatial ensemble average of the 64 traces for each burst by nonlinear regression, with the maximum of gain in the FFT and the phase at that gain providing the initial guesses for phase $F_{m,i}$ and frequency $f_{m,i}$ of each of the components, $i = 1,...,5$. It was necessary to determine the 5 frequencies and phases serially rather than concomitantly owing to failure of convergence of the nonlinear regression when more than one frequency was included. The decomposition into signal $S_m(t)$ and clutter $C_{m,i}(t)$ was based on the hypothesis that the burst represented the asymptotic convergence of the cortical dynamics to a limit cycle (hence the temporal AM and FM) under perturbation by noise, which was aborted before completion of the convergence, and that persisting local activity or other spatially coherent limit cycle activities unrelated to the CS+ and CS- would obscure the desired signal, if they were not concomitantly matched with digital adaptive filters.

Our results (Freeman and Viana Di Prisco, 1986) showed that the information we sought was in a spatial pattern of oscillation $A_{m,1}(8,8)$, which contained approximately 60% of the variance on the average, and which lay in the frequency range of 30 - 80 Hz termed the "gamma" range (Bressler and Freeman, 1980), in analogy to the high end of the x-ray spectrum. A common wave form $S_m(t)$was found in each segment, and the spatial pattern of its amplitude $A_{m,1}(x,y)$ converged to a reproducible shape each time that a learned odorant was present (Figure 3). In principle this form of information is simple. It is like a frame in a black-and-white movie, in which the carrier wave is the light wave, each pattern is formed by the highs and lows of the intensity of the light, and successive patterns follow in olfaction at the rate of respiration.

The 64x1 column vector for the dominant component of amplitude for each burst in a set of 60 bursts defined a point in 64 space. The three odorant conditions gave rise to clusters, which computed by several techniques (Sammon, 1969; Grajski et al., 1986; Freeman and Grajski, 1987; Grajski and Freeman, 1989). Stepwise discriminant analysis is exemplified for two subjects in Figure 4 to show the projection of sets of m points into the plane defined by the two discriminant functions for three classes. Incorporation of the second and third components of the EEG segments (parts of the clutter) failed to improve the classification.

The finding that the central "code" for olfaction was spatial was predicted by Adrian (1950) The role of the receptors forming a sheet of neurons in the nasal cavity is to transform a chemical odor into a spatial pattern of action potentials, much as a retinal pattern of light is transformed to a pattern of ganglion cell activity. This pattern is transmitted to the bulb by topographically ordered axons that impose a new spatial pattern in the bulb with each inhalation. Evidence for the sensory-dependent patterns comes from metabolic labeling [e.g. Lancet et al. 1982]. The sensory-dependent neural activity from the input guides the formation of the burst of activity accompanying each inhalation. But there were three aspects that were surprising, and each of these aspects that had not been predicted revealed significant properties of the perceptual process in the bulb.

4. Statistical relations of pulses to dendritic waves

First, the EEG burst information was uniformly distributed over the entire olfactory bulb for each odorant. This was determined by repeating the classification algorithm while deleting randomly selected channels on multiple runs, and finding that no one channel contributed more or less than any other to the goodness of classification, but that the goodness decreased in proportion to the number deleted. By inference every neuron participated in every perception, even if and perhaps especially if it did not fire, because

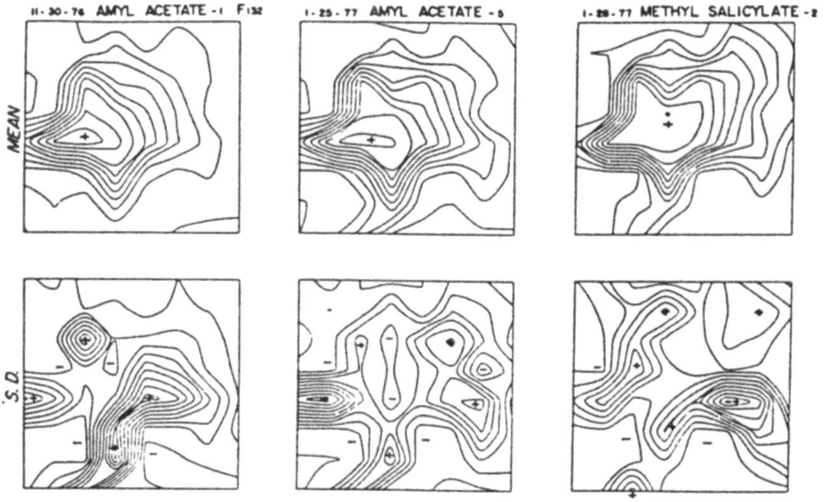

Figure 3. Examples are shown from the olfactory bulb of a rabbit of spatial patterns of burst amplitude for the mean and standard deviation (S.D.) of 10 segments after initial exposure to a CS+, several weeks later after over-training, and after serial conditioning to a new CS+.

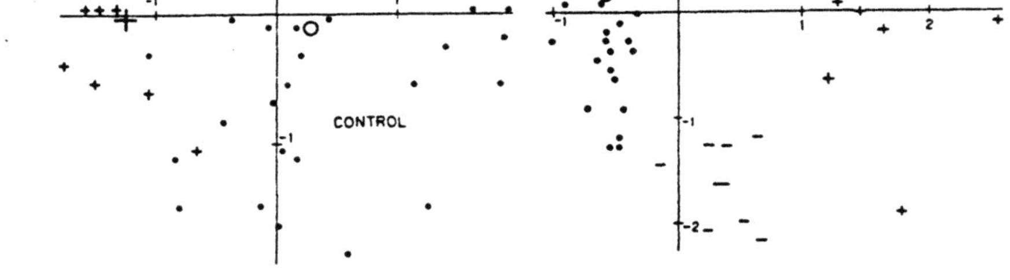

Figure 4. Two examples are shown of discriminant analysis applied to sets of bursts from rabbits trained to discriminate two odorants, indicating the variability of the spatial patterns within the clusters.

a spatial pattern required both high and low. This finding is in opposition to the expectation, based on single unit recording (Moulton, 1976) and metabolic labeling (Lancet et al., 1982), that odorant discrimination is based on the selective activation of bulbar neurons that receive input from odorant-specific receptors. Certainly that has been experimentally verified as the basis for sensory activation of the bulb, but the perceptual readout of the bulb is dominated by the cooperative, macroscopic order parameter that is manifested in the EEG (Freeman, 1991). This is the hierarchical level at which perception occurs. Moreover, we and many other investigators have attempted to demonstrate odorant specificity in the discharge rates of action potentials from single neurons. These attempts have not been conclusive. Because each EEG segment reflects the activity of many thousands of neurons, so we have concluded that the information relating to odorants is carried by assemblies of millions of neurons, and it is not reliably detectable in the activity of the handful of neurons that can be simultaneously accessed by recording from multiple microelectrodes.

There was a close statistical relationship between the neural pulses, which carry the bulbar output, and the local mean field manifested (but not caused or carried) by the EEGs. These electrical potentials result from the synaptic currents of neurons that flow between the cells, where the contributions of large numbers of neurons sum (Freeman, 1975, 1992). Thereby the EEGs give direct access to the conditional probability P of single neuron firing rate, p, with respect to the amplitudes of synaptic activity of the population of neurons as seen in the EEG, v, giving $P(p \cap v)$. The approach requires recording an extended trace of EEG simultaneously with a trace of pulse trains from one or a few neurons extracellularly. A total of about $N = 10{,}000$ pulses is needed, so that at an average firing rate of 10 pulses/sec the recording duration is about 20 minutes. The pulse trace is thresholded, and a unit pulse 1 msec in duration is recorded for each measure above threshold, or zero below. The mean and standard deviation (SD) of the EEG amplitudes digitized at 1 msec intervals are found. A histogram of the 10^6 values shows that the distribution, $P(v) = n_v(v)/N$, usually conforms to a Gaussian density (Figure 5a, 5b), though if there is a strong low frequency component owing to the respiratory forcing function the distribution is leptokurtic. Further analysis is best done after removing this component by high pass filtering of the EEG.

The range between +3 SD and -3 SD is divided into widths of 0.1 SD. For each EEG amplitude value in sequence the questions are asked, did a pulse occur at that time,

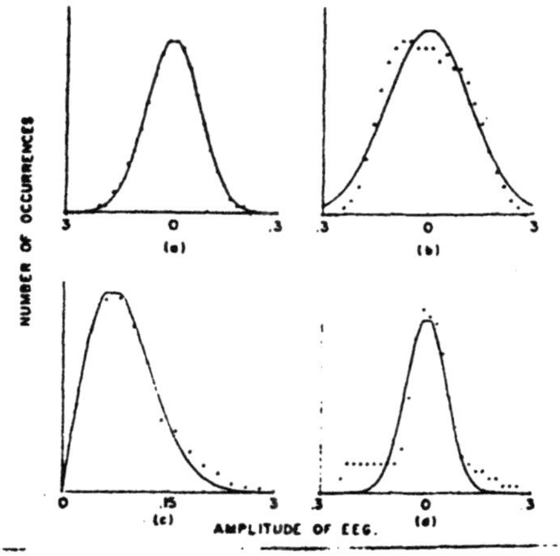

Figure 5. The dots show examples of histograms of digitized EEG amplitudes. (a) Most samples conform to a normal density distribution. (b) Records that are unusually concentrated in their spectra around a single frequency tend to have a broader peak. (c) The histogram of the envelope of the oscillatory EEG conforms to the Rayleigh distribution, which is revealed by passing white noise through a band pass filter (Freeman, 1975). (d) Records with a strong respiratory wave are leptokurtic. This forcing function is best removed by high pass filtering before statistical analysis.

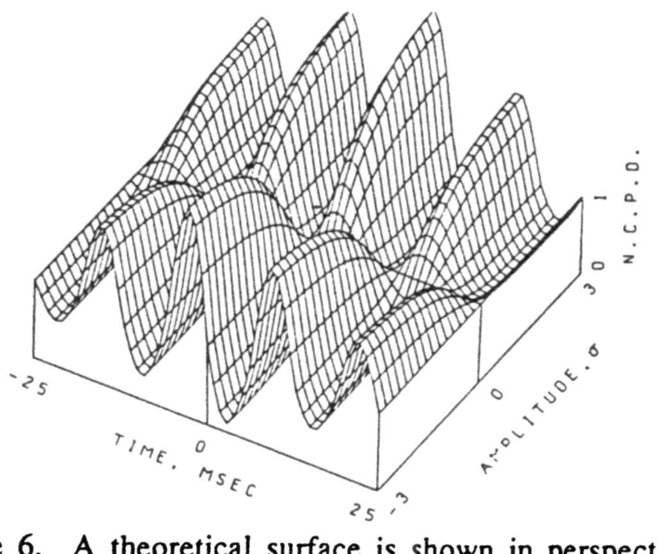

Figure 6. A theoretical surface is shown in perspective for the normalized conditional probability density of pulse formation in respect to EEG amplitude and time of occurrence (Freeman, 1975).

$P(p \cap v) = n_p(p,v) / N.$

The pulse probability density is then divided by the amplitude probability density to give the pulse probability conditional on amplitude.

$P(p \mid v) = P(p \cap v) / P(v)$

It is further necessary to ask for each amplitude occurrence, did a pulse occur in any msec preceding or following from -25 msec to +25 msec. Over the total number of occurrences n_p,

$P(p \cap v \cap T) = n_p(p,v,T) / N.$

The number of pulses in each bin of a two-dimensional table (Figure 6) is divided by the number of amplitude occurrences to give the pulse probability conditional on the EEG amplitude and time of occurrence.

$P(p \mid v \cap T) = P(p \cap v \cap T) / P(v)$

The probabilities are normalized by dividing each value by the grand mean P_o of pulse probability (Figures 6, 7).

$P_n(p \mid v \cap T) = P(p \mid v \cap T) / P_o$

to give the normalized conditional pulse probability. Two sections are taken across the table. Probabilities over the range of EEG amplitude values > 2 SD (Figure 7d, 7e) or < -2 SD (Figure 7f) are averaged to give pulse probability waves, which show that the NCPD oscillates at the frequency of the autocorrelation of the EEG and at a phase determined by the connectivity of the network (Freeman, 1975; Eeckman and Freeman, 1990). Sections across the table with respect to amplitude that are taken at the time of an extremum of amplitude of the wave (Figure 7a - 7c) yield a sigmoid curve (Freeman, 1979a; Eeckman and Freeman, 1991). It is noteworthy that pulse data that yield a strongly oscillatory pulse probability wave conditional on the EEG may show no oscillation in their autocorrelation functions (expectation densities), showing that the oscillations are a macroscopic property of the population of neurons, not a microscopic property of single neurons (Figure 8).

Second, we find that the bulbar information does not relate to the stimulus directly but instead to the meaning of the stimulus. This has been shown in several ways. The simplest is to switch a reward between two odorants, so that the previously rewarded stimulus is no longer reinforced and vice versa (Freeman and Viana Di Prisco, 1987). Both spatial patterns change, though the two odorants do not. So also does the spatial pattern for the control segments in background air. So also do all pre-existing patterns change when a new odorant is added to the repertoire (Freeman and Grajski, 1987). This lack of invariance is to be expected in a true associative memory. It shows that percepts are context-dependent and not merely stimulus-dependent (Freeman, 1991).

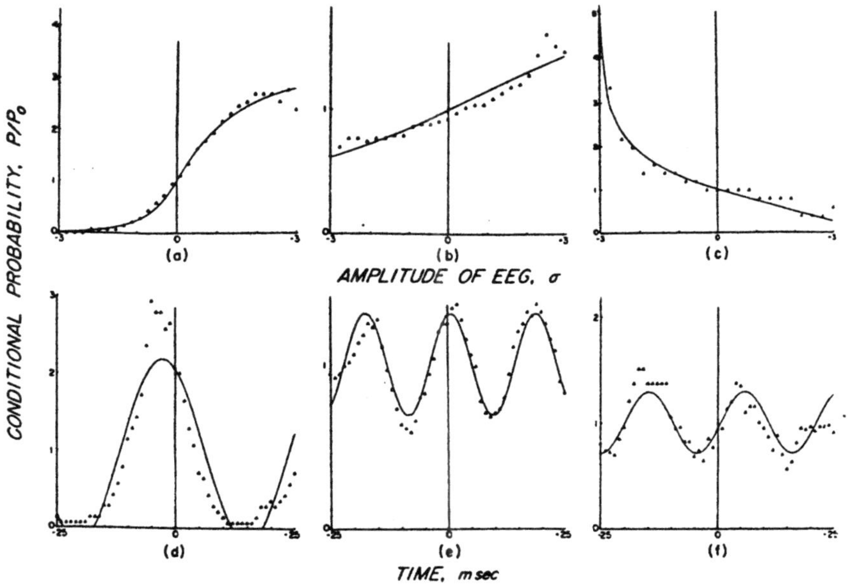

Figure 7. The dots in frames (a) to (c) show the normalized pulse probability conditional on EEG amplitude at a time lag for the maximal amplitude of the temporal oscillations shown in frames (d) through (f) as derived from concomitant pulse and EEG recordings in the olfactory bulb and cortex (Freeman, 1975).

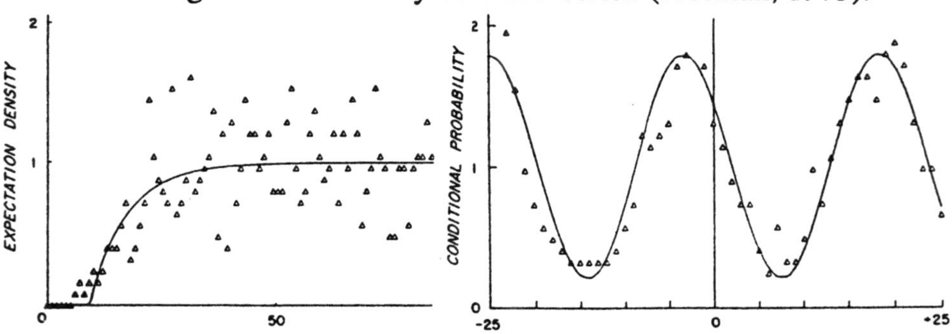

Figure 8. A comparison is made between the autocorrelation of a pulse train (the expectation density, above) and the normalized conditional pulse probability wave (below). The triangles show the data. The absolute and relative refractory periods are followed by aperiodic fluctuations in post-pulse correlation function. In contrast, the same data reveal an 80% modulation in firing probability at the frequency of the concomitantly recorded EEG. Hence the pulse probability wave is a macroscopic property of the population that is accessed through the EEG, and it is not a property of the single neuron (Freeman, 1975).

Third, the carrier wave is aperiodic. That is, it does not show oscillations at single frequencies, but instead has wave forms that are erratic and unpredictable in successive segments, nor are the time series of any two segments ever the same, irrespective of odorants. Yet the same wave form appears on all the channels in each segment, although of course at different amplitudes and values of phase with respect to the average phase. The possibility that this seemingly random wave form could occur by chance almost simultaneously on all channels is vanishingly small. There are no mechanisms by which this common activity can be imposed in this spectral range onto the whole bulb by receptors or by centrifugal pathways from the forebrain and brainstem. Moreover, each bulbar event has a unique spatial gradient in the phase of the oscillation (Freeman and Baird, 1987), which demonstrates its origin within the bulb by self-organization.

From these findings we conclude that the olfactory activity is characteristically chaotic. The conclusion is further supported by the finding that the clutter components $A_{m,i}(8x8)$, $i = 2, \dots, 5$ have the same amplitude and phase patterns as the dominant component $A_{m,1}(8x8)$, implying that the carrier wave form is a unitary event and is only arbitrarily decomposed into the modified Fourier components at discrete frequencies (Freeman and Grajski, 1987). The significance is that chaotic systems can change suddenly and completely from one global activity pattern to another upon small inputs, owing to their sensitivity to initial conditions. Further, we find that experimental inactivation of the main pathway from the bulb to the olfactory cortex causes the cortical activity to go silent both in action potentials and EEGs, whereas bulbar activity displays periodic oscillation with each inhalation (Freeman, 1975; Gray and Skinner, 1988). On recovery from the interruption of the pathway, the normal action potentials and EEGs return. These findings demonstrate that the background pulse and EEG activities are global properties, not local. They imply that the macroscopic activity of the bulb and olfactory cortex as manifested and measured through the EEG orders the activity of individual neurons throughout the system. The chaotic activity is not the local sum of the "noise" of autonomous, oscillating neurons, nor is it a silent equilibrium that is perturbed by noise, but it is activity that is controlled and directed by the system, so as to maintain continual readiness to jump to any desired perceptual state at any time (Freeman, 1991).

5. Modeling neural dynamics of action potentials and EEG

These results open major opportunities for development of new descriptive models by giving us several key insights into the dynamical processes to be simulated. We are assured that the proper element for our model is the local population and not the single neuron. This simplifies modeling, because complex dendritic trees of the multitudinous neurons in a local neighborhood can be modeled as a single integrator. The amplitude of output is transformed to the density of pulses. The relationship is not linear and time-varying as it is for single neurons, but instead it has the form of a sigmoid curve between the limits of axonal thresholds and maximal firing frequencies for the population (Figures 6, 7). Single neurons spend 99% or more of their lives just below their equilibriums, and most of their complexities are left at the hierarchical level of the neuron.

Bulbar output is transformed by spatial integration in the pathway to the next stage (Figure 9). This operation removes the sensory specific activity and the uncorrelated discharges of single neurons, and thereby extracts the spatially coherent activity that

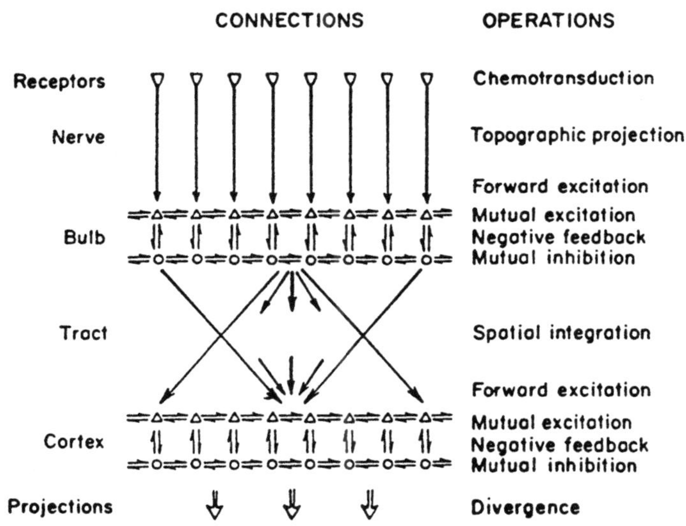

Figure 9. The olfactory system has three main layers of neurons forming 2-dimensional sheets. The receptors transmit by axons in the primary olfactory nerve with a degree of spatially topographic order. The bulbar neurons transmit to the prepyriform cortex by axons in the lateral olfactory tract, which is characterized by broad divergence from the bulb and convergence to the cortex. This implies that each cortical neuron receives and integrates the output of a broadly distributed set of bulbar neurons. This spatial integration ensures that the bulbar signal received by the cortex is the spatially coherent, macroscopic activity that has the common instantaneous frequency over the whole bulb.

constitutes the perceptual construct. The randomness of the pulse trains of individual neurons is due to the fact that each transmits to thousands of of other neurons and receives from thousands of others not the same, so that the feedback operator is described by a one dimensional diffusion term. This creates the "flat" pulse density over the bulbar population equivalent to spatially uniform white noise, against which the spatially coherent activity due to cooperative interaction stands out on spatial integration.

Oscillations manifested in the EEG arise only when an excitatory population is coupled into a loop with an inhibitory population to form negative feedback loops (Figure 9). The oscillations are periodic in a model of the bulb, as we find to be the case in the experimentally isolated bulb. Chaos in the model for the olfactory system arises when the bulbar loop is interconnected with the olfactory cortical feedback loop, so that each excites the other. Each has its own characteristic period, but they differ and cannot agree. Neither can escape the other, so that persistent aperiodic oscillation results. If the two parts are disconnected, the chaos in the model disappears, as it does in the experimental animals, when the bulb and cortex are disconnected (Freeman, 1987a).

The bulb and the cortex are each simulated by an array of local oscillators, that are interconnected between the excitatory elements by simulated synapses, so that they excite each other (Figure 9). These connections couple the oscillators into a layer, and they ensure that the whole array oscillates with a common wave form. Input and output connections are in parallel, one pair for each local oscillator. The mutually excitatory synapses between the oscillators are selectively strengthened during learning an "odorant" by presentation of examples of a class of stimuli, leading to the formation of a Hebb nerve cell assembly (Viana Di Prisco, 1984) consisting of groups of local oscillators that are co-excited by the stimuli. A global command is required in the model to "form an assembly", which is enabled by the reinforcement of an unconditioned stimulus (Gray, Freeman and Skinner, 1986). Multiple classes of stimuli are formed in sequential training sessions, leading to formation of multiple assemblies that are separated by simulated habituation (Freeman, Yao and Burke, 1988; Yao and Freeman, 1990; Yao et al., 1991).

The result is that the array of coupled oscillators generates a reproducible spatial pattern of amplitude of a common chaotic wave form, whenever an example of a learned class of stimuli is presented to the model (Freeman, 1979b,c). That pattern serves to identify and classify the stimulus presented. We say that for each learned class of stimuli the model has a wing of a global chaotic attractor with a basin of attraction. In dynamical parlance this means that the olfactory system (and its model) has certain preferred patterns of activity, any one of which it naturally falls into if given the opportunity. That opportunity is provided by the presence of any stimulus in a class that it has learned to respond to, whether or not the example was included in the original training set. A stimulus of this class provides the input and starting conditions that are needed to place the system into the basin of attraction, so named in analogy to a bowl in which a ball will roll to the bottom and stay there. The basin defines the range of generalization for a stimulus of that class.

Evidence for this dynamical process of perception has now been accumulated for the olfactory system in rabbit, rat and cat (Freeman, 1991), and for the visual system in monkey (Freeman and van Dijk, 1987) and cat (Gray et al., 1989).

6. Summary

Several lines of evidence show that the "spontaneous" background activity of populations of neurons in cortex during normal behavior is not stochastic, as long believed, but instead is an expression of deterministic chaos. The neurons in cortical columns comprise populations that sum their dendritic currents over numbers on the order of 10,000, resulting in a macroscopic state variable, the local mean field potential known as the electroencephalogram or EEG. The microscopic activity of the individual neurons consists of axonal pulse trains that are almost devoid of temporal structure. In contrast, although EEG traces have the statistical properties of random variables and are aperiodic and locally unpredictable, they are spatially coherent over extensive cortical areas. Their phase structures shows that the spatial patterns are self-organized. Their aperiodic wave forms serve as carriers for perceptual information. This chaotic activity depends on the integrity of long feedback pathways interconnecting large cortical areas, each of which is an oscillator by itself, but is not chaotic. The pulse trains of individual neurons are largely determined by the macroscopic state of the populations acting as an order parameter that emerges from the microscopic state. The cortex is exquisitely sensitive to minute inputs and displays very rapid global state transitions during acts of perception. Despite the immense numbers of neurons involved in the maintenance of chaotic background activity, the macroscopic degrees of freedom are low, far less than the total of the individual neurons. The new conception emerges that this brain "noise" that is manifested by the EEG reveals brain "signals" in its spatial patterns.

References

Adrian ED (1950) The electrical activity of the mammalian olfactory bulb. Electroencephalogr. clin. Neurophys. 2: 377-388.

Babloyantz A, Destexhe A (1986) Low-dimensional chaos in an instance of epilepsy. Proceedings of the National Academy of Sciences USA 83: 3513-3517.

Basar E (1980) EEG - Brain Dynamics. Amsterdam, Elsevier

Basar E (1990) Chaos in Brain Function. Berlin, Springer-Verlag.

Bressler SL, Freeman WJ (1980) Frequency analysis of olfactory system EEG in cat, rabbit and rat. Electroencephalography and clinical Neurophysiology 50: 19-24.

Eeckman FH, Freeman WJ (1990) Correlations between unit firing and EEG in the rat olfactory system. Brain Res. 528: 238-244.

Eeckman FH Freeman WJ (1991) Asymmetric sigmoid nonlinearity in the rat olfactory system. Brain Research 557: 13-21.

Freeman WJ (1975) Mass Action in the Nervous System. New York, Academic Press

Freeman WJ (1979a) Nonlinear gain mediating cortical stimulus-response relations. Biological Cybernetics 33:237-247.

Freeman WJ (1979b) Nonlinear dynamics of paleocortex manifested in the olfactory EEG. Biological Cybernetics 35: 21-37.

Freeman WJ (1979c) EEG analysis gives model of neuronal template-matching mechanism for sensory search with olfactory bulb. Biological Cybernetics 35.:221-234.

Freeman WJ (1987a) Simulation of chaotic EEG patterns with a dynamic model of the olfactory system. Biolological Cyberbernetics 56:139-150.

Freeman WJ (1987b) Techniques used in the search for the physiological basis of the EEG. ,In: ,Gevins A, Remond A (eds). Handbook,Electroencephalography and clinical Neurophysiology Vol 3A, Part 2, Ch. 18. Amsterdam, Elsevier. pp. 583-664.

Freeman WJ (1991) The physiology of perception. Scientific American 264: 78-85.

Freeman, WJ (1992) Tutorial in Neurobiology: From Single Neurons to Brain Chaos. International Journal of Bifurcation and Chaos 2: 451-482.

Freeman WJ, Baird B (1987) Relation of olfactory EEG to behavior: Spatial analysis: Behavioral. Neurosci. 101:393-408.

Freeman WJ, Grajski, K.A. (1987) Relation of olfactory EEG to behavior: Factor analysis: Behavioral. Neurosci. 101: 766-777.

Freeman WJ., Van Dijk B (1987) Spatial patterns of visual cortical fast EEG during conditioned reflex in a rhesus monkey. Brain Research: 422: 267-276.

Freeman WJ, Viana Di Prisco, G. (1986) Relation of olfactory EEG to behavior: Time series analysis. Behavioral Neuroscience 100:753-763.

Freeman WJ, Yao Y, Burke B. (1988) Central pattern generating and recognizing in olfactory bulb: A correlation learning rule. Neural Networks 1: 277-288.

Grajski KA, Breiman L, Viana Di Prisco G, Freeman WJ (1986) Classification of EEG spatial patterns with tree-structured methodology. IEEE Trans. Biomed. Engineering 33: 1076-1086.

Grajski KA, Freeman WJ (1989) Spatial EEG correlates of non-associative and associative learning in rabbits. Behavioral Neuroscience 103 790-804.

Gray CM, Freeman WJ, Skinner JE (1986) Chemical dependencies of learning in the rabbit olfactory bulb: acquisition of the transient spatial-pattern change depends on norepinephrine. Behavioral Neuroscience 100: 585-596.

Gray CM, Koenig P, Engel A, Singer W (1989) Oscillatory responses in cat visual cortex exhibit intercolumnar synchronization which reflects global stimulus properties. Nature 338: 334-337.

Gray CM, Skinner JE (1988) Centrifugal regulation of neuronal activity in the olfactory bulb of the waking rabbit as revealed by reversible cryogenic blockade. Exper. Brain Res. 69: 378-386.

Haken H, Stadler M (1990) Synergetics of Cognition. Berlin, Springer-Verlag.

Lancet D, Greer CA, Kauer JS, Shepherd, GM (1982) Mapping of odor-related neuronal activity in the olfactory bulb by high-resolution 2-deoxyglucose autoradiography. Proceedings, National Academy of Sciences 79: 670-674.

Moulton DG (1976) Spatial patterning of responses to odors in the peripheral olfactory system. Physiological Reviews 56:578-593.

Sammon JW (1969) A nonlinear mapping for data structure analysis. IEEE Transactions on Computers 18: 401-409.

Skarda CA, Freeman WJ (1987) How brains make chaos to make sense of the world. Brain and Behavioral Science 10: 161-195.

Thompson JMT, Stewart HB (1986) Nonlinear Dynamics and Chaos. New York, Wiley.

Viana Di Prisco G (1984) Hebb synaptic plasticity. Progress in. Neurobiology 22: 89-102.

Yao Y, Freeman WJ (1990) Model of biological pattern recognition with spatially chaotic dynamics. Neural Networks 3: 153-170.

Yao Y, Freeman WJ, Burke B, Yang Q (1991) Pattern recognition by a distributed neural network: An industrial application. Neural Networks 4: 103-121.

NATO ASI Series F

Including Special Programmes on Sensory Systems for Robotic Control (ROB) and on Advanced Educational Technology (AET)

Vol. 1: Issues in Acoustic Signal - Image Processing and Recognition. Edited by C. H. Chen. VIII, 333 pages. 1983. *(out of print)*

Vol. 2: Image Sequence Processing and Dynamic Scene Analysis. Edited by T. S. Huang. IX, 749 pages. 1983.

Vol. 3: Electronic Systems Effectiveness and Life Cycle Costing. Edited by J. K. Skwirzynski. XVII, 732 pages. 1983. *(out of print)*

Vol. 4: Pictorial Data Analysis. Edited by R. M. Haralick. VIII, 468 pages. 1983.

Vol. 5: International Calibration Study of Traffic Conflict Techniques. Edited by E. Asmussen. VII, 229 pages. 1984.

Vol. 6: Information Technology and the Computer Network. Edited by K. G. Beauchamp. VIII, 271 pages. 1984.

Vol. 7: High-Speed Computation. Edited by J. S. Kowalik. IX, 441 pages. 1984.

Vol. 8: Program Transformation and Programming Environments. Report on a Workshop directed by F. L. Bauer and H. Remus. Edited by P. Pepper. XIV, 378 pages. 1984.

Vol. 9: Computer Aided Analysis and Optimization of Mechanical System Dynamics. Edited by E. J. Haug. XXII, 700 pages. 1984. *(out of print)*

Vol. 10: Simulation and Model-Based Methodologies: An Integrative View. Edited by T. I. Ören, B. P. Zeigler, M. S. Elzas. XIII, 651 pages. 1984.

Vol. 11: Robotics and Artificial Intelligence. Edited by M. Brady, L. A. Gerhardt, H. F. Davidson. XVII, 693 pages. 1984.

Vol. 12: Combinatorial Algorithms on Words. Edited by A. Apostolico, Z. Galil. VIII, 361 pages. 1985.

Vol. 13: Logics and Models of Concurrent Systems. Edited by K. R. Apt. VIII, 498 pages. 1985.

Vol. 14: Control Flow and Data Flow: Concepts of Distributed Programming. Edited by M. Broy. VIII, 525 pages. 1985. *Reprinted as Springer Study Edition 1986.*

Vol. 15: Computational Mathematical Programming. Edited by K. Schittkowski. VIII, 451 pages. 1985.

Vol. 16: New Systems and Architectures for Automatic Speech Recognition and Synthesis. Edited by R. De Mori, C.Y. Suen. XIII, 630 pages. 1985. *(out of print)*

Vol. 17: Fundamental Algorithms for Computer Graphics. Edited by R. A. Earnshaw. XVI, 1042 pages. 1985. *Reprinted as Springer Study Edition 1991.*

Vol. 18: Computer Architectures for Spatially Distributed Data. Edited by H. Freeman and G. G. Pieroni. VIII, 391 pages. 1985. *(out of print)*

Vol. 19: Pictorial Information Systems in Medicine. Edited by K. H. Höhne. XII, 525 pages. 1986.

Vol. 20: Disordered Systems and Biological Organization. Edited by E. Bienenstock, F. Fogelman Soulié, G. Weisbuch. XXI, 405 pages.1986

Vol. 21: Intelligent Decision Support in Process Environments. Edited by E. Hollnagel, G. Mancini, D. D. Woods. XV, 524 pages. 1986.

Vol. 22: Software System Design Methods. The Challenge of Advanced Computing Technology. Edited by J. K. Skwirzynski. XIII, 747 pages. 1986. *(out of print)*

Vol. 23: Designing Computer-Based Learning Materials. Edited by H. Weinstock and A. Bork. IX, 285 pages. 1986. *(out of print)*

Vol. 24: Database Machines. Modern Trends and Applications. Edited by A. K. Sood and A. H. Qureshi. VIII, 570 pages. 1986.

NATO ASI Series F

Including Special Programmes on Sensory Systems for Robotic Control (ROB) and on Advanced Educational Technology (AET)

Vol. 25: Pyramidal Systems for Computer Vision. Edited by V. Cantoni and S. Levialdi. VIII, 392 pages. 1986. *(ROB)*

Vol. 26: Modelling and Analysis in Arms Control. Edited by R. Avenhaus, R. K. Huber and J. D. Kettelle. VIII, 488 pages. 1986. *(out of print)*

Vol. 27: Computer Aided Optimal Design: Structural and Mechanical Systems. Edited by C. A. Mota Soares. XIII, 1029 pages. 1987.

Vol. 28: Distributed Operating Systems. Theory und Practice. Edited by Y. Paker, J.-P. Banatre and M. Bozyiğit. X, 379 pages. 1987.

Vol. 29: Languages for Sensor-Based Control in Robotics. Edited by U. Rembold and K. Hörmann. IX, 625 pages. 1987. *(ROB)*

Vol. 30: Pattern Recognition Theory and Applications. Edited by P. A. Devijver and J. Kittler. XI, 543 pages. 1987.

Vol. 31: Decision Support Systems: Theory and Application. Edited by C. W. Holsapple and A. B. Whinston. X, 500 pages. 1987.

Vol. 32: Information Systems: Failure Analysis. Edited by J. A. Wise and A. Debons. XV, 338 pages. 1987.

Vol. 33: Machine Intelligence and Knowledge Engineering for Robotic Applications. Edited by A. K. C. Wong and A. Pugh. XIV, 486 pages. 1987. *(ROB)*

Vol. 34: Modelling, Robustness and Sensitivity Reduction in Control Systems. Edited by R.F. Curtain. IX, 492 pages. 1987.

Vol. 35: Expert Judgment and Expert Systems. Edited by J. L. Mumpower, L. D. Phillips, O. Renn and V. R. R. Uppuluri. VIII, 361 pages. 1987.

Vol. 36: Logic of Programming and Calculi of Discrete Design. Edited by M. Broy. VII, 415 pages. 1987.

Vol. 37: Dynamics of Infinite Dimensional Systems. Edited by S.-N. Chow and J. K. Hale. IX. 514 pages. 1987.

Vol. 38: Flow Control of Congested Networks. Edited by A. R. Odoni, L. Bianco and G. Szegö. XII, 355 pages. 1987.

Vol. 39: Mathematics and Computer Science in Medical Imaging. Edited by M. A. Viergever and A. Todd-Pokropek. VIII, 546 pages. 1988.

Vol. 40: Theoretical Foundations of Computer Graphics and CAD. Edited by R. A. Earnshaw. XX, 1246 pages. 1988. *(out of print)*

Vol. 41: Neural Computers. Edited by R. Eckmiller and Ch. v. d. Malsburg. XIII, 566 pages. 1988. *Reprinted as Springer Study Edition 1989, 1990.*

Vol. 42: Real-Time Object Measurement and Classification. Edited by A. K. Jain. VIII, 407 pages. 1988. *(ROB)*

Vol. 43: Sensors and Sensory Systems for Advanced Robots. Edited by P. Dario. XI, 597 pages. 1988. *(ROB)*

Vol. 44: Signal Processing and Pattern Recognition in Nondestructive Evaluation of Materials. Edited by C. H. Chen. VIII, 344 pages. 1988. *(ROB)*

Vol. 45: Syntactic and Structural Pattern Recognition. Edited by G. Ferraté, T. Pavlidis, A. Sanfeliu and H. Bunke. XVI, 467 pages. 1988. *(ROB)*

Vol. 46: Recent Advances in Speech Understanding and Dialog Systems. Edited by H. Niemann, M. Lang and G. Sagerer. X, 521 pages. 1988.

NATO ASI Series F

Including Special Programmes on Sensory Systems for Robotic Control (ROB) and on Advanced Educational Technology (AET)

Vol. 47: Advanced Computing Concepts and Techniques in Control Engineering. Edited by M. J. Denham and A. J. Laub. XI, 518 pages. 1988. *(out of print)*

Vol. 48: Mathematical Models for Decision Support. Edited by G. Mitra. IX, 762 pages. 1988.

Vol. 49: Computer Integrated Manufacturing. Edited by I. B. Turksen. VIII, 568 pages. 1988.

Vol. 50: CAD Based Programming for Sensory Robots. Edited by B. Ravani. IX, 565 pages. 1988. *(ROB)*

Vol. 51: Algorithms and Model Formulations in Mathematical Programming. Edited by S. W. Wallace. IX, 190 pages. 1989.

Vol. 52: Sensor Devices and Systems for Robotics. Edited by A. Casals. IX, 362 pages. 1989. *(ROB)*

Vol. 53: Advanced Information Technologies for Industrial Material Flow Systems. Edited by S. Y. Nof and C. L. Moodie. IX, 710 pages. 1989.

Vol. 54: A Reappraisal of the Efficiency of Financial Markets. Edited by R. M. C. Guimarães, B. G. Kingsman and S. J. Taylor. X, 804 pages. 1989.

Vol. 55: Constructive Methods in Computing Science. Edited by M. Broy. VII, 478 pages. 1989.

Vol. 56: Multiple Criteria Decision Making and Risk Analysis Using Microcomputers. Edited by B. Karpak and S. Zionts. VII, 399 pages. 1989.

Vol. 57: Kinematics and Dynamic Issues in Sensor Based Control. Edited by G. E. Taylor. XI, 456 pages. 1990. *(ROB)*

Vol. 58: Highly Redundant Sensing in Robotic Systems. Edited by J. T. Tou and J. G. Balchen. X, 322 pages. 1990. *(ROB)*

Vol. 59: Superconducting Electronics. Edited by H. Weinstock and M. Nisenoff. X, 441 pages. 1989.

Vol. 60: 3D Imaging in Medicine. Algorithms, Systems, Applications. Edited by K. H. Höhne, H. Fuchs and S. M. Pizer. IX, 460 pages. 1990. *(out of print)*

Vol. 61: Knowledge, Data and Computer-Assisted Decisions. Edited by M. Schader and W. Gaul. VIII, 421 pages. 1990.

Vol. 62: Supercomputing. Edited by J. S. Kowalik. X, 425 pages. 1990.

Vol. 63: Traditional and Non-Traditional Robotic Sensors. Edited by T. C. Henderson. VIII, 468 pages. 1990. *(ROB)*

Vol. 64: Sensory Robotics for the Handling of Limp Materials. Edited by P. M. Taylor. IX, 343 pages. 1990. *(ROB)*

Vol. 65: Mapping and Spatial Modelling for Navigation. Edited by L. F. Pau. VIII, 357 pages. 1990. *(ROB)*

Vol. 66: Sensor-Based Robots: Algorithms and Architectures. Edited by C. S. G. Lee. X, 285 pages. 1991. *(ROB)*

Vol. 67: Designing Hypermedia for Learning. Edited by D. H. Jonassen and H. Mandl. XXV, 457 pages. 1990. *(AET)*

Vol. 68: Neurocomputing. Algorithms, Architectures and Applications. Edited by F. Fogelman Soulié and J. Hérault. XI, 455 pages. 1990.

Vol. 69: Real-Time Integration Methods for Mechanical System Simulation. Edited by E. J. Haug and R. C. Deyo. VIII, 352 pages. 1991.

Vol. 70: Numerical Linear Algebra, Digital Signal Processing and Parallel Algorithms. Edited by G. H. Golub and P. Van Dooren. XIII, 729 pages. 1991.

NATO ASI Series F

Including Special Programmes on Sensory Systems for Robotic Control (ROB) and on Advanced Educational Technology (AET)

Vol. 71: Expert Systems and Robotics. Edited by T. Jordanides and B.Torby. XII, 744 pages. 1991.

Vol. 72: High-Capacity Local and Metropolitan Area Networks. Architecture and Performance Issues. Edited by G. Pujolle. X, 536 pages. 1991.

Vol. 73: Automation and Systems Issues in Air Traffic Control. Edited by J. A. Wise, V. D. Hopkin and M. L. Smith. XIX, 594 pages. 1991.

Vol. 74: Picture Archiving and Communication Systems (PACS) in Medicine. Edited by H. K. Huang, O. Ratib, A. R. Bakker and G. Witte. XI, 438 pages. 1991.

Vol. 75: Speech Recognition and Understanding. Recent Advances, Trends and Applications. Edited by P. Laface and Renato De Mori. XI, 559 pages. 1991.

Vol. 76: Multimedia Interface Design in Education. Edited by A. D. N. Edwards and S. Holland. XIV, 216 pages. 1992. *(AET)*

Vol. 77: Computer Algorithms for Solving Linear Algebraic Equations. The State of the Art. Edited by E. Spedicato. VIII, 352 pages. 1991.

Vol. 78: Integrating Advanced Technology into Technology Education. Edited by M. Hacker, A. Gordon and M. de Vries. VIII, 185 pages. 1991. *(AET)*

Vol. 79: Logic, Algebra, and Computation. Edited by F. L. Bauer. VII, 485 pages. 1991.

Vol. 80: Intelligent Tutoring Systems for Foreign Language Learning. Edited by M. L. Swartz and M. Yazdani. IX, 347 pages. 1992. *(AET)*

Vol. 81: Cognitive Tools for Learning. Edited by P. A. M. Kommers, D. H. Jonassen, and J. T. Mayes. X, 278 pages. 1992. *(AET)*

Vol. 82: Combinatorial Optimization. New Frontiers in Theory and Practice. Edited by M. Akgül, H. W. Hamacher, and S. Tüfekçi. XI, 334 pages. 1992.

Vol. 83: Active Perception and Robot Vision. Edited by A. K. Sood and H. Wechsler. IX, 756 pages. 1992.

Vol. 84: Computer-Based Learning Environments and Problem Solving. Edited by E. De Corte, M. C. Linn, H. Mandl, and L. Verschaffel. XVI, 488 pages. 1992. *(AET)*

Vol. 85: Adaptive Learning Environments. Foundations and Frontiers. Edited by M. Jones and P. H. Winne. VIII, 408 pages. 1992. *(AET)*

Vol. 86: Intelligent Learning Environments and Knowledge Acquisition in Physics. Edited by A. Tiberghien and H. Mandl. VIII, 285 pages. 1992. *(AET)*

Vol. 87: Cognitive Modelling and Interactive Environments. With demo diskettes (Apple and IBM compatible). Edited by F. L. Engel, D. G. Bouwhuis, T. Bösser, and G. d'Ydewalle. IX, 311 pages. 1992. *(AET)*

Vol. 88: Programming and Mathematical Method. Edited by M. Broy. VIII, 428 pages. 1992.

Vol. 89: Mathematical Problem Solving and New Information Technologies. Edited by J. P. Ponte, J. F. Matos, J. M. Matos, and D. Fernandes. XV, 346 pages. 1992. *(AET)*

Vol. 90: Collaborative Learning Through Computer Conferencing. Edited by A. R. Kaye. X, 260 pages. 1992. *(AET)*

Vol. 91: New Directions for Intelligent Tutoring Systems. Edited by E. Costa. X, 296 pages. 1992. *(AET)*

Vol. 92: Hypermedia Courseware: Structures of Communication and Intelligent Help. Edited by A. Oliveira. X, 241 pages. 1992. *(AET)*

Vol. 93: Interactive Multimedia Learning Environments. Human Factors and Technical Considerations on Design Issues. Edited by M. Giardina. VIII, 254 pages. 1992. *(AET)*

NATO ASI Series F

Including Special Programmes on Sensory Systems for Robotic Control (ROB) and on Advanced Educational Technology (AET)

Vol. 94: Logic and Algebra of Specification. Edited by F. L. Bauer, W. Brauer, and H. Schwichtenberg. VII, 442 pages. 1993.

Vol. 95: Comprehensive Systems Design: A New Educational Technology. Edited by C. M. Reigeluth, B. H. Banathy, and J. R. Olson. IX, 437 pages. 1993. *(AET)*

Vol. 96: New Directions in Educational Technology. Edited by E. Scanlon and T. O'Shea. VIII, 251 pages. 1992. *(AET)*

Vol. 97: Advanced Models of Cognition for Medical Training and Practice. Edited by D. A. Evans and V. L. Patel. XI, 372 pages. 1992. *(AET)*

Vol. 98: Medical Images: Formation, Handling and Evaluation. Edited by A. E. Todd-Pokropek and M. A. Viergever. IX, 700 pages. 1992.

Vol. 99: Multisensor Fusion for Computer Vision. Edited by J. K. Aggarwal. XI, 456 pages. 1993. *(ROB)*

Vol. 100: Communication from an Artificial Intelligence Perspective. Theoretical and Applied Issues. Edited by A. Ortony, J. Slack and O. Stock. XII, 260 pages. 1992.

Vol. 101: Recent Developments in Decision Support Systems. Edited by C. W. Holsapple and A. B. Whinston. XI, 618 pages. 1993.

Vol. 102: Robots and Biological Systems: Towards a New Bionics? Edited by P. Dario, G. Sandini and P. Aebischer. XII, 786 pages. 1993.

Vol. 103: Parallel Computing on Distributed Memory Multiprocessors. Edited by F. Özgüner and F. Erçal. VIII, 332 pages. 1993.

Vol. 104: Instructional Models in Computer-Based Learning Environments. Edited by S. Dijkstra, H. P. M. Krammer and J. J. G. van Merriënboer. X, 510 pages. 1993. *(AET)*

Vol. 105: Designing Environments for Constructive Learning. Edited by T. M. Duffy, J. Lowyck and D. H. Jonassen. VIII, 374 pages. 1993. *(AET)*

Vol. 106: Software for Parallel Computation. Edited by J. S. Kowalik and L. Grandinetti. IX, 363 pages. 1993.

Vol. 107: Advanced Educational Technologies for Mathematics and Science. Edited by D. L. Ferguson. XII, 749 pages. 1993. *(AET)*

Vol. 108: Concurrent Engineering: Tools and Technologies for Mechanical System Design. Edited by E. J. Haug. XIII, 998 pages. 1993.

Vol. 109: Advanced Educational Technology in Technology Education. Edited by A. Gordon, M. Hacker and M. de Vries. VIII, 253 pages. 1993. *(AET)*

Vol. 110: Verification and Validation of Complex Systems: Human Factors Issues. Edited by J. A. Wise, V. D. Hopkin and P. Stager. XIII, 704 pages. 1993.

Vol. 111: Cognitive Models and Intelligent Environments for Learning Programming. Edited by E. Lemut, B. du Boulay and G. Dettori. VIII, 305 pages. 1993. *(AET)*

Vol. 112: Item Banking: Interactive Testing and Self-Assessment. Edited by D. A. Leclercq and J. E. Bruno. VIII, 261 pages. 1993. *(AET)*

Vol. 113: Interactive Learning Technology for the Deaf. Edited by B. A. G. Elsendoorn and F. Coninx. XIII, 285 pages. 1993. *(AET)*

Vol. 114: Intelligent Systems: Safety, Reliability and Maintainability Issues. Edited by O. Kaynak, G. Honderd and E. Grant. XI, 340 pages. 1993.

Vol. 115: Learning Electricity and Electronics with Advanced Educational Technology. Edited by M. Caillot. VII, 329 pages. 1993. *(AET)*

NATO ASI Series F

Including Special Programmes on Sensory Systems for Robotic Control (ROB) and on Advanced Educational Technology (AET)

Vol. 116: Control Technology in Elementary Education. Edited by B. Denis. IX, 311 pages. 1993 *(AET)*

Vol. 118: Program Design Calculi. Edited by M. Broy. VIII, 409 pages. 1993.

Vol. 119: Automating Instructional Design, Development, and Delivery. Edited by. R. D. Tennyson. VIII, 266 pages. 1994 *(AET)*

Vol. 120: Reliability and Safety Assessment of Dynamic Process Systems. Edited by T. Aldemir, N. O. Siu, A. Mosleh, P. C. Cacciabue and B. G. Göktepe. X, 242 pages. 1994.

Vol. 121: Learning from Computers: Mathematics Education and Technology. Edited by C. Keitel and K. Ruthven. XIII, 332 pages. 1993. *(AET)*

Vol. 122: Simulation-Based Experiential Learning. Edited by D. M. Towne, T. de Jong and H. Spada. XIV, 274 pages. 1993. *(AET)*

Vol. 123: User-Centred Requirements for Software Engineering Environments. Edited by D. J. Gilmore, R. L. Winder and F. Détienne. VII, 377 pages. 1994.

Vol. 124: Fundamentals in Handwriting Recognition. Edited by S. Impedovo. IX, 496 pages. 1994.

Vol. 125: Student Modelling: The Key to Individualized Knowledge-Based Instruction. Edited by J. E. Greer and G. I. McCalla. X, 383 pages. 1994. *(AET)*

Vol. 126: Shape in Picture. Mathematical Description of Shape in Grey-level Images. Edited by Y.-L. O, A. Toet, D. Foster, H. J. A. M. Heijmans and P. Meer. XI, 676 pages. 1994.

Vol. 127: Real Time Computing. Edited by W. A. Halang and A. D. Stoyenko. XXII, 762 pages. 1994.

Vol. 129: Human-Machine Communication for Educational Systems Design. Edited by M. D. Brouwer-Janse and T. L. Harrington. X, 342 pages. 1994.

Vol. 130: Advances in Object-Oriented Database Systems. Edited by A. Dogac, M. T. Özsu, A. Biliris and T. Sellis. XI, 515 pages. 1994.

Vol. 131: Constraint Programming. Edited by B. Mayoh, E. Tyugu and J. Penjam. VII, 452 pages. 1994.

Vol. 132: Mathematical Modelling Courses for Engineering Education. Edited by Y. Ersoy and A. O. Moscardini. X, 246 pages. 1994.

Vol. 133: Collaborative Dialogue Technologies in Distance Learning. Edited by M. F. Verdejo and S. A. Cerri. XIV, 296 pages. 1994.

Vol. 134: Computer Integrated Production Systems and Organizations. The Human-Centred Approach. Edited by F. Schmid, S. Evans, A. W. S. Ainger and R. J. Grieve. X, 347 pages. 1994.

Vol. 135: Technology Education in School and Industry. Emerging Didactics for Human Resource Development. Edited by D. Blandow and M. J. Dyrenfurth. XI, 367 pages. 1994. *(AET)*

Vol. 136: From Statistics to Neural Networks. Theory and Pattern Recognition Applications. Edited by V. Cherkassky, J. H. Friedman and H. Wechsler. XII, 394 pages. 1994.

Springer-Verlag and the Environment

We at Springer-Verlag firmly believe that an international science publisher has a special obligation to the environment, and our corporate policies consistently reflect this conviction.

We also expect our business partners – paper mills, printers, packaging manufacturers, etc. – to commit themselves to using environmentally friendly materials and production processes.

The paper in this book is made from low- or no-chlorine pulp and is acid free, in conformance with international standards for paper permanency.

MIX
Papier aus verantwortungsvollen Quellen
Paper from responsible sources
FSC® C105338

If you have any concerns about our products,
you can contact us on
ProductSafety@springernature.com

In case Publisher is established outside the EU,
the EU authorized representative is:
Springer Nature Customer Service Center GmbH
Europaplatz 3, 69115 Heidelberg, Germany

Printed by Libri Plureos GmbH
in Hamburg, Germany